fourth edition

foundation of
ALLIED HEALTH SCIENCES

an

introduction to

chemistry

and

cell biology

›FREDERICK C. ROSS›
DELTA COLLEGE

WCB **Wm. C. Brown Publishers**

Dubuque, IA   Bogotá   Buenos Aires   Caracas   Chicago   Guilford, CT   London
Madrid   Mexico City   Seoul   Singapore   Sydney   Taipei   Tokyo   Toronto

Project Team

Editors *Colin Wheatley/Kristine Noel*
Developmental Editor *Kelly Drapeau*
Production Editor *Marla K. Irion*
Marketing Manager *Tom Lyon*
Cover Designer *Kaye Farmer*/Interior Designer *Barb Hodgson*
Art Editor *Jennifer L. Osmanski*
Photo Editor *Nicole Widmyer*
Advertising Coordinator *Heather Wagner*
Permissions Coordinator *Mavis M. Oeth*

Wm. C. Brown Publishers

President and Chief Executive Officer *Beverly Kolz*
Vice President, Director of Editorial *Kevin Kane*
Vice President, Sales and Market Expansion *Virginia S. Moffat*
Vice President, Director of Production *Colleen A. Yonda*
Director of Marketing *Craig S. Marty*
National Sales Manager *Douglas J. DiNardo*
Executive Editor *Michael D. Lange*
Advertising Manager *Janelle Keeffer*
Production Editorial Manager *Renée Menne*
Publishing Services Manager *Karen J. Slaght*
Royalty/Permissions Manager *Connie Allendorf*

A Times Mirror Company

Brief Contents

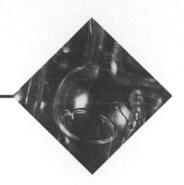

Contents

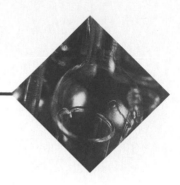

Preface

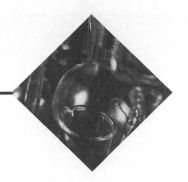

Many students find they are underprepared to take courses leading to a career in the allied health sciences. This textbook is designed to provide the science background that is a prerequisite to anatomy and physiology courses. The book is written for students; it is our intention to write something that students find helpful and interesting.

This text should help you understand various chemical and biological principles. At the beginning of each chapter is a "Purpose" section containing some hints about how the chapter fits in with the rest of the book. It is a signpost that shows you where you are going and why. If you pay careful attention to the purpose, you will know when you have attained your goal, and you will be able to gain some insight into why this goal was set.

Following the "Purpose" section, we present a thought-provoking situation entitled "Clinical Viewpoint." This section is a short article, story, or scenario based on actual occurrences or research (laboratory or clinical) that pertain to the material presented in the chapter. The intent is to: (1) provide topical information on the subject, (2) show practical applications, (3) integrate the concepts of the course with the actual material, and hopefully, (4) integrate the chapter material into both your personal and professional lives. We hope these "Clinical Viewpoints" better enable you to see life through the eyes of an allied health professional.

Each chapter is subdivided into topics with headings. These subdivisions are not chosen by chance, but are logical chunks of material chosen to make learning more manageable.

You might find the new vocabulary hard to handle. To prevent you from becoming too discouraged as you approach this "foreign language," a new term is printed in **boldface.** As an additional help, each of these new terms is defined for you three times in the text: first, in the narrative when the term becomes a functional part of biological thought; second, at the end of the chapter in which it first appears in the section marked "Glossary"; and third, in a total glossary at the end of the book. As you review a chapter, mentally define each of the new terms. If you are unsure of the meaning of these terms, check the definitions in the book.

You will notice that there is a phonetic spelling following each glossary word. This can be helpful if you will learn how to read the symbols.

An unmarked vowel (a, e, i, o, u) at the end of a syllable will have the long sound, as in the word "prey" = PRA. An unmarked vowel followed by a consonant has the short sound, as in the phonetic spelling of the word "cell" = SEL.

A vowel in the middle of a syllable may have a mark over it to indicate short or long sound. A straight bar (ā) indicates the long sound, and a small arc (ă), the short sound. The word "amylase" = am'ĭ-lās shows these two marks plus a slash (') that tells us to accent the first syllable. Some phonetic spellings may have a double slash (") as well as a single slash ('). The double slash also indicates an accented syllable—but not as heavily accented as with the single slash, as in ob"sir-va'shun.

A number of illustrations occur throughout the text; these illustrations should do more than just attract your attention. Each has been carefully chosen to help you understand a point or relate that point to something you already know. Use these illustrations and their captions to learn and understand the ideas presented.

A set of five videotapes contains over 50 animations of physiological processes integral to the study of allied health sciences. These videotapes, entitled WCB Life Science Animations (LSA), cover such topics as chemistry and genetics. A videotape icon appears in the appropriate figure legends to alert the reader to these animations.

Figure 2.10
LSA 1   Formation of an Ionic Bond
Figure 5.1
LSA 2   Journey into a Cell

Figure 5.7
LSA 4   Cellular Secretion
Figure 5.9
LSA 3   Endocytosis
Figure 7.3
LSA 11   ATP as an Energy Carrier
Figure 7.9
LSA 7   Electron Transport Chain
Figure 7.11
LSA 5   Glycolysis
Figure 7.12
LSA 6   Oxidative Respiration
Figure 8.6
LSA 15   DNA Replication

Figure 8.8
LSA 16   Transcription of a Gene
Figure 8.11
LSA 17   Protein Synthesis
Figure 9.1
LSA 12   Mitosis
Figure 10.1
LSA 13   Meiosis
Figure 10.15
LSA 14   Crossing Over
Figure 10.16
LSA 14   Crossing Over
Figure 11.2
LSA 40   A, B, O Blood Types

Each chapter ends with a summary. As you finish your study of a chapter, read the summary sentence-by-sentence; making sure that there is no new information in the summary. If something is new to you, you have not thoroughly mastered the entire chapter.

Following the chapter summary is a series of review questions. These questions can be used in a variety of ways. You might use them to help channel your attention as you study a chapter or as a review to indicate how well you know the material. Each of these questions is directly answered in the chapter narrative or in the illustrations.

In order to help students with calculations and mathematical conversions, a handy reference guide is provided inside the cover of the text, in Box 3.1, as well as in the Laboratory Manual.

A Laboratory Manual is available for courses that implement hands-on experience in scientific inquiries. The exercises will guide you through various techniques of research and problem-solving methods.

A Study Guide for this textbook is available through your college bookstore under the title *Student Study Guide to Accompany Foundation of Allied Health Sciences,* fourth edition. This Study Guide will help you master course material by acting as a tutorial, review, and guide to testing proficiency. If you don't see a copy on your bookstore's shelves, ask the bookstore manager to order a copy for you.

New to this edition are multimedia correlations. Throughout the text, you will find a videotape icon next to many figure legends. The icon indicates that there is a corresponding animation from the *WCB Life Science Animation Videotape Series.* The above chart lists all the figures that have corresponding animations.

At the end of a few chapters there is a reference made to the CD-ROM entitled *The Dynamic Human. The Dynamic Human CD-ROM* illustrates the important relationships between anatomical structures and their functions in the human body. Realistic computer visualization and three-dimensional visualizations are the premier features of this CD-ROM.

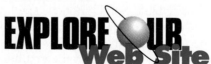

http://www.wcbp.com
http://www.wcbp.com/lifescience/dynamic_human

I would like to thank Paula S. Sandy, Frederick Community College, for reviewing this text.

Science and Life

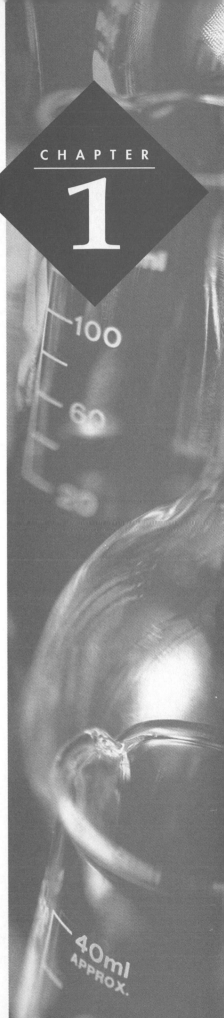

CHAPTER OUTLINE

PURPOSE

This chapter introduces the significance of a scientific background to the allied health sciences. It discusses the nature of science and the importance of knowing how science differs from other areas of study. In particular, it discusses the scientific method and how it is used to gain new information. Since the majority of this text deals with the activities of living cells, there is a discussion of some of the fundamental characteristics of living things at the end of the chapter.

CLINICAL VIEWPOINT

Take ten minutes to look through your local newspaper and find advertisements for an over-the-counter drug that you have in your medicine cabinet. Note the claims that are made for it. Read the literature that accompanies the drug package. Are there any factual discrepancies? Are there any implied actions that are not substantiated by the literature? Can you read and understand the literature?

LEARNING OBJECTIVES

- Understand the difference between science, nonscience, and pseudoscience
- Know the sequence of events in the scientific method
- Recognize the limitations of the scientific method
- Recognize that pseudoscience appears to be scientific but can be used to mislead
- Know the characteristics used to differentiate between living and nonliving things
- Understand that many advances in the quality of life are the result of biological science
- Be able to identify and list the universal characteristics of living things

THE ROLE OF SCIENCE IN HEALTH CAREERS

As you prepare for a career in the allied health sciences, it is important to develop an understanding of the way in which science works. The health sciences are founded on scientific principles, and also include many social and psychological skills that are valuable in motivating and dealing with clients. This text introduces basic scientific knowledge and principles that are important to your further study. One of the first ideas explored is the difference between a scientific approach to understanding our world and other approaches that are philosophically valid but not scientific. In addition, invalid approaches are used by some people to mislead the public by creating images that appear to be scientific but are not.

Most of today's important questions have philosophical, social, and scientific aspects. None of these approaches individually presents a solution to most problems. For example, a large body of scientific evidence indicates that cigarette smoking causes significant health problems. The cost of dealing with these problems is borne by society in general as increased health care costs. One solution to this problem is to make smoking cigarettes illegal. This "solution," however, may be philosophically or socially unacceptable. Science can provide information about the effects of cigarette smoking on human health, but society must answer the more fundamental social and philosophical questions—how should society control the behavior of its members, and which controls are acceptable? It is important to recognize that science has a role to play but is not the answer to all our problems. If we are going to understand the role of science in health care fields, we need to become acquainted with how scientists perceive the world and what factors influence their thinking.

It is important to understand the scientific method since you will be dealing with clients that have a wide range of education and many misconceptions about procedures, medications, or advice given by members of the health care industry. To increase the likelihood that clients will take maximum advantage of their health care services and comply with its directives, it will be imperative that you have a good understanding of what information is "good" and what is "bad." As a member of the health care team it will be your responsibility to communicate effectively with the lay public, research laboratory personnel, children, and highly educated fellow professionals. A solid understanding of your field will enable you to become a well-respected member of this professional community.

SCIENCE AND THE SCIENTIFIC METHOD

The word *science* is a noun derived from a Latin term (*scientia*) meaning *to have knowledge* or *to know* (table 1.1). However, humans have accumulated a vast amount of "knowledge" using a variety of methods, some by scientific methods and some by other methods.

Science is really distinguished by *how* knowledge is acquired, rather than by the act of accumulating facts. **Science** is actually a process or way of arriving at a solution to a problem or understanding an event in nature that involves testing possible solutions. The process has become known as the *scientific method*. The **scientific method** is a way of gaining information (facts) about the world by forming possible solutions to questions followed by rigorous testing to determine if the proposed solutions are valid (VALID = meaningful, convincing, sound, satisfactory, confirmed by others). Scientists are in the business of distinguishing between situations that are merely correlated (happen at the same time) and those that are correlated and show *cause-and-effect relationships*. When an event occurs as the result of a known reason, a cause-and-effect relationship exists. Many events are correlated but not all correlations show a cause-and-effect relationship. Knowing that a cause-and-effect relationship exists enables us to make predictions about what will happen should that same set of circumstances occur in the future. This process has been so successful that others have adopted the method to help them answer questions and make predictions in their field of interest.

Table 1.1 Branches of Science	
Physical Sciences	**Biological Sciences**
Physics	Botany (plants)
Chemistry	Zoology (animals)
Geology	Microbiology (microscopic organisms)
Astronomy	Bacteriology (bacteria)
Geography	Immunology (defense mechanisms)
	Mycology (fungi)
	Virology (viruses)
	Phycology (algae)

What scientists learn by using this approach may help them solve a particular practical problem, such as how to prevent the spread of cold and flu viruses. It may also advance their understanding of an important concept, such as evolution, but have little immediate practical value. The scientific method requires a systematic search for information and a continual checking and rechecking to see if previous ideas are still supported by new information. If the new evidence is not supportive, scientists discard or change their original ideas. Scientific information undergoes constant reevaluation, criticism, and modification.

People who use the scientific method follow the thought processes and activities outlined in table 1.2. As with your own thought processes, the minds of scientists bounce from thought to thought and from category to category as they wrestle with the problem at hand. Keep in mind that scientists try not to "reinvent the wheel"; therefore, they do not always start at the beginning. The sequence presented in table 1.2 is idealistic and a simplification of a very complex series of events.

Observation

Scientific inquiry usually begins with an observation that an event has occurred repeatedly. An **observation** occurs when we use our senses (smell, sight, hearing, taste, touch) or an extension of our senses (microscope, tape recorder, X-ray machine, thermometer) to record an event. Observation is more than just taking note of something. You may hear a sound or see something without really observing. Scientists learn how to increase their level of awareness. Do you know what music is being played in a shopping mall? You hear it but you don't observe. What color was the car that just drove past? You saw it but you didn't observe. When scientists talk about their observations, they are referring to careful, thoughtful recognition of an event—not just a casual notice.

The information gained by direct observation of the event is called **empirical evidence** (EMPIRIC = based on experience; Gr. *empirikos* = experience). Empirical evidence is capable of being verified or disproved by further observation. If the event only occurs once or cannot be repeated in an artificial situation, it is impossible to use the scientific method to gain further information about the event and explain it.

Questioning and Exploration

As scientists gain more empirical evidence about the event, they begin to develop *questions* about it. How does this happen? What causes it to occur? When will it take place again? Can I control the event to my benefit? The formation of the question is not as simple as it might seem because the way the question is asked will determine how you go about answering it. A question that is too broad or

Table 1.2 The Scientific Method

EVENT	ACTIVITY	EXAMPLE
Observation	Recognize something has happened and that it occurs repeatedly. (Empirical evidence is gained from experience or observation.)	Students in a classroom are stricken with a disease that causes red rashes on their faces. This same situation has been described in several schools in your region. Skin cultures taken from the students indicate that there are some unusual bacteria present.
Question Formulation	Write many different kinds of questions about the observations, evaluate the questions, and keep the ones that will be answerable.	Is the disease psychosomatic (i.e., is this a case of hysteria in which there is nothing organically wrong)? Is the rash caused by a bacterium? Is the disease caused by a virus?
Exploration of Alternative Resources	Go to the library to obtain information about this observation. Also, talk to others who are interested in the same problem. Visits to other researchers or communication via letter, FAX, or computer will help determine if your question is a good one if others have already explored the topic.	A search of the medical literature reveals that physicians who used antibiotic X in similar circumstances reported cures even though they never found a bacterium to be present. Attend scientific meetings where this disease outbreak will be discussed. Contact scientists who are reported to be interested in the same problem.
Hypothesis Formation	Pose a possible answer to your question. Be sure that it is testable and that it accounts for all the known information. Recognize that your hypothesis may be wrong.	Antibiotics do not usually affect viruses. Further, the disease has been reported elsewhere which tends to rule out psychosomatic disease. Therefore, your hypothesis is that the disease is caused by a bacterium and that antibiotic X can cure the disease by controlling the rate of growth of the bacterial population.
Experimentation	Set up an experiment that will allow you to test your hypothesis, using a control group and an experimental group. Be sure to collect and analyze the data carefully.	To test the cause-and-effect relationship between administering antibiotic X and curing the illness, you set up two groups. A control group will be given a placebo (a pill with no active ingredient). The experimental group will receive pills containing antibiotic X. The pills will look identical and will be coded so that neither the person receiving the pill nor the person administering the pill will know which individuals receive the medication and which individuals receive the placebo. This is called a "double-blind" test.
		After five days you collect the data and find that 90% of those receiving antibiotic X no longer have the rash. By contrast, only 10% of those receiving the placebo have recovered.
		You conclude that the disease is not psychosomatic and that a bacterium is probably the cause.
		You publish your results and others in the country report back that they have had similar results.
Theory Formation	Repeat the experiment and share information with others over a long period of time. Should your information continue to be considered valid and consistent with other closely related research, the scientific community will recognize that a theory has been established or that your information is consistent with existing theories.	Your results support the generally held theory that many kinds of diseases are caused by microorganisms. This generalization is called the *germ theory of disease*.
Law Formation	If your findings are seen to fit with many other major blocks of information that tie together many different kinds of scientific information, it will be recognized by the scientific community as being consistent with current scientific laws. If it is a major new finding, a new law may be formulated.	Your experimental results are consistent with the *biogenetic law* that states that all living things come from previously living things. Your results strongly suggest that the disease was caused by the multiplication of certain bacteria, and that the antibiotic stopped their multiplication.

too complex may be impossible to answer; therefore, a great deal of effort is put into asking the question in the right way. In some situations, this can be the most time-consuming part of the scientific method; asking the right question is critical to how you look for answers.

Let's say, for example, if you observed that men are often bald while women are seldom bald, you could ask several kinds of questions:

1. a—Is baldness related to the kinds of occupations men and women have?
   b—Does wearing hats cause baldness?

2. a—Are there biochemical differences between men and women that cause larger numbers of men to be bald?
   b—Does the presence of the male hormone, testosterone, cause baldness to be more common in men?

Obviously, the second of each pair of questions is much easier to answer than the first even though the two questions are attempting to obtain similar information.

Once the question is written, scientists *explore other sources of knowledge* to arrive at an acceptable answer. They turn first to the research of others to avoid wasting time and energy answering an already-answered question. This usually means a trip to the library, time spent on a computer with Internet, or contact with fellow scientists interested in the same field of study. Even if their particular question has not already been answered, scientific literature and fellow scientists can provide insight into the problem that will help in its solution. It is during this time that a hypothesis is formed.

The Formation and Testing of Hypotheses

A **hypothesis** is a possible answer to a question or an explanation of an observation. A good hypothesis is able to explain the observation, allow one to predict future events relating to that same observation, and be testable. Just as writing a good scientific question is important, hypothesis formation is critical and may be difficult. If the hypothesis does not account for all the observed facts in the situation, doubt will be cast on the work and may eventually invalidate the hypothesis. Doubt may also surround a hypothesis that is not testable. If a possible explanation is not supported by the evidence, it would only be hearsay and no more useful than mere speculation. Keep in mind that a hypothesis is an educated guess based on observations and information gained from other knowledgeable sources. Scientists try to disprove a hypothesis, not prove they are right. If you cannot disprove something, it increases your confidence that the hypothesis is probably correct, but it does not prove it. It could be that there may be another alternative hypothesis that explains the situation (they have not thought of it yet), or they have not made the observations that indicate their hypothesis is wrong. To test the soundness of a hypothesis, scientists begin the next step in the scientific method—experimentation.

An **experiment** is a re-creation of an event or occurrence in a way that enables a scientist to support or disprove a hypothesis. This can be difficult because a particular event may involve many separate occurrences. For example, the maintenance of teeth free from cavities (dental caries) involves a great number of factors, including genetics, eating habits, nutrition, and brushing. It might seem that developing an understanding of the factors involved in disease-free teeth would be an impossible task. To help unclutter such situations, scientists have devised what is known as a controlled experiment. A **controlled experiment** allows scientists to compare two situations that are identical in all but one respect. The situation used as the basis for comparison is called the **control group,** while the other is called the **experimental group.** The single factor allowed to be different in the experimental group but controlled in the other group is called the **variable.** The situation with tooth care can be broken down into many simple questions, as discussed earlier. Each question provides the basis upon which experimentation occurs. Each experiment provides information about a small part of the total problem of dental care. For example, to test if the mineral fluoride is important in preventing dental caries, an experiment can be performed in which one group (experimental group) receives a dietary fluoride supplement and the other (control group) does not. Both groups would be identical in all other respects, except the experimental group would receive the fluoride supplement. After the experiment, the new data (facts) are analyzed. If there is no difference in the amount of dental caries in the two groups, the variable evidently does not have a cause-and-effect relationship. However, if there is a difference, it is likely that the variable is responsible for the difference between the control and experimental groups. In this case, it has been shown that the addition of fluoride to the diet does reduce the likelihood of dental caries. While most people think of "laboratory experiments" as being conducted under extremely controlled conditions, many must be "field experiments." These are more difficult to control. In some situations, conducting controlled experiments has been impossible. In these situations, the hypotheses have been upheld by making more observations that support the original hypothesis. For example, the bacterium *Treponema pallidum* has been determined to be the cause of the sexually transmitted disease syphilis only through repeated observation of the organisms in people with the symptoms of the disease. Never has this bacterium been grown in a laboratory.

Any experiment needs to be repeated many times to be validated, since scientists encourage challenges to their work and admit that no experiment is perfect. In our example, this means that the same type of experiment needs to be conducted on different populations of people in various parts of the world, and that large numbers of individuals need to be involved in each group. The larger the group, the more comfortable a scientist is that the results are valid. This is often difficult to attain in the health field because a limited number of individuals display a specific disease or abnormality. Furthermore, scientists will apply statistical tests to the results to help decide if the results obtained (1) are **valid** (meaningful; fit with other knowledge), (2) are **reliable** (give the same results repeatedly), (3) are the result of random events, or (4) show cause-and-effect. Random events can give the impression of having a cause-and-effect relationship and that the hypothesis is valid when in fact it is not. If there is a cause-and-effect relationship, the hypothesis will have predictive value. For example, some water supplies naturally contain fluoride. If the control group drinks naturally fluoridated water, there will be no recognizable difference between the experimental and control groups because both groups are getting fluoride. During experimentation, scientists learn new information and formulate new questions that can lead to even more experiments. Some scientists speculate that one good experiment can result in a hundred new questions and experiments. The discovery of the structure of the DNA molecule by Watson and Crick has resulted in thousands of experiments and has stimulated the development of the field of molecular biology (figure 1.1). Similarly, the discovery of molecules that control pain has resulted in much research about how these molecules work and which ones might be used for health purposes.

Often the development of experiments involves ethical questions. In order to establish a drug's effectiveness in humans, it is necessary to have control and experimental groups in which the experimental group receives the drug and the control group does not. Is it ethical to withhold treatment from a group of people because they are part of a control group? For example, is it necessary to test the drug AZT, which is used to treat people with the AIDS virus, in this way? Experimental surgical procedures need to be developed on living patients. Is it ethical to ask a patient to undergo a procedure that may do him or her considerable harm even though the information gained from the procedure would be of great help to future generations?

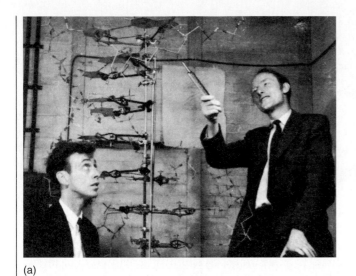

(a)

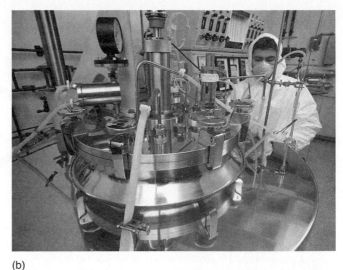

(b)

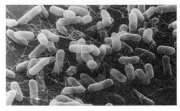

(c)

FIGURE 1.1 The growth of knowledge.
James D. Watson and Francis W. Crick are theoretical scientists who determined in 1953 the structure of the DNA molecule, which contains the genetic information of a cell. (a) This photograph shows the model of DNA they constructed. The discovery of the structure of the DNA molecule was followed by much research into how the molecule codes information, how it makes copies of itself, and how the information is put into action. Ultimately, these lines of research have led to altering the DNA of bacteria so that they produce useful materials such as vitamins, proteins, and antibiotics. (b) Genetically altered bacteria can be grown in special vats and the useful materials harvested. (c) The bacterium *E. coli* is commonly found in the human intestine.

Theories and Laws

If the processes of questioning and experimentation continue and evidence consistently supports the original hypothesis and other closely-related hypotheses, the scientific community begins to see how these hypotheses and facts fit together into a broad pattern. When this happens, a theory comes into existence.

A **theory** is a plausible, scientifically acceptable generalization that is the result of years of questioning, experimentation, and data collection. Unfortunately the word theory is often used in popular culture to refer to an unsubstantiated claim, for example, "He has a theory that eating large quantities of vitamin C will prevent cancer." Obviously this use of the word theory is very different from what is meant by a scientific theory.

An example of a biological theory is the germ theory of disease. This theory states that certain diseases, called *infectious* diseases, are caused by microorganisms that are capable of being transmitted from one individual to another. As you can see, this is a very broad statement. It is the result of years of questioning, experimentation, and pulling data together. While a hypothesis is an answer to a specific question, a theory encompasses the answers to many complex questions. As a result, there are fewer theories than hypotheses.

Another example of a theory is the atomic theory, which states that all matter is made up of small particles called atoms. Both the germ theory and atomic theories are generally accepted by most scientists and are fundamental to the development of entire areas of science. Chemistry is based on the assumption that matter is made of many kinds of atoms, and public health and other medical scientists rely heavily on the germ theory of disease to explain how infectious diseases are spread.

Just because a theory has been formulated does not mean that testing stops. In fact, many scientists see this as a challenge and exert great effort to disprove theories. Occasionally a theory may be found to be incorrect or to need modification.

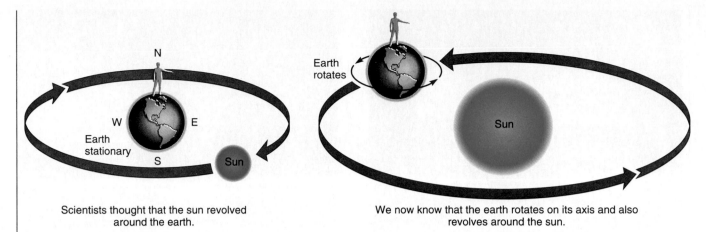

FIGURE 1.2 Science must be willing to challenge previous beliefs.

Science always needs to be aware that new discoveries may force a reinterpretation of previously held beliefs. Early scientists thought that the sun revolved around the earth in a clockwise direction. This was certainly a reasonable theory at the time. Subsequently we have learned that the earth revolves around the sun in a counterclockwise direction while at the same time rotating on its axis in a counterclockwise direction. It is this rotation of the earth on its axis that gives us the impression that the sun is moving.

At one time, the theory of the structure of the universe had the earth at the center with sun, moon, and stars revolving around it. People observed that the sun rose in the east and traveled across the sky to set in the west. Since scientists could not feel the earth moving, it seemed perfectly logical that the sun traveled around the earth. When it was understood that the earth rotated on its axis, a completely new theory of the organization of our solar system and the universe was developed (figure 1.2). Although this theory seems easy to understand today, it was not readily accepted at the time of its discovery, and required major changes in the way people thought.

The germ theory has been modified to include several different kinds of disease-causing organisms, including bacteria, viruses, fungi, and protozoa. Because each of these kinds of organisms has different characteristics, their methods of transmission are somewhat different. Yet the basic theory that disease-causing microorganisms can be spread from one person to another remains valid.

If a theory survives this skeptical approach and continues to be supported by experimental evidence, it may become a scientific law. A **scientific law** is a uniform or constant rule of nature. The biogenetic law, which states that all living things come from preexisting living things, is an example. Scientific laws are even more general than theories and they encompass the answers to even more complex questions. Therefore, there are relatively few scientific laws.

SCIENCE, NONSCIENCE, AND PSEUDOSCIENCE

Fundamental Attitudes in Science

As you can see from this discussion of the scientific method, a scientific approach to the world requires a certain way of thinking. There is an insistence on ample supporting evidence by numerous studies rather than easy acceptance of strongly stated opinions. Scientists must separate opinions from statements of fact. A scientist is a healthy skeptic.

Careful attention to detail is also important. Because scientists publish their findings, and their colleagues examine their work, there is a strong desire to conduct careful work that can be easily defended. This does not mean that scientists do not speculate and state opinions, but great care is taken to clearly distinguish fact from opinion.

There is also a strong ethic of honesty. Scientists are not saints, but the fact that science is conducted out in the open in front of one's peers tends to reduce the incidence of dishonesty. The scientific community strongly condemns and severely penalizes those who perform shoddy science, falsify data, or steal another's ideas. Any of these infractions will lead to the loss of one's professional position and reputation.

There is a tendency for the general public to hold science in awe because they do not always understand the concepts and ideas being put forth by scientists. This unfortunately is often paired with a sense that science is infallible, or that science can solve all the problems of the world. However, science is in a constant state of development and mistakes are made; therefore, as new information is gathered and old mistaken ideas are clarified, our understanding of the world changes.

Many early anatomists and physiologists had what appears to us to be rather strange ideas of how the body works. At one time, it was thought that the blood ebbed and flowed like the tides. Eventually William Harvey made some careful observations that demonstrated that the blood in surface veins of the skin proceeded in only one direction. He blocked off the flow of blood in a surface vein in two places and observed that the middle section of the vein did not fill with blood (figure 1.3).

Scientists are often asked to provide a solution to a problem—and the public wants the solution to be risk-free. This is impossible. Medical advances have allowed millions of people to live longer, more productive lives, but with each advance there is a risk. For example, immunization of children against childhood diseases has saved millions of lives, but some individuals have severe reactions to vaccines or may contract the disease from the vaccine. This number is very small and is considered a small risk to take for the vast amount of good that is done.

FROM EXPERIMENTATION TO APPLICATION

The scientific method has helped us to understand and control many aspects of our natural world. Some information is extremely important in understanding the structure and functioning of things but appears at first glance to have little practical value. For example, an understanding of the life cycle of a star or how meteors travel through the universe may be very important for those who are trying to answer questions about how the universe was formed, but it is of little value to the average citizen. However, as our knowledge has increased, the time between first discovery to practical application has decreased significantly (box 1.1).

Scientists known as *genetic engineers*, have altered the chemical code system of small organisms (microorganisms) so that they may produce many new drugs such as antibiotics, hormones, and enzymes. The ease with which these complex chemicals are produced would not have been possible had it not been for the information gained from the basic research conducted by the theoretical sciences of microbiology, molecular biology, and genetics (*see* figure 1.2). Our understanding of how organisms genetically control the manufacture of proteins has led to the large scale production of enzymes. Some of these chemicals can more gently and efficiently remove necrotic (dead or decaying) tissue from burned skin.

As another example, Louis Pasteur was interested in the theoretical problem of whether life could be generated from nonliving material. Much of his theoretical work led to practical applications in disease control. His theory that there are microorganisms that cause diseases and decay led to the development of vaccinations against rabies and the development of pasteurization for the preservation of foods (figure 1.4).

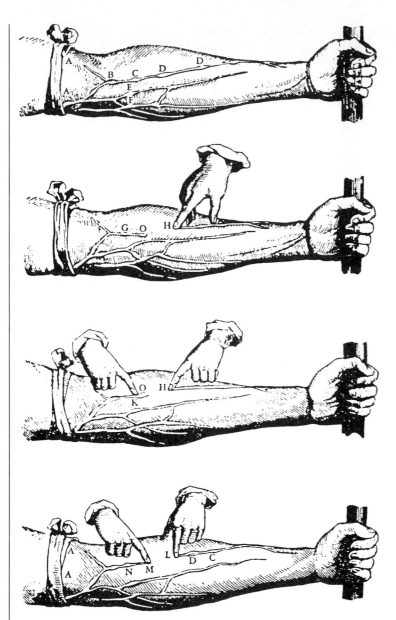

FIGURE 1.3 William Harvey and the circulation of blood.
William Harvey was able to show that blood flowed in only one direction in the veins of the body. In the figures shown here he demonstrated that blood moved toward the central body and that valves present in the veins prevented the blood from flowing from the central body into the arm.

Source: William Harvey, *An Anatomical Disquisition on the Motion of the Heart and Blood in Animals*, London, 1628.

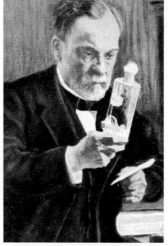

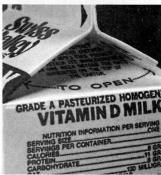

FIGURE 1.4 Louis Pasteur and pasteurized milk.
Louis Pasteur (1822–1895) performed many experiments while he studied the question of the origin of life, one of which led directly to the food-preservation method now known as pasteurization.

Science and Nonscience

The differences between science and nonscience are often based on the assumptions and methods used to gather and organize information and, most importantly, the testing of these assumptions. The difference between a scientist and a nonscientist is that a scientist continually challenges and tests the principles and laws to determine a cause-and-effect relationship, whereas a nonscientist may not feel that this is important.

BOX 1.1

Edward Jenner and the Control of Smallpox

Edward Jenner first developed the technique of vaccination in 1795. This was the result of a twenty-six-year study of two diseases: cowpox and smallpox. Cowpox was known as *vaccinae*. From this word evolved the present terms *vaccination* and *vaccine*. Jenner *observed* that milkmaids developed pocklike sores after milking cows infected with cowpox, but they rarely became sick with smallpox. He asked the *question*, Why don't milkmaids get smallpox? He developed the *hypothesis* that the mild reaction milkmaids had to cowpox protected them from the often fatal small-pox. This led him to perform an *experiment* in which he transferred puslike material from the cowpox to human skin and discovered that *vaccinated* people were protected from smallpox. When these results became known, public reaction was mixed. Some people thought that vaccination was the work of the devil. Many European rulers supported Jenner by encouraging their subjects to be vaccinated. Napoleon and the Empress of Russia were very influential and, in the United States, Thomas Jefferson had some members of his family vaccinated.

Many years later, following the *development of the germ theory* of disease, it was discovered that both cowpox and smallpox are caused by viruses that are very similar in structure. Exposure to the cowpox virus allows the body to develop immunity against the cowpox virus and the smallpox virus at the same time. In 1979, almost two hundred years after Jenner developed his vaccination, the Centers for Disease Control and Prevention in the United States and the World Health Organization of the United Nations declared that smallpox was extinct.

BOX TABLE 1.1 Recommended Childhood Immunization Schedule*—United States, January 1995

Vaccine	Birth	2 Months	4 Months	6 Months	12 Months	15 Months	18 Months	4–6 Years	11–12 Years	14–16 Years
Hepatitis B	HB-1									
		HB-2		HB-3						
Diphtheria, Tetanus, Pertussis		DTP	DTP	DTP	DTP or DTaP at ≥ 15 months			DTP or DTaP	Td	
H. influenzae type b		Hib	Hib	Hib	Hib					
Poliovirus		OPV	OPV	At least 2 OPV						
Measles, Mumps, Rubella				MMR				MMR or MMR		

*Recommended vaccines are listed under the routinely recommended ages. Shaded bars indicate range of acceptable ages for vaccination. While the above information is current and accurate, there is additional information from the CDC that clarifies these age ranges and notes special precautions and recommendations. Please refer to this publication for further details.

Sources: Advisory Committee on Immunization Practices, American Academy of Pediatrics, and American Academy of Family Physicians, as appeared in *Morbidity and Mortality Weekly Report*. Centers for Disease Control, Vol. 43, nos. 51 & 52, p. 960, January 6, 1995.

Once you understand the scientific method, you won't have any trouble identifying astronomy, chemistry, physics, and biology as sciences. But what about economics, sociology, anthropology, history, philosophy, and literature? All of these fields may make use of certain laws that are derived in a logical way, but they are also nonscientific in some ways. Some things are beyond science and cannot be approached using the scientific method. Art, literature, theology, and philosophy are rarely thought of as sciences. They are concerned with beauty, human emotion, and speculative thought rather than with facts and verifiable laws. On the other hand, physics, chemistry, geology, and biology are almost always considered sciences. Music is an area of study in a middle ground where scientific approaches may be used to some extent. "Good" music is certainly unrelated to science, but the study of how the human larynx generates the sound of a song is based on scientific principles (figure 1.5). Any serious student of music

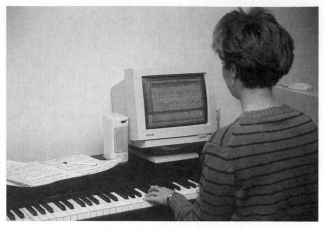
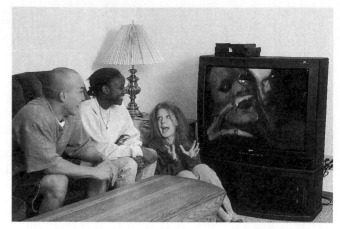

FIGURE 1.5 The science and nonscience of electronic movie music.
Not many people realize that electronic music was first created in the late 1800s. Some of those early instruments are still used in the production of movie sound tracks, especially science fiction and horror movies. While scientists are not in the business of evaluating whether such music is "good" or not, they have certainly contributed to the understanding of (1) the physics of how the sounds are created, (2) the anatomy and physiology of how the sound stimulates nerve endings in the ear, (3) the biochemistry of how the nerve impulses travel through the body and affect the various body structures such as tear glands (crying), muscles (tension during a fear response), hormone levels (pounding in your chest), and vocalizations (screaming!).

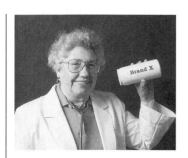

FIGURE 1.6 "Nine out of ten doctors surveyed recommend Brand X."
It is obvious that there are many things wrong with this statement. First of all, is the person in the white coat a physician? Second, if only ten doctors were asked, the sample size is too small. Third, only selected doctors might have been asked to participate. Finally, the question could have been asked in such a way as to obtain the desired answer: "Would you recommend Brand X over Dr. Pete's snake oil?" (*see* table 1.2).

will study the anatomy of the human voice box and how the vocal cords vibrate to generate sound waves. Similarly, economics makes use of mathematical models and established economic laws to help make predictions about future economic conditions. However, the regular occurrence of unpredicted economic changes indicates that economics is far from scientific, since the reliability of predictions is a central criterion of science. Anthropology and sociology also have many aspects that are scientific in nature, but they cannot be considered to be true sciences because many of the generalizations they have developed cannot be tested by repeated experimentation. They also do not show a significantly high degree of cause-and-effect or have poor predictive value.

Pseudoscience

Pseudoscience (*pseudo* = false) takes on the flavor of science but is not supportable as valid or reliable. Often, the purpose of pseudoscience is to confuse or mislead. The area of nutrition is one that is flooded with pseudoscience (figure 1.6 and table 1.3). We all know that we must obtain certain nutrients like amino acids, vitamins, and minerals from the food that we eat or we may become ill. Many scientific experiments have been performed that reliably demonstrate the validity of this information. However, in most cases, it has not been demonstrated that the nutritional supplements so vigorously advertised are as useful or desirable as advertised. Rather, selected bits of scientific information (amino acids, vitamins, and minerals are essential to good health) have been used to create the feeling that additional amounts of these nutritional supplements are necessary or that they can improve your health. In reality, the average person eating a varied diet will obtain all of these nutrients in adequate amounts, and nutritional supplements are not required.

In addition, many of these products are labeled as organic or natural, with the implication that they have greater nutritive value because they are organically grown (grown without pesticides or synthetic fertilizers) or because they come from nature. The poisons curare, strychnine, and nicotine are all organic molecules that are produced in nature by plants that could be grown organically, but we wouldn't want to include them in our diet.

Table 1.3 Professional Science Degrees and Titles

DEGREE	EDUCATION	TITLE
A.S. (Associate of Science)	2 years community or junior college; focus on introductory course in science in general (ex., Biology, Chemistry, Physics).	Mr. Mrs. Ms.
A.A.S. (Associate Degree in Applied Science)	2 years community or junior college; focus on courses of study such as nursing, dental hygiene, radiography, and respiratory therapy and requires Biology, Chemistry, and Physics.	Mr. Mrs. Ms.
B.S. (Bachelor of Science)	4–5 years college or university; major course work in a specific area (ex., Biology) with minor course work in related field (ex., Chemistry) along with general education courses (ex., English, Math, Government).	Mr. Mrs. Ms.
M.S. (Master of Science)	2–3 years past Bachelor's degree, college or university; major course work in a specific area (ex., Bacteriology) with minor course work in related field (ex., Biochemistry); lab research project may be required and production of thesis research paper.	Mr. Mrs. Ms.
Ph.D. (Doctor of Philosophy)	4–5 years past Bachelor's degree, university; major course work in a specific area (ex., Exotoxin Production of the *Streptococcaceae*) with major research project required and production of Doctoral Dissertation paper.	Doctor
M.D. (Medical Doctor including general practitioners and specialists)	4–5 years past Bachelor's degree, university; concentrated course work and clinical experience in the practice of medicine.	Doctor
D.D.S. (Doctor of Dental Science)	4–5 years past Bachelor's degree, university; concentrated course work and clinical experience in the practice of dentistry.	Doctor
Ed.D. (Doctor of Education)	4–5 years past Bachelor's degree, university; major course work in a specific area (ex., Learning Theory as Applied to Adult Learners) with major research project required and production of Doctoral Dissertation paper.	Doctor

Limitations of Science

By definition, science is a way of thinking and seeking information to solve problems. Therefore, the scientific method can be applied only to questions that have a factual basis. Questions concerning morals, value judgments, social issues, and attitudes cannot be answered using the scientific method. What makes a painting great? What is the best type of music? Which wine is best? What color should I paint my car? These questions are related to values, beliefs, and tastes; therefore, the scientific method cannot be used to answer them.

Just because scientists say something is true does not necessarily make it true. Everyone makes mistakes, and quite often, as new information is gathered, old laws must be changed or discarded. For example, at one time scientists were sure that the sun went around the earth. They observed that the sun rose in the east and traveled across the sky to set in the west. Since scientists could not feel the earth moving, it seemed perfectly logical that the sun traveled around the earth. Once they understood that the earth rotated on its axis, they began to understand that the rising and setting of the sun could be explained in other ways. A completely new concept of the relationship between the sun and the earth developed (*see* figure 1.2).

Although this kind of study seems rather primitive to us today, this change in thinking about the sun and the earth was a very important step in understanding the universe and how the various parts are related to one another. This background information was built upon by many generations of astronomers and space scientists, and finally led to space exploration.

Many people view science as a powerful tool that will come up with answers to the major problems of our time. This is not necessarily true. Most of the problems we face are generated by the behavior and desires of people. Famine, drug abuse, and pollution are human-caused and must be resolved by humans. Science may provide some tools for the social planners, politicians, and ethical thinkers, but science does not have, nor does it attempt to provide, all the answers to the problems of the human race. Science is merely one of the tools at our disposal.

CHARACTERISTICS OF LIFE

As a person preparing for a career in the health field, it is important to have a thorough knowledge of how living things work and what constitutes life. But what does it mean to be alive? You would think that this question could be answered very easily. However, this question is more than just a theoretical one, since it has become necessary in recent years to construct some legal definitions of what life is—when it begins and ends. The legal definition of death is important, since it may determine whether or not a person will receive life insurance benefits or if body parts may be used in transplants. In the case of heart transplants, the person donating the heart may be legally *dead* but the heart certainly isn't because it can be removed while it still has *life.* In other words, there are different kinds of death. There is the death of the whole living unit and the death of each cell within the living unit. A person actually *dies* before every cell has died. Death, then, is the absence of life, but that still doesn't tell us what life is. At this point, we won't try to define life but we will describe some of the basic characteristics of living things.

The ability to manipulate energy and matter is unique to living things. Just how this is accomplished can be used to better understand how living things differ from nonliving things. Living things show four characteristics that the nonliving do not: (1) metabolic processes, (2) generative processes, (3) responsive processes, and (4) control processes.

Metabolic processes (METABOLISM = Gr. *metaballein,* to turn about, change, alter) are the total of all chemical reactions taking place within an organism. There are three essential aspects of metabolism: (1) *nutrient uptake,* (2) *nutrient processing,* and (3) *waste elimination.* All living things expend energy to take in nutrients (raw materials) and energy from their environment. Many animals take in these materials by eating or swallowing other organisms. Microorganisms and plants absorb raw materials into their cells to maintain their lives. Once inside, nutrients enter a network of chemical reactions. These reactions process nutrients in order to manufacture new parts, make repairs, and reproduce. However, not all materials entering a living thing are valuable to it. There may be portions of nutrients that are valuable, but the rest may be useless or even harmful. In that situation, organisms eliminate waste. Heat energy may also be considered a waste product.

The second group of characteristics of life are known as the generative processes. **Generative processes** are reactions that result in an increase in the size of an individual organism—*growth;* or an increase in the number of individuals in a population of organisms—*reproduction.* During growth, living things add to their structure, repair parts, and store nutrients for later use. However, growth cannot go on indefinitely because as organisms get larger, they become inefficient. Living things respond to this problem by reproducing. Reproduction is one of the most important life functions, because it is the only way that living things can perpetuate themselves. There are a number of different ways that organisms can reproduce and guarantee their continued existence.

Survival also depends on the organism's ability to react to external and internal changes in its environment. The group of characteristics involved are called the **responsive processes.** Three types of responsive processes have been identified: *irritability, individual adaptation,* and *population adaptation (evolution).* Irritability is an individual's rapid response to a stimulus, such as a knee-jerk reflex. This type of response occurs only in the individual receiving the stimulus and is rapid because the mechanism that allows the response to occur (i.e., muscles, bones, and nerves) is already in place. Individual adaptation is also an individual response, but is slower since it requires the activation of genetic information. For example, when a person moves from sea level to a high altitude he or she may initially suffer from altitude sickness or experience shortness of breath. After some time, the person's ability to carry oxygen in the blood increases because more red blood cells are produced, and the symptoms go away. Population adaptation is also known as evolution. Evolution is a slow change in the genetic makeup of a *population* of organisms. This enables a group of organisms to adapt and better survive threatening changes in their environment over many generations.

The **control processes** of *coordination* and *regulation* constitute the fourth characteristic of life. Control processes are mechanisms that ensure an organism will carry out all metabolic activities in the proper sequence (coordination) and the proper rate (regulation). All the chemical reactions of an organism are coordinated and linked together in specific pathways. The orchestration of all the reactions ensures that there will be specific stepwise handling of nutrients needed to maintain life. The molecules responsible for coordinating these reactions are known as enzymes. **Enzymes** are molecules produced by organisms that are able to increase and control the rate at which life's chemical reactions occur. Enzymes also regulate the amount of nutrients processed into other forms.

In addition to the four basic processes that are typical of living things, it is important to point out that living things have some basic structural similarities. All living things are composed of complex, structural units called **cells.** These cells have an outer limiting membrane or sheet-like material consisting of complex molecular arrangements and internal structural units that have specific functions. Some living things, like you, consist of trillions of cells with specialized abilities that interact to provide the independent functioning unit called an **organism.** Typically in large multicellular organisms like humans, cells cooperate with one another in units called **tissues.** Groups of tissues (muscle, nervous) are organized into larger units known as **organs,** and in turn, into **organ systems** (circulatory) (figure 1.7). Other organisms, like bacteria or yeasts, fulfill all four life processes within a single cell. Nonliving materials like rocks, water, or gases do not share a structurally complex common subunit. Table 1.4 summarizes the differences between living and nonliving things.

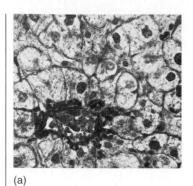

(a)

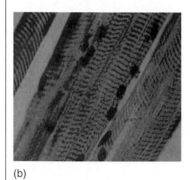

(b)

FIGURE 1.7 Organization of a complex organism.

The basic building block of all living things is the cell. (a) These are typical human liver *cells*. While the components of these cells are not "alive," they function together as a "living" thing. (b) When cells with similar structure and function work together to serve a common purpose they are called a *tissue*. This microscopic photograph shows the cells of human skeletal muscle. (c) When various tissues work together they form *organs*, a human heart. (d) Organs in turn can work together as *organ systems*, the human circulatory system. (e) When all the organ systems are interconnected and function as a whole, they become an *organism*.

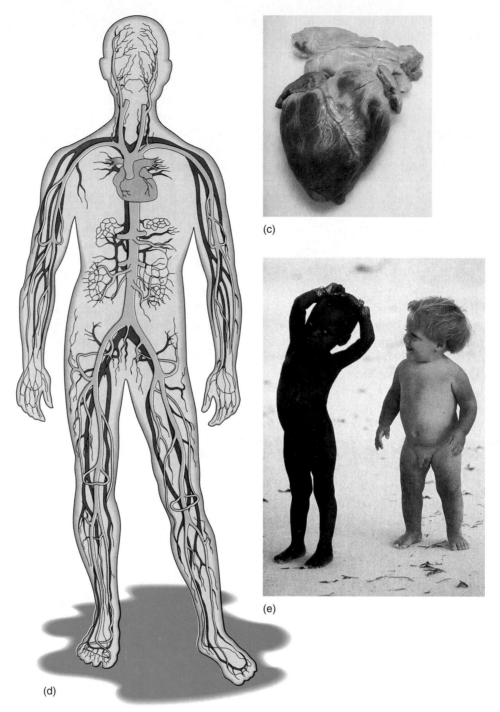

(c)

(d)

(e)

Table 1.4

Characteristics of Life. Living and nonliving things differ in a number of ways. Some of these differences are shown here.

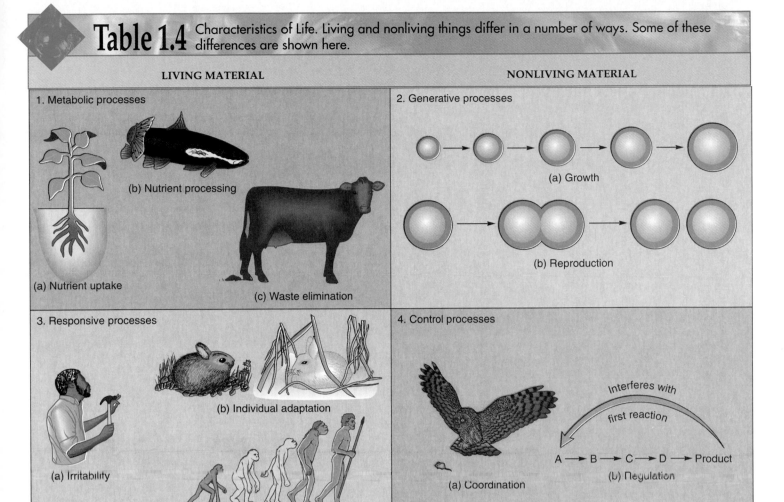

LIVING MATERIAL

1. Metabolic processes

(a) Nutrient uptake

(b) Nutrient processing

(c) Waste elimination

3. Responsive processes

(a) Irritability

(b) Individual adaptation

(c) Population adaptation (evolution)

NONLIVING MATERIAL

2. Generative processes

(a) Growth

(b) Reproduction

4. Control processes

(a) Coordination

Interferes with first reaction

A → B → C → D → Product

(b) Regulation

SUMMARY

Science and nonscience can be distinguished by the kinds of laws and rules that are constructed to unify the body of knowledge. Science involves the continuous testing of rules and principles by the collection of new facts. In science these rules are usually arrived at by using the scientific method—observation, questioning, exploring resources, hypothesis formation, experimentation, theory formation, and law formation. If the rules are not testable or if no rules are used, it is not science. Pseudoscience uses scientific appearances to mislead.

Living things show the characteristics of (1) metabolic processes, (2) generative processes, (3) responsive processes, and (4) control processes.

In addition to these functional characteristics, living things have a structural unit called a cell.

QUESTIONS

1. List two characteristics of a good hypothesis.
2. What is the difference between science and nonscience? Give examples.
3. Why is testing so important in science?
4. How do you identify pseudoscience?
5. List four characteristics of living things.
6. Explain what is meant by "cause-and-effect."
7. List three misunderstandings that were clarified by additional study and research.
8. The scientific method cannot be used to deny or prove the existence of God. Why?
9. What are controlled experiments? Why are they necessary to support a hypothesis?
10. List the steps in the scientific method.

CHAPTER GLOSSARY

cells (selz) The basic structural units that make up all living things.

control group (con-trōl' grūp) The situation used as the basis for comparison in a controlled experiment.

control processes (con-trōl pros'es-es) Mechanisms that ensure that an organism will carry out all metabolic activities in the proper sequence (coordination) and the proper amount (regulation).

controlled experiment (con-trōl'd ek-sper'ĭ-ment) An experiment that allows for a comparison of two events that are identical in all but one respect.

empirical evidence (em-pir'ĭ-cal ev-ĭ-dens) The information gained by observing an event.

enzymes (en'zīms) Molecules produced by organisms that are able to control the rate at which chemical reactions occur.

experiment (ek-sper'ĭ-ment) A re-creation of an event in a way that enables a scientist to gain valid and reliable empirical evidence.

experimental group (ek-sper'ĭ-men'tal grūp) The situation in a controlled experiment that is identical to the control group in all respects but one.

generative processes (jen'uh-ra"tiv pros'es-es) Actions that increase the size of an individual organism (growth), or increase the number of individuals in a population (reproduction).

hypothesis (hi-poth'e-sis) A possible answer to or explanation of a question that accounts for all the observed facts and is testable.

metabolic processes (me-ta-bol'ik pros'es-es) The total of all chemical reactions within an organism; for example, nutrient uptake and processing, and waste elimination.

observation (ob-sir-vā-shun) The process of using the senses or extensions of the senses to record events.

organ (or'gun) A structure composed of two or more kinds of tissues.

organism (or'gah-nizm) An independent living unit.

organ system (or'gun sis'tem) A group of organs that perform a particular function.

pseudoscience (su-do-si'ens) The use of the appearance of science to mislead. The assertions made are not valid or reliable.

reliable (re-li'a-bul) Giving the same result on successive trials.

responsive processes (re-spon'siv pros'es-es) Those abilities to react to external and internal changes in the environment; for example, irritability, individual adaptation, and evolution.

science (si'ens) A process or way of arriving at a solution to a problem or understanding an event in nature involving hypotheses formation and testing.

scientific law (si-en-tif'ik law) A uniform or constant feature of nature supported by several theories.

scientific method (si-en-tif'ik meth'ud) A way of gaining information (facts) about the world around you involving observation, hypothesis formation, experimentation, theory formation, and law formation.

theory (the'o-re) A plausible, scientifically acceptable generalization supported by several hypotheses and experimental trials.

tissue (tish'u) A group of similar cells that performs a specific function; ex., bone.

valid (va'lid) Meaningful data that fits into the framework of scientific knowledge.

variable (var'e-a-bul) The single factor that is allowed to be different.

Chemical Principles for Allied Health

CHAPTER OUTLINE

PURPOSE

In order to understand the structure and activities of living organisms, you must know something about the materials from which they are made. In this chapter we will discuss the structure of matter and the energy it contains. As you read this chapter, you should consciously try to build a vocabulary that will help you describe matter. The study of linguistics (the Sapir-Whorf Hypothesis) teaches that language shapes thought. People think in the words and related concepts our language gives us. It is easier to conceive of something if we have a word for it. Words or terminology help give substance to ideas.

CLINICAL VIEWPOINT

Sodium chloride (NaCl) is commonly referred to as salt. This chemical is essential to all life. Each molecule is composed of an atom of sodium (Na) bonded to an atom of chlorine (Cl). The average adult has between 160 to 175 grams of salt in their body, about 6 ounces worth. An estimated 200 milligrams of NaCl is lost through perspiration and other body fluids each day. In developed countries, meats usually contain enough salt to replace this loss without using supplements. However, cultures primarily eating cereals, vegetables, and grains must add salt to their diet in order to replace that lost each day. Salt is also used to prevent foods from spoiling, as in salt pork, fish, and jerky. Prior to the invention of refrigeration, salt was so important that in some cultures it was used as money. The term "salary" is descended from Roman times when the soldiers who guarded salt shipments were paid in salt, i.e., they earned "salarium" and they were "worth their salt."

LEARNING OBJECTIVES

- Understand that all matter is composed of atoms of different elements
- Know the basic structure of an atom
- Recognize how isotopes differ from one another
- Differentiate among ionic, covalent, and hydrogen bonds
- Describe the relationships among acids, bases, salts, and the pH scale

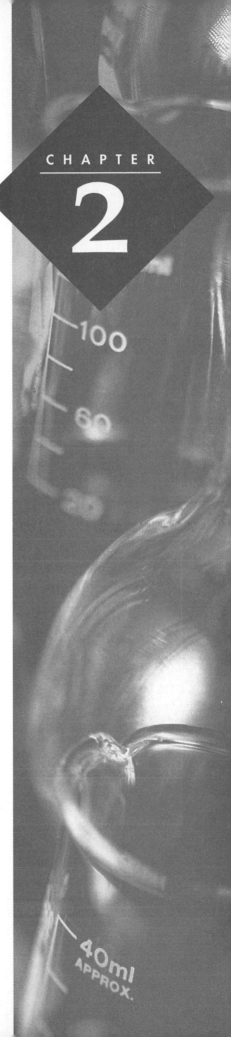

All living things are composed of and use chemicals. There are more than 100,000 chemicals used by organisms for communication, defense, aggression, reproduction, and various other activities. Chemicals are also known as *matter*. **Matter** is anything that has weight (mass) and also takes up space (volume). Mass is how much matter there is in an object, while weight refers to the amount of force with which that object is attracted by gravity. For example, a textbook is composed of the same amount of matter whether you measure its mass on the Earth or on the Moon. However, since the force of gravity is greater on the Earth, the book will weigh more on Earth than it would on the Moon. Both mass and volume depend on the amount of matter you are dealing with; the greater the amount, the greater its mass and volume, provided the temperature and pressure of the environment stays the same.

Characteristics that are independent of the amount of matter include density and activity. **Density** is the weight of a certain volume of material; it is frequently expressed as grams per cubic centimeter. For example, a cubic centimeter of lead is very heavy in comparison to a cubic centimeter of aluminum. Lead has a higher density than aluminum. The activity of matter depends almost entirely on its composition.

All matter has a certain amount of **energy,** something an object has that enables it to do work (box 2.1). This chapter will focus on two types of energy, kinetic and potential. **Kinetic energy** is energy of motion. The energy an object has that can become kinetic energy is called **potential energy.** You might think of potential energy as stored energy. When we talk of chemical energy, we are really talking about potential energy in chemicals. This energy can be released as kinetic energy to do work such as performing chemical reactions, i.e., change the way atoms are attached to one another. An object that appears to be motionless does not necessarily lack energy. Its individual molecules will still be moving, but the object itself appears to be stationary. An object on top of a mountain may be motionless, but still may contain significant amounts of potential energy. One of the important scientific laws of chemistry, the *Law of Conservation of Energy* or the **First Law of Thermodynamics,** states that energy can be neither created nor destroyed; it can only be changed from one form to another. The amount of energy that a molecule has is related to how fast it moves. **Temperature** is a measure of this velocity, or energy of motion. The higher the temperature, the faster the molecules are moving.

The three **states of matter**—solid, liquid, and gas—can be explained by thinking of the relative amounts of energy possessed by the molecules of each. A **solid** contains molecules packed tightly together. The molecules vibrate in place and are strongly attracted to each other. They are moving rapidly and constantly bump into each other. The amount of kinetic energy in a solid is less than that in a liquid of the same material. A **liquid** has molecules still strongly attracted to each other, but slightly farther apart. Since they are moving more rapidly, they sometimes slide past each other as they move. This gives the flowing property to a liquid. Still more energetic are the molecules of a **gas.** The attraction the gas molecules have for each other is overcome by the speed with which the individual molecules move. Since they are moving the fastest, their collisions tend to push them farther apart and so a gas expands to fill its container. A common example of a substance that displays the three states of matter is water. Ice, liquid water, and water vapor are all composed of the same chemical—H_2O. The molecules are moving at different speeds in each state because of the difference in kinetic energy. Considering the amount of energy in the molecules of each state of matter helps us explain changes such as freezing and melting. When a liquid becomes a solid, its molecules lose some of their energy; when it becomes a gas, its molecules gain energy.

Gravity

The weakest and most familiar force in the universe. The electromagnetic force is millions of times stronger; however, *gravity* is a significant force when a body is extremely large. It is the force that keeps the Moon in motion around the Earth and pulls smaller objects toward it.

Electromagnetism

The force holding electrons close to the nucleus in atoms. *Electromagnetism* is as responsible for the shape of the world as gravity. It is the force that holds atoms together in combinations to form molecules.

The Strongest Force

While electromagnetism holds combinations of atoms together and the electrons of atoms to the nucleus, the *strong force* holds the particles of the nucleus (protons and neutrons) itself together. It is 137 times stronger than the electromagnetic force. It affects only the particles in the nucleus, and not particles such as electrons, normally found outside the atomic nucleus and operates at exceedingly short distances.

The Weak Force

While the strong force holds a nucleus together, the *weak force* acts in certain situations to push it apart. The weak force is responsible for certain types of radioactivity, known as beta radiation.

Fifth Force

A force that may exist. Its existence has not yet been confirmed. It is thought to slightly counteract gravity.

Sixth Force

A force that may exist. Its existence has not yet been confirmed. It is thought to slightly increase the force of gravity.

All matter is composed of one or more types of substances called *elements.* **Elements** are the basic building blocks from which all things are made. Elements are units of matter that cannot be broken down into materials that are more simple by ordinary chemical reactions. You already know the names of some of these elements: oxygen, iron, aluminum, silver, carbon, and gold. The sidewalk, water, air, and your body are all composed of various types of elements combined or interacting with one another in various ways. The **periodic table of the elements** (*see* box 2.3) lists all the elements. Don't worry. You will not have to know the entire table. Only about 12 are dealt with in this text. Each unit of a particular element is called an **atom.** Under certain circumstances, atoms of elements join together during a chemical reaction to form units called **compounds.** A compound is a material formed from two or more elements in which the elements are always combined in the same proportions. Each unit of a particular compound is called a **molecule.** A molecule of a particular compound, for example table sugar ($C_{12}H_{22}O_{11}$), *always* contains 12 atoms of the element carbon, 22 atoms of the element hydrogen, and 11 atoms of the element oxygen. In most cases, elements and compounds are found as **mixtures** (box 2.2). A mixture is matter that contains two or more substances NOT in set proportions. For example, salt water can be composed of varying amounts of NaCl and H_2O. If the components of the mixture are distributed equally throughout it is called a *homogenous solution.* **Solutions** are homogenous mixtures in which the particles are the size of atoms or small molecules.

In order to understand living things we must understand how elements act and we need to understand what they are composed of. The smallest part of an element that still acts like that element is called an atom and retains all the traits of that element. When we use a **chemical symbol** such as Al for aluminum or C for carbon, it represents one atom of that element. The atom is constructed of three major particles; two of them are in a central region called the **atomic nucleus.** The third type of particle is in the region surrounding the nucleus (figure 2.1). The weight, or mass, of the atom is concentrated in the nucleus, which is composed of neutrons and protons. One major group of particles located in the nucleus

STRUCTURE OF THE ATOM

BOX 2.2

Another Type of Mixture—Suspension

A **suspension** is similar to a solution, but the dispersed particles are larger than molecular size. A suspension has particles that eventually settle out and are no longer equally dispersed in the system. Dust particles suspended in the air are an example of a suspension. The dust settles out and collects on tables and other furniture. Another type of mixture is a **colloid.** This system contains dispersed particles that are larger than molecules but still small enough that they do not settle out. Even though colloids are composed of small particles that are mixed together with a liquid such as water, they do not act like solutions or a suspension. In a colloidal system, the dispersed particles form a spongelike network that holds the water molecules in place. One unique characteristic of a colloid is that it can become more or less solid depending on the temperature. When the temperature is lowered, the mixture becomes solidified; as the temperature is increased, it becomes more liquid. We speak of these as the *gel* (solid) and *sol* (liquid) phases of a colloid. A gelatin dessert is a good example of a colloidal system. If you heat the gelatin, it becomes liquid as it changes to the sol phase. If you cool it again, it goes back to the gel phase and becomes solid. Environmental changes other than temperature can also cause colloids to change their phase. In living cells, this sol/gel transformation can cause the cell to move.

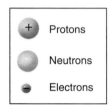

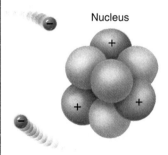

FIGURE 2.1 Atomic structure. The nucleus of the atom contains the protons and the neutrons, which are the massive particles of the atom. The electrons, much less massive, are in constant motion about the nucleus.

is the **neutrons;** they were named *neutrons* to reflect their lack of electrical charge. **Protons,** the second type of particle in the nucleus, have a positive electrical charge. **Electrons,** found in the area surrounding the nucleus, have a negative charge.

An atom is neutral in charge when the number of positively charged protons is balanced by the number of negatively charged electrons. You can determine the number of either of these two particles in a balanced atom if you know the number of the other particle. For instance, hydrogen with one proton would have one electron, carbon with six protons would have six electrons, and oxygen with eight electrons would have eight protons.

The atoms of each kind of element have a specific number of protons. It is the number of protons that determines the identity of the element. For example, carbon always has six protons. No other element has that number. Oxygen always has eight protons. The **atomic number** of an element is the number of protons in an atom of that element; therefore, each element has a unique atomic number. Since oxygen has eight protons, its atomic number is eight. The mass of a proton is 1.67×10^{-24} grams. Since this is an extremely small mass and is awkward to express, it is said to be equal to one **atomic mass unit,** abbreviated **AMU.** One AMU is actually 1/12 of the mass of a particular carbon atom, but is very close to the mass of each proton (table 2.1).

Although all atoms of the same element have the same number of protons, they do not always have the same number of neutrons. In the case of oxygen, over 99% of the atoms have eight neutrons, but there are others with more or fewer neutrons. Each atom of the same element with a different number of neutrons is called an **isotope** of an element.

The most common isotope of oxygen has eight neutrons, but another isotope of oxygen has nine neutrons. We can determine the number of neutrons by comparing the masses of the isotopes. The **mass number** of an atom is the number of protons plus the number of neutrons in the nucleus. The mass number is customarily used to compare different isotopes of the same element. An oxygen isotope with a mass number of sixteen AMUs is composed of eight protons and eight neutrons and is identified as ^{16}O. Oxygen 17, or ^{17}O, has a mass of seventeen AMUs. Eight of these units are due to the eight protons that every oxygen atom has; the rest of the mass is due to nine neutrons (17 – 8 = 9). Figure 2.2 shows different isotopes of hydrogen.

Table 2.1 Comparison of Atomic Particles			
	PROTONS	**ELECTRONS**	**NEUTRONS**
Location	Nucleus	Outside nucleus	Nucleus
Charge	Positive (+)	Negative (–)	None (neutral)
Number present	Identical to the atomic number	Equal to number of protons	Mass number minus atomic number
Mass	1 AMU	1/1,836 AMU	1 AMU

The periodic table of the elements (box 2.3) lists all the elements in order of increasing atomic number (number of protons). In addition, this table lists the mass number of each element. You can use these two numbers to determine the number of the three major particles in an atom—protons, neutrons, and electrons. Look at the periodic table and find helium in the upper right-hand corner (He). Two is its atomic number; thus, every helium atom will have two protons. Since the protons are positively charged, the nucleus will have two positive charges that must be balanced by two negatively charged electrons. The atomic mass of helium is given as 4.003. This is the calculated average mass of a group of helium atoms. Most of them have a mass of four—two protons and two neutrons. Generally, you will need to work only with the most common isotope, so the mass number should be rounded to the nearest whole number. If it is a number like 4.003, use 4 as the most common mass. If the mass number is a number like 39.95, use 40 as the nearest whole number. Look at several atoms in the periodic table. You can easily determine the number of protons and the number of neutrons in the most common isotopes of almost all of these atoms.

Since isotopes differ in the number of neutrons they contain, the isotopic forms of a particular element differ from one another in some of their characteristics. For example, there are many isotopes of iodine. The most common isotope of iodine is ^{127}I; it has a mass number of 127. A different isotope of iodine is ^{131}I; its mass number is 131 and it is **radioactive.** This means that it is not stable and that its nucleus disintegrates, releasing energy and particles. The energy can be detected by using photographic film or a Geiger counter. If a physician suspects that a patient has a thyroid gland that is functioning improperly, ^{131}I may be used to help confirm the diagnosis. The thyroid normally collects iodine atoms from the blood and uses them in the manufacture of the body-regulating chemical thyroxine. If the thyroid gland is working properly to form thyroxine, the radioactive iodine will collect in the gland, where its presence can be detected. If no iodine has collected there, the physician knows that the gland is not functioning correctly and can take steps to help the patient.

The number and position of the electrons in an atom are responsible for the way atoms interact with each other. Electrons are the negatively charged particles of an atom that balance the positive charges of the protons in the atomic nucleus. The mass of an electron is a tiny fraction of the mass of a proton. This mass is so slight that it usually does not influence the AMU of an element. But electrons are important even though they do not have a major effect on the mass of the element. The number and location of the electrons in any atom determines the kinds of chemical reactions it may undergo. Living things all have the ability to manipulate matter and energy, i.e., direct these chemical reactions.

When atoms or molecules interact with each other and rearrange to form new combinations, we say that they have undergone a **chemical reaction.** A chemical reaction usually involves a change in energy as well as some rearrangement in

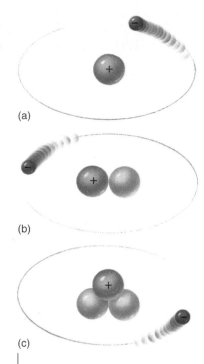

(a)

(b)

(c)

FIGURE 2.2 Isotopes of hydrogen.
(a) The most common form of hydrogen is the isotope that is 1 AMU. It is composed of one proton and no neutrons. (b) The isotope deuterium is 2 AMU and has one proton and one neutron. (c) Tritium, 3 AMU, has two neutrons and one proton. Each of these isotopes of hydrogen also has one electron, but since the mass of an electron is so small, they do not contribute significantly to the mass as measured in AMU.

CHEMICAL REACTIONS

Chemical Principles for Allied Health   23

Box 2.3 The Periodic Table of the Elements

Traditionally, elements are represented in a shorthand form by letters. For example, the symbol for water, H_2O, shows that a molecule of water consists of two atoms of hydrogen and one atom of oxygen. These chemical symbols can be found on any periodic table of elements. Using this table, we can determine the number and position of the various parts of atoms. Notice that the atoms numbered 3, 11, 19, and so on, are in column one. The atoms in this column act in a similar way since they all have one electron in their outermost layer. In the next column, Be, Mg, Ca, and so on, act alike because these metals all have two electrons in their outermost electron layer. Similarly, atoms 9, 17, 35, and so on, all have seven electrons in their outer layer.

Knowing how fluorine, chlorine, and bromine act, you can probably predict how iodine will act under similar conditions. At the far right in the last column, argon, neon, and so on, all act alike. They all have eight electrons in their outer electron layer. Atoms with eight electrons in their outer electron layer seldom form bonds with other atoms.

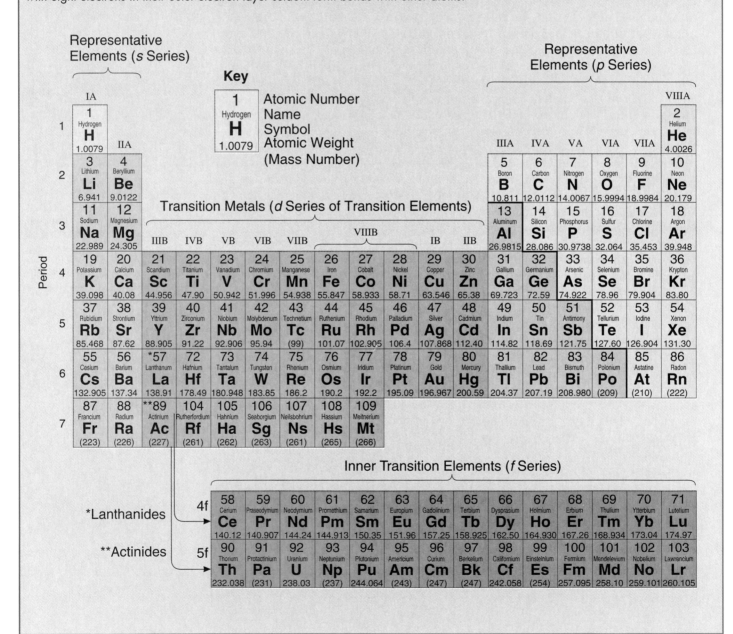

FIGURE 2.3 Chemical equations.
The three equations here use
chemical shorthand to indicate that
there has been a rearrangement of
the chemical bonds in the reactants

$$HCl + NaOH \rightarrow NaCl + H_2O$$
$$C_6H_{12}O_6 + 6\ O_2 \rightarrow 6\ H_2O + 6\ CO_2 + energy$$
$$C_6H_{12}O_6 + C_6H_{12}O_6 \rightarrow C_{12}H_{22}O_{11} + H_2O$$

to form the products. Along with the rearrangement of the chemical bonds, there has been a
change in the energy content. Notice the numbers in front of the formula for water (H_2O). That
number indicates that there are a total of 6 waters formed in this reaction. If there is no such
number preceding a formula, it is assumed that the number is one (1) of that kind of unit.

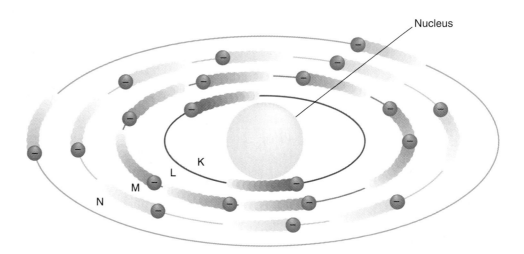

FIGURE 2.4 The Bohr atom.
Several decades ago we thought
that electrons revolved around
the nucleus of the atom in
particular paths, or tracks. Each
track was labeled with a letter: K,
L, M, N, and so on. Each track
was thought to be able to hold a
specific number of electrons
moving at a particular speed.
These electron tracks were
described as quanta of energy.

the molecular structure. We frequently use a chemical shorthand to express what is
going on. An arrow ($\rightarrow$) indicates that a chemical reaction is occurring. The arrow-
head points to the materials that are produced by the reaction; we call these the
products. On the other side of the arrow, we generally show the materials that are
going to react with each other; we call these the ingredients of the reaction or the
reactants. Some of the most fascinating information we have learned recently
concerns the way in which living things manipulate chemical reactions to release
or store chemical energy. This material is covered in detail in chapters 5 and 6. Figure 2.3 shows the chemical shorthand used to indicate several reactions. The chemical shorthand is called an *equation.* Look closely at the equations and identify the
reactants and products in each. Four of the most important chemical reactions that
occur in organisms are: (1) hydrolysis (breaking a molecule using a water molecule; (2) dehydration synthesis (combining smaller molecules by extracting the
equivalent of water molecules from the parts); (3) oxidation-reduction (reactions
that may release or store energy); (4) acid-base; and (5) phosphorylation. These will
be discussed in more detail in later chapters.

Electron Distribution

Electrons are constantly moving at great speeds and tend to be found in specific regions some distance from the nucleus (figure 2.4). The position of an electron at any
instant in time is determined by several factors. First, since protons and electrons are
of opposite charge, electrons are attracted to the protons in the nucleus of the atom.
Second, counterbalancing this is the force created by the movement of the electrons,
which tends to cause them to move away from the nucleus. Third, the electrons repel
one another because they have identical charges. The balance of these three forces
creates a situation in which the electrons of an atom tend to remain in the neighbor-
hood of the nucleus but are distributed apart from one another. Electron distribution
is not random, but electrons are likely to be found in certain locations.

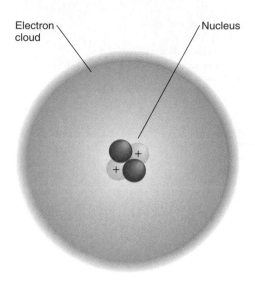

Figure 2.5 The electron cloud. The electrons are moving so fast around the nucleus that they can be thought of as forming a cloud around it, rather than an orbit or track. You might think of the electron cloud as hundreds of photographs of an atom. Each photograph shows where an electron was at the time the picture was taken. But when the next picture is taken, the electron is somewhere else. Although we are able to determine where an electron is at a given time, we do not know the path it uses to go from there to where it is the next time we determine its position.

When chemists first described the atom, they tried to account for the fact that electrons seemed to be traveling at one of several different speeds about the atomic nucleus. Electrons did not travel at intermediate speeds. Because of this, it was thought that electrons followed a particular path, or orbit, similar to the orbits of the planets about the sun.

The model of an atom shown in figure 2.4 is called the Bohr atom because Niels Bohr, a Danish physicist, advanced the theory that electrons move in discrete circular orbits about a nucleus. In the Bohr model, the electrons with the greatest amount of energy are farther from the nucleus. Think of swinging a weight on an elastic strap. As you swing the weight around your head, it makes a path a certain distance from you. If you swing it harder to make it go faster, to give it more energy, the path is a bigger circle a greater distance from your head. It was thought that there were only certain paths that electrons could follow. No electrons were thought to be found between two shell paths. The speeds or paths are now called *quanta* (singular *quantum*), meaning a certain amount of energy. From the collection of early experimental data, it was thought that only two electrons could exist in the first quantum, or *shell* closest to the nucleus, eight electrons could occupy the second shell, eight (or sometimes eighteen) the third shell, and so on. These shells, also known as *energy levels*, were labeled *K, L, M,* and so forth.

The Modern Model of the Atom

Several decades ago, as more experimental data were gathered and interpreted, we began to think of the *K* shell not as a particular pathway, but as a region or space within which electrons were likely to be. In this more modern model of the atom, each region or **orbital** is able to hold a maximum of two electrons. Each orbital is designated with a number that indicates the major energy level and a letter that indicates the kind of space the electrons occupy. The first orbital is lowest in energy and is designated as *1s*. The *1* indicates it is the first energy level from the nucleus and the *s* is used to help us remember that the space is spherical in shape. (Originally the *s* indicated something entirely different but a lucky happenstance allows us to use it to remember the spherically shaped space.) Thus, the electrons in a helium atom would be located in the area described as an electron cloud in figure 2.5. The area is labeled the *1s* orbital, and that orbital is full with its two electrons.

If an atom has more than two electrons, not all of these have the same amount of energy. Neon, for example, has ten electrons. The first two we would say are located in the first energy level, just as the two in the helium atom. They

FIGURE 2.6 The second energy level of electrons. The electrons on the second energy level all have about the same amount of energy, but more energy than the electrons in the first energy level. The electrons are most likely to be located in the four regions labeled 2s, 2px, 2py, and 2pz.

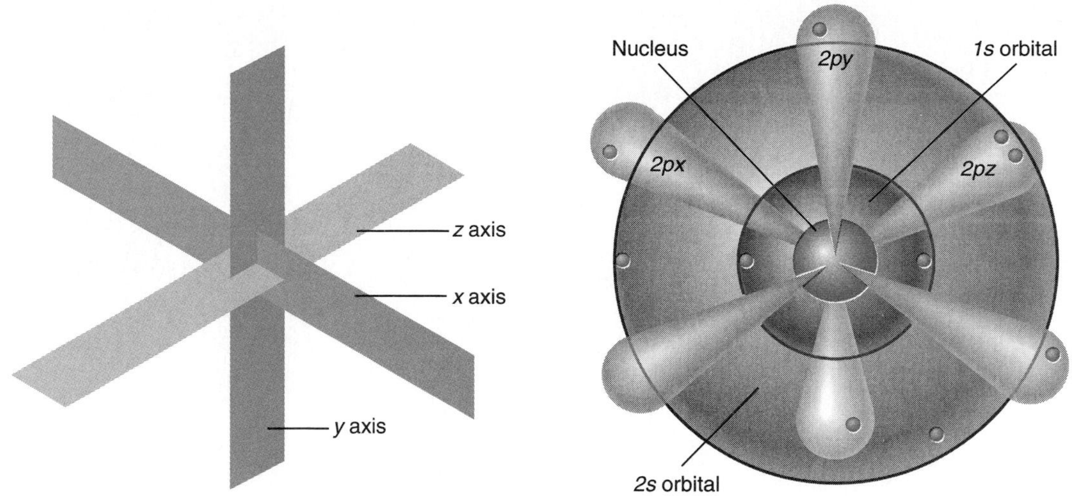

are designated as being in the *1s* orbital. The rest of the electrons—the other eight—would be in a higher, second energy level. (This second energy level is similar to the Bohr model of atomic structure with eight electrons located on the second orbit or path.) All eight of these electrons, however, do not have exactly the same energy and they are not likely to occupy the same spatial area.

We now think that two of these eight electrons have an amount of energy that makes it likely that they will occupy a special area of the second energy level, designated as the *2s* orbital. The 2 indicates that it is the second energy level and the *s* helps us remember that the shape of the space the electrons occupy is spherical. The other six electrons have slightly more energy and they tend to occupy three areas as far away from each other as possible, but still on the second energy level. You might think of these three areas as propeller-shaped areas on the *x, y,* and *z* axes (figure 2.6). Each propeller-shaped area can hold a maximum of two electrons, so the eight electrons of the *L* shell of the Bohr atomic model can now be more accurately described as being located in one spherical area and three propeller-shaped areas at right angles to each other. By convention, we indicate these areas as the *2s,* the *2px,* the *2py,* and the *2pz* areas.

The third energy level (formerly called the *M* shell) contains electrons that have a greater amount of energy than those in the second energy level. These electrons are distributed in four different orbitals, which are designated as the *3s, 3px, 3py,* and *3pz* (figure 2.7). You can see how cluttered the graphic representation of the atom in figure 2.7 becomes when you try to account for the number and location of all its protons, neutrons, and electrons. This will become even more difficult as we deal with larger and larger atoms. A simpler way to represent the atom is shown in figure 2.8. The arrows on the diagram represent the electrons. In order to diagram the structure of an atom and place the electrons in their proper orbitals, you must start filling the spaces at the *1s* level and move outward. Each orbital is filled with two electrons. If the atom contains more than two electrons, proceed to the second energy level. At the second energy level there are four different orbitals (*2s, 2px, 2py, 2pz*). The *2s* is filled with electrons first, before any additional electrons are placed in the *p* orbitals. After you have filled the *2s* orbital, begin adding electrons one at a time to each of the three *p* orbitals. An electron is added to the *2px,* a second is added to the *2py,* and a third to the *2pz.* Additional electrons are then added in this same sequence until each orbital contains two electrons. Then you can continue to the third energy level and beyond using the same pattern.

An atom such as potassium, with nineteen protons and nineteen electrons, would have two electrons in the first energy level (*1s*). In the second energy level,

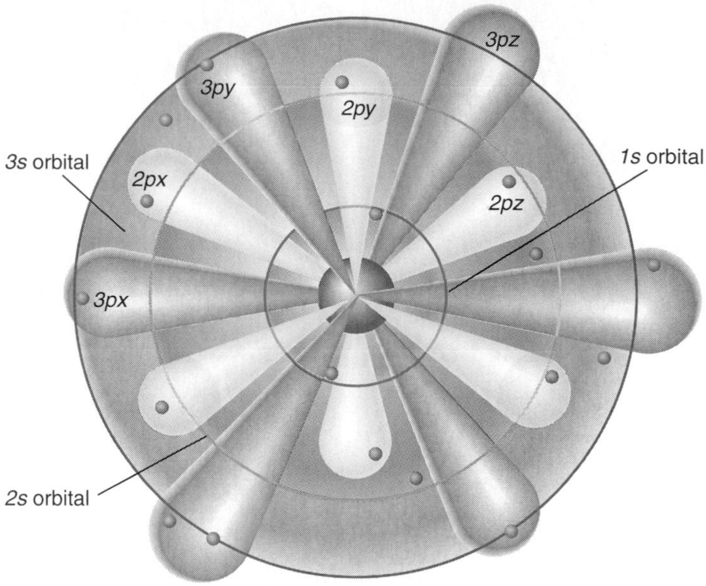

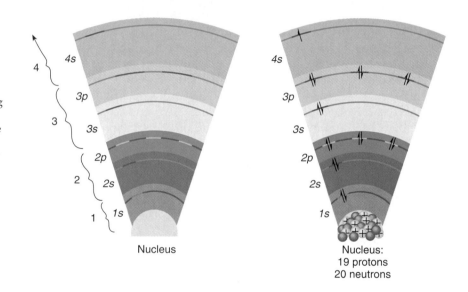

Figure 2.7 The third energy level of electrons.
The electrons in these outer clouds all have about the same amount of energy. The areas where they are located are labeled *3s, 3px, 3py,* and *3pz.*

Figure 2.8 Electron configuration.
This chart is like a theater seating chart. The lines represent places where electrons can be. Each line can hold a maximum of two electrons. The electrons are most likely to be in the lower energy levels. They will go in an empty area of the same energy level before they will occupy an area that already has a negative electron in it. The filled-in chart on the right is of the atom potassium, number 19.

there would be two electrons in the *2s* orbital; two electrons in each of the *2p* orbitals; two electrons in the *3s* orbital; two in each of the *3px, 3py,* and *3pz* orbitals; and one electron in the *4s* orbital.

Ions

Now that you know the rules for positioning electrons in their proper orbitals, it would be convenient if all atoms always followed these rules. Remember that atoms are electrically neutral when they have equal numbers of protons and electrons. Certain atoms, however, are able to exist with an unbalanced charge, i.e., the number of protons is not equal to the number of electrons. These unbalanced, or charged, atoms are called **ions.** The ion of sodium is formed when one of the eleven electrons of the sodium atom escapes. Let's look at the electron distribution to help explain how and why this happens. The sodium nucleus is composed of eleven positive charges (protons) insulated from each other by twelve neutrons. (The most common isotope of sodium is sodium 23, which has twelve neutrons.) The eleven electrons that balance the charge are most likely positioned as follows: two electrons in the

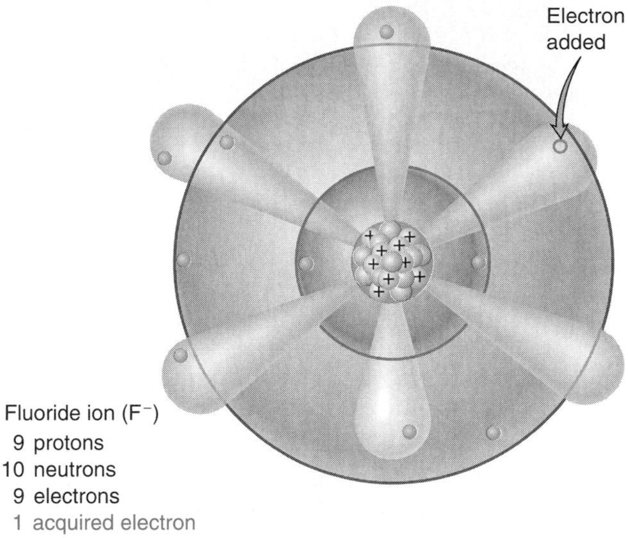

FIGURE 2.9 Fluoride ion.
When the fluorine atom accepts
an additional electron, it becomes
a negative ion. Negative ions are
indicated with a minus sign and
often end in -ide.

Fluoride ion (F⁻)
9 protons
10 neutrons
9 electrons
1 acquired electron

first energy level, eight in the second energy level, and one in the third energy level. Focus your attention on the outermost electron. It has more energy than any of the other electrons. But because it is farther from the nucleus than any other electron, it is not as strongly attracted to the positive charges in the nucleus. This is similar to gravitational attraction—the closer to earth an object is, the greater the gravitational pull. Since this electron is the least attracted to the nucleus and has the most kinetic energy, when conditions are right it might escape from the sodium atom. What remains when the electron leaves the atom is called the *ion*. In this case, the sodium ion is now composed of the eleven positively charged protons and the twelve neutral neutrons—but it has only ten electrons. The fact that there are eleven positive and only ten negative charges means that there is an excess of one positive charge. We still use the chemical symbol Na to represent the ion, but we add the ⁺ to indicate that it is no longer a neutral atom, but an electrically charged ion (i.e., Na⁺). It is easy to remember that a positive ion is formed because it loses negative electrons.

The sodium ion is relatively stable because its outermost energy level is full. A sodium atom will lose one electron from its third major energy level so that the second energy level becomes outermost and is full of electrons. Similarly, magnesium loses two electrons from its third major energy level so that the second major energy level, which is full with eight electrons, becomes outermost. When a magnesium atom (Mg) loses two electrons, it becomes a magnesium ion (Mg⁺⁺). The periodic table of the elements is arranged so that all atoms in the first column become ions in a similar way. That is, when they form ions, they do so by losing one electron. Each becomes a ⁺ ion. Atoms in the second column of the periodic table become ⁺⁺ ions when they lose two electrons. Those atoms at the extreme right of the periodic table of the elements do not become ions; they tend to be stable as atoms. These atoms are called *inert* or *noble* because of their lack of activity. They seldom react because their protons and electrons are equal in number and they have a full outer energy level; therefore, they are not likely to lose electrons.

The column to the left of these gases contains atoms that lack a full outer energy level. They all require an additional electron. Fluorine with its nine electrons would have two in the *K* shell (*1s* orbital) and seven in the *L* shell (two in *2s*, two in *2px*, two in *2py*, and one in *2pz*). The second major energy level can hold a total of eight electrons. You can see that one additional electron could fit into the *2pz* orbital. Whenever the atom of fluorine can, it will accept an extra electron so that its outermost energy level is full. When it does so, it no longer has a balanced charge. When it accepts an extra electron, it has one more negative electron than positive protons; thus, it has become a negative ion (F⁻) (figure 2.9).

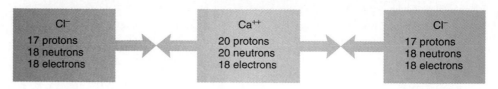

FIGURE 2.10

Calcium chloride.
This combination of a calcium ion
and two chloride ions makes up the
compound calcium chloride. The
formula of the compound is CaCl$_2$.
Notice that the overabundance of
two positive charges on the calcium ion is offset by the two chloride
ions, each of which has an overabundance of only one negative charge.

Cl⁻	Ca⁺⁺	Cl⁻
17 protons	20 protons	17 protons
18 neutrons	20 neutrons	18 neutrons
18 electrons	18 electrons	18 electrons

Similarly, chlorine will form a $^-$ion. Oxygen, in the next column, will accept two electrons and become a negative ion with two extra negative charges (O$^=$). If you know the number and position of the electrons, you are better able to hypothesize whether or not an atom will become an ion and, if it does, whether it will be a positive ion or a negative ion. You can use the periodic table of the elements to help you determine an atom's ability to form ions. This information is useful as we see how ions react to each other.

CHEMICAL BONDS

There are a variety of physical and chemical forces that act on atoms and make them attractive to each other. Each of these results in a particular arrangement of atoms or association of atoms. The forces that combine atoms and hold them together are called **chemical bonds.** Bonds are formed in an attempt to stabilize atoms energetically, i.e., complete their outer shells. There are several types of chemical bonds. They differ from each other with respect to the kinds of attractive forces holding the atoms together. The bonding together of atoms results in the formation of a compound. This compound is composed of a specific number of atoms (or ions) joined to each other in a particular way and is represented by a **chemical formula.** We generally use the chemical symbols for each of the component atoms when we designate a compound. Sometimes there will be a small number behind the chemical symbol. This number indicates how many atoms of that particular element are used in the compound. The group of chemical symbols and numbers is termed an **empirical formula;** it will tell you what elements are in a compound and also how many atoms of each element are required. For example, CaCl$_2$ tells us that the compound of calcium chloride is composed of one calcium atom and two chlorine atoms (figure 2.10). A **structural formula** is a drawing that shows the number and spatial arrangement of atoms within the molecule.

The properties of a compound are very different from the properties of the atoms that make up the compound. Table salt is composed of the elements sodium and chlorine bound together. Both sodium and chlorine are very poisonous when they are by themselves. Yet, when they are combined as table salt, the compound is a nontoxic substance, essential for living organisms.

Ionic Bonds

When positive and negative ions are near each other, they are mutually attracted because of their opposite charges. This attraction between ions of opposite charge results in the formation of a stable group of ions. This attraction is termed an **ionic bond.** Compounds that form as a result of attractions between ions are called *ionic compounds* (figure 2.10) and are very important in living systems. When an ionic compound such as table salt is mixed with water to form a solution, these bonds are not strong enough to be maintained and the compound falls apart or **dissociates** into its ions.

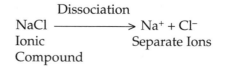

When the water is removed, the separated ions may come close enough to one another again to re-form ionic bonds. When this occurs the compound is re-formed. Compounds that dissociate in water are able to conduct electricity and are called **electrolytes.** Electrolytes can be strong or weak, depending on the percentage of ionic bonded molecules that dissociate when they are placed in water. Sodium chlorine is a strong electrolyte because essentially 100% of the molecules dissociate in water. On the other hand acetic acid (vinegar) is a weak electrolyte because only about 0.5% of the molecules dissociate. We can categorize these ionic compounds into three different groups.

Acids, Bases, and Salts

Acids and bases are two classes of biologically important compounds. Their characteristics are determined by the nature of their chemical bonds. When acids are dissociated in water, hydrogen ions (H^+) are set free. The hydrogen ion is positive because it has lost its electron and now has only the positive charge of the proton. An **acid** is any ionic compound that releases a hydrogen ion in a solution. You can think of an acid, then, as a substance able to donate a proton to a solution. However, this is only part of the definition of an acid. We also think of acids as compounds that act like the hydrogen ion—they attract negatively charged particles. An example of a common acid with which you are probably familiar is the sulfuric acid (H_2SO_4) in your automobile battery. Sulfuric acid is a *strong electrolyte* or *acid* whereas the acid vinegar is a *weak electrolyte* or *acid* as mentioned above.

A **base** is the opposite of an acid in that it is an ionic compound that releases a group known as a **hydroxyl ion,** or OH^- group. This group is composed of an oxygen atom and a hydrogen atom bonded together, but with an additional electron. The hydroxyl ion is negatively charged. It is a base because it is able to donate electrons to the solution. A base can also be thought of as any substance that is able to attract positively charged particles. A very strong base used in oven cleaners is NaOH, sodium hydroxide. Sodium hydroxide is a *strong electrolyte* or *base*. (Notice that free ions are always written with the type and number of their electrical charge as a superscript.)

The degree to which a solution is acidic or basic is represented by a quantity known as **pH.** The pH scale is a measure of hydrogen ion concentration. A pH of seven indicates that the solution is neutral and has an equal number of H^+ ions and OH^- ions to balance each other. As the pH number gets smaller, the number of hydrogen ions in the solution increases. A number higher than seven indicates that the solution has more OH^- than H^+. As the pH number gets larger, the number of hydroxyl ions increases (figure 2.11).

An additional group of biologically important ionic compounds is called the *salts*. **Salts** are compounds that do not release either H^+ or OH^-; thus, they are neither acids nor bases. They are generally the result of the reaction between an acid and a base in a solution. For example, when an acid such as HCl is mixed with NaOH in water, the H^+ and the OH^- combine with each other to form water, H_2O. The remaining ions (Na^+ and Cl^-) join to form the salt NaCl.

$$HCl + NaOH \longrightarrow (Na^+ + Cl^- + H^+ + OH^-) \longrightarrow NaCl + H_2O$$

The chemical process that occurs when acids and bases react with each other is called **neutralization,** or an *acid-base reaction*. The acid no longer acts as an acid (it has been neutralized) and the base no longer acts like a base.

As you can see from figure 2.11, not all acids or bases produce the same pH. Some compounds release hydrogen ions very readily and cause low pHs, the strong acids. Hydrochloric acid (HCl) and sulfuric acid (H_2SO_4) are examples of strong acids. Many other compounds give up their hydrogen ions grudgingly and therefore do not change the pH very much. They are the weak acids.

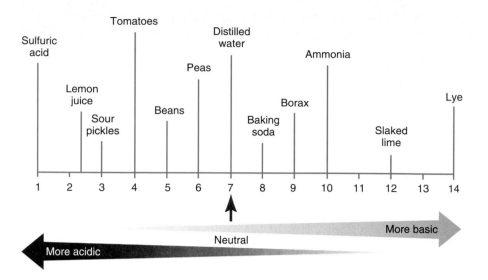

FIGURE 2.11 The pH scale. The concentration of acid (proton donor or electron acceptor) is greatest when the pH number is lowest. As the pH number increases, the concentration of base (proton acceptor or electron donor) increases. At a pH of 7.0, the concentrations of H^+ and OH^- are equal.

Carbonic acid (H_2CO_3) and many organic acids found in living things are weak acids. Similarly, there are strong bases like sodium hydroxide (NaOH) and weak bases like sodium bicarbonate ($NaHCO_3$).

Buffers

In certain situations, it is important that the pH of a solution not be able to change significantly. This is especially true in biological systems where the proper pH can influence the activity of enzymes and other biological chemicals. Mixtures of chemicals that operate to maintain a constant pH in a solution are called **buffers.** Many different kinds of buffers have been developed that are used in many chemical and biological situations. Living things have natural buffers that help them maintain a constant pH. Buffers are mixtures containing a *weak acid* and the *salt of a weak acid.* The salt of a weak acid is the negatively charged ion formed after dissociation.

$$H_2CO_3 \longrightarrow H^+ + HCO_3^-$$

| Weak Carbonic | Hydrogen | Salt of |
| Acid | Ion | Weak Acid |

The weak acid will release hydrogen ions and the salt of a weak acid will remove hydrogen ions.

One of the most interesting buffer systems in the human body is in the blood. This buffer system consists of weak carbonic acid, H_2CO_3, and a bicarbonate salt that releases bicarbonate ions, HCO_3^-. These materials are normally dissolved in the blood plasma. If the blood has an increase of H^+ ions, these ions are able to combine with the bicarbonate ions to form carbonic acid; thus, the excess hydrogen ions are absorbed, and the pH does not change. If hydroxyl ions are added to the system, they will join with the hydrogen ions to form water. However, the hydrogen ions will be replaced because some carbonic acid will separate into hydrogen ions and bicarbonate ions. This mixture of carbonic acid and bicarbonate ions maintains the stability of the pH in the blood. The double-headed arrows in the following reaction indicate that the reaction can go in either direction. If excess hydrogen ions are present, the reaction shifts to the left; if the solution is becoming too basic, it shifts to the right, and hydrogen ions are released.

$$CO_2 + H_2O \longleftrightarrow H_2CO_3 \longleftrightarrow H^+ + HCO_3^-$$

| | Carbonic | Bicarbonate |
| | Acid | Ion |

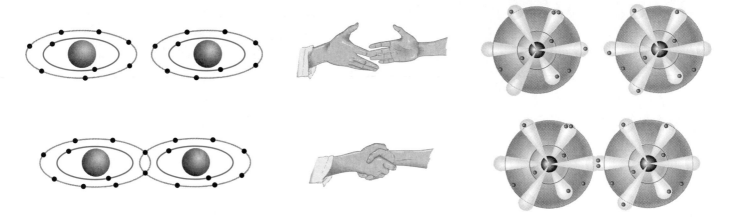

FIGURE 2.12 Covalent bonds.
When two atoms come sufficiently close to each other that the locations of the outermost electrons overlap, an electron from each one can be shared to "fill" that outermost energy-level area. When two people shake hands, they need to be close enough to each other so that their hands can overlap to form a handshake. At the left, using the Bohr model, the L-shells of the two atoms overlap, and so each shell appears to be full. Using the modern model at the right, the propeller-shaped orbitals of the second energy level of each atom overlap, so that each propeller appears to have a full orbital. Notice that just as it takes two hands to form a handclasp, it takes two electrons to form a covalent bond.

Covalent Bonds

In addition to ionic bonds, there is a second strong chemical bond known as a *covalent bond*. A **covalent bond** is formed by two atoms that share a pair of electrons. This sharing can occur when two atoms have orbitals that overlap one another. A covalent bond should be thought of as belonging to each of the atoms involved. You can visualize the bond as people shaking hands: the people are the atoms, the hands are electrons to be shared, and the handshake is the combining force (figure 2.12). Generally, this sharing of a pair of electrons is represented by a single straight line between the atoms involved. The reason covalent bonds form relates to the arrangement of electrons within the atoms. There are many elements that do not tend to form ions. They will not lose electrons, nor will they gain electrons. Instead, these elements get close enough to other atoms that have unfilled outer orbitals and share electrons with each other. If the two elements have orbitals that overlap, the electrons can be shared. By sharing electrons, the unfilled outer energy levels of each atom will be filled. Both atoms become more stable as a result of the formation of this covalent bond.

Molecules are defined as the smallest particles of chemical compounds. They are composed of a specific number of atoms arranged in a particular pattern. For example, a molecule of water is composed of one oxygen atom bonded covalently to two atoms of hydrogen. The shared electrons are in the second energy level of oxygen, and the bonds are almost at right angles to each other. Now that you realize how and why bonds are formed, it makes sense that only certain numbers of certain atoms will bond with each other to form molecules. Chemists also use the term *molecule* to mean the smallest naturally occurring part of an element or compound. Using this definition, one atom of iron is a molecule because one atom is the smallest natural piece of the element. Hydrogen, nitrogen, and oxygen tend to form into groups of two atoms. Molecules of these elements are composed of two atoms of hydrogen, two atoms of nitrogen, and two atoms of oxygen, respectively. When covalently bonded molecules are mixed with water, the component atoms are bound so tightly that they do not dissociate from one another. Therefore, when sugar is mixed with water, each molecule ($C_6H_{12}O_6$) remains intact. Covalently bonded solutions are generally not good electrolytes.

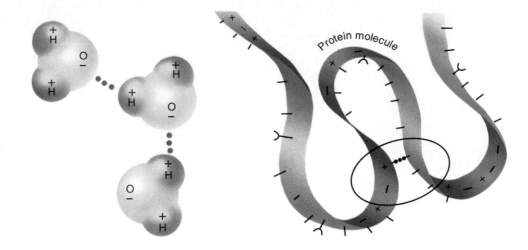

FIGURE 2.13 Hydrogen bonds. Water molecules arrange themselves so their positive portions are near the negative portions of other water molecules. The attractions are indicated as three dots. The large protein molecule here also has polar areas. When the molecule is folded so that the partially positive areas are near the partially negative areas, a slight attraction forms that tends to keep it folded.

Hydrogen Bonds

Molecules that are composed of several atoms sometimes have an uneven distribution of charge. This may occur because the electrons involved in the formation of bonds may be located on one side of the molecule. This makes that side of the molecule slightly negative and the other side slightly positive. One side of the molecule has possession of the electrons more than the other side. When a molecule is composed of several atoms that have this uneven charge distribution, the whole molecule may show a positive side and a negative side. We sometimes think of such a molecule as a tiny magnet with a positive pole and a negative pole. This polarity of the molecule may influence how the molecule reacts with other molecules. When several of these *polar molecules* are together, they orient themselves so that the slightly positive end of one is near the slightly negative end of another. This attraction between two molecules is called a **hydrogen bond.** Hydrogen bonds hold molecules together; they do not bond atoms together. Since hydrogen has the least attractive force for electrons when it is combined with other elements, the hydrogen electron tends to spend more of its time encircling the other atom's nucleus than its own. The result is the formation of a polar molecule. When the negative pole of this molecule is attracted to the positive pole of another similar polar molecule, the hydrogen will usually be located between the two molecules. Since the hydrogen serves as a bridge between the two molecules, this weak bond has become known as a *hydrogen bond.*

We usually represent this attraction as three dots between the attracted regions. This weak bond is not responsible for forming molecules, but it is important in determining how groups of molecules are arranged. Water, for example, is composed of polar molecules that form hydrogen bonds (figure 2.13, left). Because of this, individual water molecules are less likely to separate from each other. They need a large input of energy to become separated. This is reflected in the relatively high boiling point of water in comparison to other substances such as rubbing alcohol. In addition, when a very large molecule, such as a protein or DNA (which is long and threadlike), has parts of its structure slightly positive and other parts slightly negative, these two areas will attract each other and result in coiling or folding of the chain of molecules in particular ways (figure 2.13, right).

All matter is composed of atoms, which contain a nucleus of neutrons and protons. The nucleus is surrounded by moving electrons. There are many kinds of atoms, called elements. These differ from one another by the number of protons and electrons they contain. Each is given an atomic number, based on the number of protons in the nucleus and an atomic mass number, determined by the total number of protons and neutrons. Atoms of an element that have the same atomic number but differ in their atomic mass number are called isotopes. Some isotopes are radioactive, which means that they fall apart releasing energy and smaller, more stable particles. Atoms may be combined into larger units called molecules. Two kinds of chemical bonds allow molecules to form—ionic bonds and covalent bonds. A third bond, the hydrogen bond, is a weaker bond that holds molecules together and may also help large molecules maintain a specific shape.

Energy can neither be created nor destroyed, but it can be converted from one form to another. Potential energy and kinetic energy can be interconverted. When energy is converted from one form to another, some of the useful energy is lost. The amount of kinetic energy that the molecules of various substances contain determines whether they are solids, liquids, or gases. The random motion of molecules, which is due to their kinetic energy, results in their distribution throughout available space.

An ion is an atom that is electrically unbalanced. Ions interact to form ionic compounds, such as acids, bases, and salts. Those compounds that release hydrogen ions when dissolved in water are called acids; those that release hydroxyl ions are called bases. A measure of the hydrogen ions present in a solution is known as the pH of the solution. Molecules that interact and exchange parts are said to undergo chemical reactions. The changing of chemical bonds in a reaction may release energy or require the input of additional energy.

1. How many protons, electrons, and neutrons are there in a neutral atom of potassium having a mass number of thirty-nine?

2. Diagram an atom showing the positions of electrons, protons, and neutrons.

3. Name three kinds of chemical bonds that hold atoms or molecules together. How do these bonds differ from one another?

4. Diagram two isotopes of oxygen.

5. What does it mean if a solution has a pH number of three, twelve, two, seven, or nine?

6. What relationship does kinetic energy have to the three states of matter? homogenous solutions? chemical bonds?

7. Define the following terms: AMU, atomic number, orbital, second energy level, and covalent bond.

8. Define the term *chemical reaction* and give an example.

9. What is the difference between an atom and an element? between a molecule and a compound?

10. How do acids, bases, and salts differ from one another?

acid (ă'sid) Any compound that releases a hydrogen ion (or other ion that acts like a hydrogen ion) in a solution.

atom (ă'tom) The smallest part of an element that still acts like that element.

atomic mass unit (AMU) (ă-tom'ik mas yu-nit) A unit of measure used to describe the mass of atoms and is equal to 1.67×10^{-24} grams, approximately the mass of one proton.

atomic nucleus (ă-tom'ik nu'kle-us) The central region of the atom.

atomic number (ă-tom'ik num'ber) The number of protons in an atom.

base (bās) Any compound that releases a hydroxyl group in a solution (or other ion that acts like a hydroxyl group).

buffer (bŭ'fer) A mixture of a weak acid and the salt of a weak acid that operates to maintain a constant pH.

chemical bonds (kem'ĭ-kal bonds) Forces that combine atoms or ions and hold them together.

chemical formula (kem'ĭ-kal form'yu-lah) Symbols used to represent each of the component atoms when we designate a compound.

chemical reaction (kem'ĭ-kal re-ak'shun) The formation or rearrangement of chemical bonds, usually indicated in an equation by an arrow from the reactants to the products.

chemical symbol (kem'ĭ-kal sim'bol) "Shorthand" used to represent one atom of an element, such as Al for aluminum or C for carbon.

colloid (kol'oid) A mixture that contains dispersed particles larger than molecules but small enough that they do not settle out.

compound (kom'pound)   A kind of matter that consists of a specific number of atoms (or ions) joined to each other in a particular way and held together by chemical bonds.

covalent bond (ko-va'lent bond)   The attractive force formed between two atoms that share a pair of electrons.

density (den'sĭ-te)   The weight of a certain volume of a material.

dissociation (dis-so'she-a'shun)   The separation of ions from an ionically bonded compound when it is mixed with water to form a solution.

electrolyte (e-lek'tro-līt)   Solutions containing dissolved inorganic ions, such as sodium, potassium, and chloride, and capable of conducting electricity.

electrons (e-lek'trons)   The negatively charged particles moving at a distance from the nucleus of an atom that balance the positive charges of the protons.

elements (el'ĕ-ments)   Matter consisting of only one kind of atom.

empirical formula (em-pir'e-kal form'yu-lah)   A symbol that will tell what elements are in a compound and also how many atoms of each element are required.

energy (en'er-je)   The property of an object that enables it to do work.

First Law of Thermodynamics (furst law uv ther'mo-di-nam'iks)   Energy in the universe remains constant; it can neither be created nor destroyed. Also referred to as the law of conservation of energy.

formula (form'yu-lah)   The group of chemical symbols that indicate what elements are in a compound and the number of each kind of atom present. Two types are used: empirical and structural.

gas (gas)   The state of matter in which the molecules are more energetic than the molecules of a liquid, resulting in only slight attraction for each other.

hydrogen bond (hi'dro-jen bond)   Weak attractive forces between molecules; important in determining how groups of molecules are arranged.

hydroxyl ion (hi-drok'sil i'on)   A negatively charged particle (OH⁻) composed of oxygen and hydrogen atoms released from a base when dissolved in water.

ionic bond (i-on'ik bond)   The attractive force between ions of opposite charge.

ions (i'ons)   Electrically unbalanced or charged atoms.

isotopes (i'so-tōps)   Atoms of the same element that differ only in the number of neutrons.

kinetic energy (kĭ-net'ik en'er-je)   Energy of motion.

liquid (lik'wid)   The state of matter in which the molecules are strongly attracted to each other, but because they are farther apart than in a solid, they move past each other more freely.

mass number (mas num'ber)   The weight of an atomic nucleus expressed in atomic mass units (the sum of the protons and neutrons).

matter (mat'er)   Anything that has weight (mass) and also takes up space (volume).

mixture (miks'chur)   Matter that contains two or more substances NOT in set proportions.

molecule (mol'ĕ-kūl)   The smallest particle of a chemical compound; also the smallest naturally occurring part of an element or compound.

neutralization (nu'tral-ĭ-za"shun)   A chemical reaction involved in mixing an acid with a base; results in formation of a salt and water: an acid-base reaction.

neutrons (nu'trons)   Particles in the nucleus of an atom that have no electrical charge; they were named *neutrons* to reflect this lack of electrical charge.

orbital (or'bĭ-tal)   The area of an atom able to hold a maximum of two electrons.

periodic table of the elements (pĭr-e-od'ik ta-bul uv the el'ĕ-ments)   A list of all of the elements in order of increasing atomic number (number of protons).

pH   A scale used to indicate the strength of an acid or base.

potential energy (po-ten'shal en'er-je)   The energy an object has because of its position.

products (prŏ'dukts)   New molecules resulting from a chemical reaction.

protons (pro'tons)   Particles in the nucleus of an atom that have a positive electrical charge.

radioactive (ra-de-o-ak'tiv)   A term used to describe the property of releasing energy or particles from an unstable atom.

reactants (re-ak'tants)   Materials that will be changed in a chemical reaction.

salts (salts)   Ionic compounds formed from a reaction between an acid and a base.

solid (sol'id)   The state of matter in which the molecules are packed tightly together; they vibrate in place.

solution (so-lu'shun)   Homogenous mixtures in which the particles are the size of atoms or small molecules.

states of matter (stāts uv mat'er)   Physical conditions of matter (solid, liquid, and gas) determined by the relative amounts of energy of the molecules.

structural formula (struk'tūr-al form'yu-lah)   A drawing that shows the number and spatial arrangement of atoms within the molecule.

suspension (sus-pen'shun)   Similar to a solution, but the dispersed particles are larger than molecular size.

temperature (tem'per-ah-tūr)   A measure of molecular energy of motion.

Energy and Action

CHAPTER OUTLINE

PURPOSE

Matter behaves in particular ways, based on the amount of energy it possesses. This chapter provides some background information that will allow you to understand the interactions of matter and energy and explore several concepts relating to energy. The laws of thermodynamics that are basic to this understanding are dealt with early in the chapter.

The word *energy* may create many images in your mind—rockets going to the moon, nuclear explosions, a heartbeat, electricity, and many more. But exactly what is energy? Although it comes in many forms, energy is not a material thing, but is a capacity or an ability to cause something to move or to change it in some way. Let's look at the concept in some detail to see if we can get a clearer picture of this ability and how this relates to the allied health professions.

CLINICAL VIEWPOINT

Energy in the human body is frequently measured in kilocalories. We count kilocalories when we diet, and we "burn" them as we exercise. A donut contains about 350 kilocalories. It is interesting to see how much exercise or work will use up the energy provided by this one donut. Twenty minutes of walking up stairs, forty minutes of jogging, forty-two minutes of swimming, and forty-six minutes of vigorous exercise in an average individual use up about 350 kilocalories. It takes one-and three-quarters hour of walking to use this much energy, and three hours or more of activities like changing clothes. Sitting and watching television for three hours will also use up that donut.

LEARNING OBJECTIVES

- Differentiate between potential and kinetic energy
- State the first and second laws of thermodynamics and explain them
- Correctly use the terms frequency, cycle, and wavelength to describe the energy of the electromagnetic spectrum
- Describe what may happen to energy when it strikes an object
- Relate heat energy to temperature and describe how an individual generates or releases heat
- Relate the pressure of a gas with its temperature and volume
- Describe electrical energy and its conduction
- Relate force to mass, specific gravity, and density

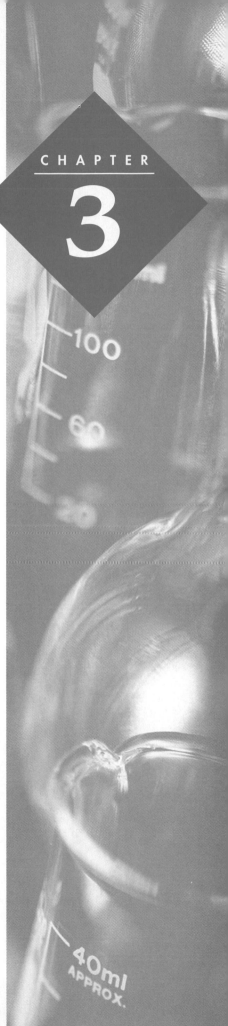

It is easy to see that a wagon rolling down a hill has energy. So does a person running down the field to catch a touchdown pass. This kind of energy is energy of motion, or kinetic energy. Energy in this case is possessed by the moving object. This same wagon or person sitting still on the top of a hill possesses another kind of energy, potential energy. Potential energy is defined as the energy an object has due to its position or condition. An object that appears to be motionless does not necessarily lack energy. Its individual molecules are still moving, but the object itself appears to be stationary. Although the wagon is motionless, it contains significant amounts of potential energy due to its position at the top of the hill. If it were to start rolling down the hill, the potential energy it contained at the top of the hill would be converted into kinetic energy (figure 3.1). Likewise, a compressed spring has potential energy due to its condition.

The **First Law of Thermodynamics** or the **Law of Conservation of Energy** states that the total amount of energy in the universe remains constant; it can neither be created nor destroyed but only transferred and transformed. One type of energy can be converted to other forms of energy. Potential energy and kinetic energy are forms that can be interconverted following the First Law of Thermodynamics. Although there may be less potential energy after such a change, there is still the same total amount of energy in the universe. Such a change does not create or destroy energy. It is merely a conversion from one form to another. Energy exists in many different forms such as chemical bonds, light, heat, sound, X rays, radio waves, and electricity. Each of these forms of energy has the ability to cause something to move or change. All forms of energy can be interconverted, just as potential energy can be changed to kinetic energy. An everyday example of how energy can be changed from one form to another is the conversion of electricity to other types of energy. The burning of coal or oil in a power plant forms heat, and that heat causes a turbine to move and generate electricity. In your home, this electrical energy is converted to other forms of energy (figure 3.2). In your body, the potential energy in the chemical bonds of molecules such as sugar can be converted into muscle movement.

Although energy can be converted from one form to another, this change is never 100% efficient. When the chemical energy in fuel is converted into the kinetic energy of motion in the steam turbine, some energy is "wasted" as heat and friction. As electrical energy is converted into light energy, some energy is converted to heat. This is a basic physical principle that applies to all energy

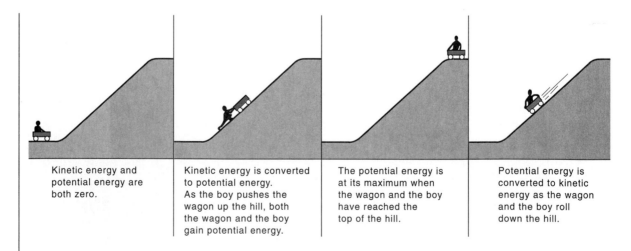

| Kinetic energy and potential energy are both zero. | Kinetic energy is converted to potential energy. As the boy pushes the wagon up the hill, both the wagon and the boy gain potential energy. | The potential energy is at its maximum when the wagon and the boy have reached the top of the hill. | Potential energy is converted to kinetic energy as the wagon and the boy roll down the hill. |

FIGURE 3.1 Kinetic and potential energy.
In this series of four illustrations, kinetic energy is converted to potential energy, and potential energy is then converted to kinetic energy.

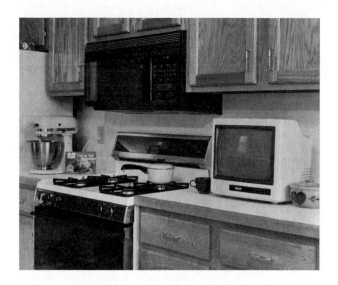

FIGURE 3.2 Energy conversion.
In a power plant the chemical energy in coal is converted to electrical energy. This electrical energy is transmitted to your home, where it can be changed into other forms of energy. Look at the picture. Can you find four types of energy conversion that occur in this kitchen?
(Answer: stove-heat energy, mixer-mechanical energy, and television-light and sound energy.)

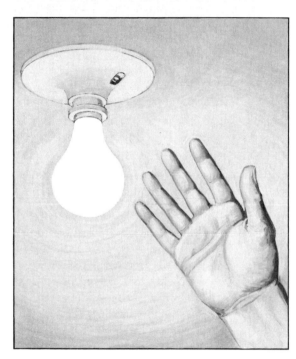

FIGURE 3.3 Second Law of Thermodynamics.
When energy is converted from one form to another, some of the energy is changed into heat. You can experience this by feeling the heat released from a lightbulb.

changes. Whenever one form of energy is converted to another form of energy, a third form is always produced, and this third form is usually heat. In cells of the human body, this transformation of potential chemical-bond energy in sugars also results in the release of heat energy. This basic principle is the **Second Law of Thermodynamics** (figure 3.3). Formally, this Law states that whenever a spontaneous event takes place, it is accompanied by an increase in the randomness or disorder of the parts involved in the event.

Various forms of energy share certain qualities. One such characteristic is that many forms of energy behave as if they were waves. Wavelike forms of energy such as radio-TV waves, X rays, microwaves, and light make up the **electromagnetic spectrum.** We think of these types of energy as moving in waves similar to ocean waves at the seashore. You can see the energy in these ocean waves as they crash onto the shore causing the sand, beach plants, rocks and other items to be moved or even destroyed. A wave in the ocean consists of a high point, the *crest,* followed by a low

ENERGY AS WAVES

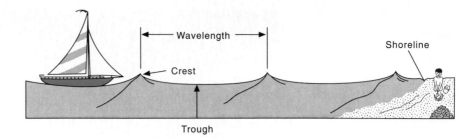

FIGURE 3.4 Properties of waves.
The ocean waves are moving toward the shore. The rate at which they arrive at the shore is known as the frequency. The distance from one crest to another is the wavelength.

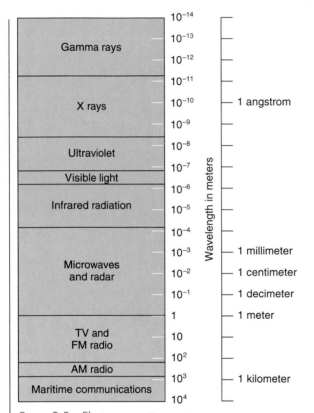

FIGURE 3.5 Electromagnetic spectrum.
Listed are various kinds of energy with a wavelike nature. The difference between one kind of energy and another is called the wavelength. A wavelength of 10^{-10} centimeters is classified as x-ray energy. A wavelength of 10^{-1} centimeters, which is a longer wave, is microwave energy.

point, the *trough,* and again rises to a high point as shown in figure 3.4. The distance from one crest to the next is a **wavelength.** If you were standing on the shore, the waves would arrive with a certain frequency, and might be expressed as the number of waves washing up on shore each minute.

Since the waves of energy are moving very rapidly, their **frequency** is measured as the number of waves produced per second. We usually express this as **cycles** (numbers of waves) **per second** in regard to the electromagnetic spectrum. The distance from one crest to the next crest of a wave of energy is very tiny. In the electromagnetic spectrum, wavelength is usually measured in **Angstrom** units (Å), which is one 100 millionth of a centimeter, or in **nanometers,** which is a billionth of a meter (box 3.1). If the speed of the waves remains the same, there is a simple relationship between wavelength and frequency. The longer the wave, the lower the frequency. Fewer of the longer waves will reach the shore each minute. Likewise, if the speed remains constant as the electromagnetic wavelength increases, the frequency decreases. Figure 3.5 lists various kinds of energy with a wavelike nature.

Each kind of energy is measured in terms of the amount of energy that strikes an object in a given time. The greater the frequency, the larger the amount of energy one encounters in a given period of time. If you listen to low frequency vibrations and compare them to higher frequency vibrations, the sound may begin to hurt your ears as the energy level reaches certain frequencies. Some individuals are so sensitive to higher frequencies of sound energy that they are unable to work around broadcast control rooms that produce these sounds. Other individuals are not able to hear such vibrations and so are unaffected by them.

Ears respond to changes in sound waves. Sound is produced by the vibration of molecules. Consequently, the ears are detecting changes in the quantity of energy and the quality of sound waves. Sound has several characteristics. Loudness, or volume, is a measure of the intensity of sound energy that arrives at the ear. Very loud sounds will literally vibrate your body, and can cause hearing loss if they are too intense. Pitch is a quality of sound that is determined by the frequency of the sound vibrations. High-pitched sounds have short wavelengths; low-pitched sounds have long wavelengths.

Noise is referred to as unwanted sound. However, noise can be more than just unpleasant sound. Research has shown that exposure to noise can cause physical, as well as mental, harm to the body. The loudness of the noise is measured by decibels (db). Decibel scales are logarithmic, rather than linear. Thus, the change from 40 db (a quiet library) to 80 db (a dishwasher or garbage disposal) represents a ten-thousandfold increase in sound loudness.

Box 3.1

Throughout the world, most scientists use a system of measurements formally known as the International System of Units, abbreviated **SI** from the French *Le Systeme International d'Unites*. The base units of measure in the SI system are:

Measurement:	Unit:	Symbol:
Length	meter	m
Mass	kilogram	kg
Time	second	s
Electric current	ampere	A
Temperature	kelvin	K
Amount of substance	mole	mol
Luminous intensity	candela	cd

You probably have not heard of some of the units listed above and may not see some that you thought would be there. That is because the SI system is different than the old metric system. While scientists in general have chosen to use the SI system, many of the Metric System units continue to be used worldwide:

Measurement:	Unit:	Symbol:
Volume	liter	L
Weight	gram	g
Length	meter	m
Temperature	Celsius	°C

There are two types of divisions in the Metric System: *sub*units and *super*units. Subunits are used for measurements smaller than the base unit. Superunits are used for measurements larger than the base unit. These divisions are indicated with a prefix in front of the four measurements noted above.

Prefix:	Symbol:	Amount:
make unit larger:		
mega-	M	a million times (1,000,000)
kilo-	k	a thousand times (1,000)
deca-	da	ten times (10)
make unit smaller:		
deci-	d	one tenth of (0.1)
centi-	c	one hundredth of (0.01)
milli-	m	one thousandth of (0.001)
micro-	μ (pronounced "mew")	one millionth of (0.000,001)
nano-	n	one billionth of (0.000,000,001)

In the metric system, the divisions are in amounts of ten. This means we can easily change divisions in the metric system. Rather than having to remember dozens of conversion factors (ex., 12 inches = 1 foot), we need only remember the number 10. By moving the decimal point the proper number of places to the right or to the left, we can convert to a larger or smaller division. To make a conversion, first determine if you want to express the information in a larger or smaller unit. If larger, you will be moving the decimal point to the left. If the new unit is to be smaller, you will move the decimal point to the right. For example, to convert 55 cm to meters, move the decimal to the left two places; i.e., 55 cm = 0.55 m. To convert 1.24 g to mg, simply move the decimal three places to the right, i.e., 1.24 g = 1240 mg.

In the United States, we use both the metric and English systems of measurements. Therefore, from time to time it is necessary to change from one to the other (also see inside of text cover).

Length:
1 in = 2.54 cm
1 ft = 30.48 cm
1 yd = 91.44 cm
0.62 mi = 1 km
1.609 km = 1 mi
0.393 in = 1 cm

Volume:
1 liq. oz = 29.57 mL
1 qt = 946.35 mL
1 gal = 3.79 L
1.056 qt = 1 L
0.95 L = 1 qt

Mass:
1 oz = 28.35 g
1 lb = 453.59 g
2.2 lb = 1 kg
28.35 g = 1 oz

Temperature:
$1\ °C = 5/9(°F–32)$
$1\ °F = (9/5 × °C) + 32$

Pressure:
1 atm = 760 torr
1 atm = 14.696 psi
1 atm = 29.921 in Hg

Energy:
$1\ eV = 1.6022 × 10^{-19}$ Joul
1 cal = 4.184 Joul
$1\ Joul = 1\ kg\ m^2 s^{-2}$
$1\ Joul = 10^7$ erg

Table 3.1 Intensity of Noise

SOURCE OF SOUND	INTENSITY IN DECIBELS (DB)
Jet aircraft at takeoff	145
Pain occurs	**140**
Hydraulic press	130
Jet airplane (160 meters/523.20 feet) overhead	120
Unmuffled motorcycle	110
Subway train	100
Farm tractor	98
Gasoline lawn mower	96
Food blender	93
Heavy truck (15 meters/yards) away	90
Heavy city traffic	90
Vacuum cleaner	85
Hearing loss after long exposure	**85**
Garbage disposal unit	80
Dishwasher	65
Normal speech	**60**
Window air conditioner	60

The frequency or pitch of a sound is also a factor in determining its degree of harm. The most common sound pressure scale for high-pitched sounds is the A scale, whose units are written "dbA." Hearing loss begins with prolonged exposure (eight hours or more) to 80 to 90 dbA levels of sound pressure. Sound pressure becomes painful at around 140 dbA and can kill at 180 dbA (table 3.1).

In addition to hearing loss, noise pollution is linked to a variety of other human ailments, ranging from nervous tension headaches to neuroses. Research has also shown that noise may cause blood vessels to constrict (reducing the blood flow to key body parts), disturbs unborn children, and sometimes causes seizures in epileptics. The U.S. EPA has estimated that noise causes about forty million U.S. citizens to suffer hearing damage or other mental or physical effects. Up to sixty-four million people are estimated to live in homes affected by aircraft, traffic, or construction noise.

ENERGY TRANSMISSION

Just as energy can be transformed from one form to another, it can also be *transmitted* from one location to another. The music that you hear on your radio is transmitted as energy in the form of radio waves from the broadcasting station to your radio. When a form of energy strikes an object, one of four things may happen: (1) it may pass through the object in the same direction as it entered; (2) it may be bent as it passes through and leaves in a different direction than it entered; (3) it may bounce off of the object; or (4) it may be absorbed by the object.

If the energy passes through the object, the object is transparent. **Transparency** is the property that allows the transmission of energy through materials. The walls in your home allow radio waves to pass through, but they are not transparent to light waves. The windows in your home, however, are transparent to both radio and light waves. Parts of your body (skin, for example), are transparent to X rays; bones are not. In some situations, the energy wave leaves an object in the same direction as it entered, or the energy wave may bend as it passes through the material.

The direction of the wave energy as it leaves an object is sometimes different than its direction of entry. This is called **refraction.** The property of refraction is the basis for the lenses in eyeglasses (figure 3.6).

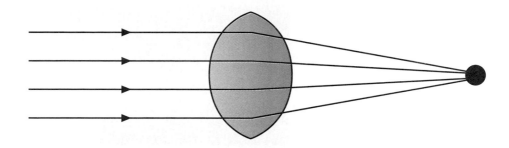

FIGURE 3.6 Refraction.
The shape of this lens causes the parallel light waves to bend as they pass through and converge at a given point. The type and shape of the material determine the amount and type of refraction as the energy passes through.

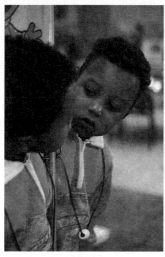

FIGURE 3.7 Reflection.
Images can be seen because light waves are reflected by the mirror.

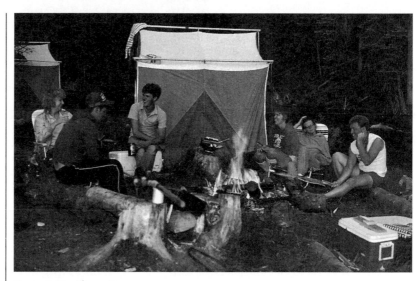

FIGURE 3.8 Absorption.
These people are warming themselves as their bodies absorb heat from the fire.

If the energy does not pass through the object but bounces off, it is reflected. **Reflection** is the property of energy bouncing off of the object it intersects. Echoes are caused by the reflection of sound waves. Other forms of energy, such as light, may also be reflected (figure 3.7).

If the energy strikes an object and remains in that object, it is absorbed. **Absorption** occurs when energy strikes a material and is retained within that material (figure 3.8).

Since energy can cause changes within the cells of the body, it is necessary to use proper techniques to safeguard against damaging the cells. Sunscreens are used to protect the skin from the sun's harmful rays. Warnings are posted to alert people with pacemakers that microwaves may be in use; the microwave energy may damage the pacemaker. Particular care must be observed when using various forms of radiation such as X rays (figure 3.9).

HEAT ENERGY

Heat, a form of energy produced by the random motion of atoms and molecules, is extremely important in living systems. It is measured in units called calories. A **calorie** is the amount of heat necessary to raise the temperature of one gram of water one degree **Celsius** (° C). Note that heat (measured in calories) and temperature (measured in Celsius) are not the same thing but are related to one another. The heat that an object possesses cannot be measured with a thermometer. What a thermometer measures is the temperature of an object. The **temperature** is really a measure of how fast the molecules of the substance are moving, and how often they bump into other molecules. This is a measure of the kinetic energy of the molecules. If heat is added to an object, the molecules will move faster. Consequently, the temperature will rise because the added heat energy will result in a

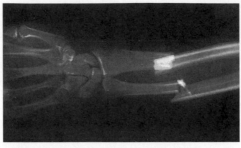

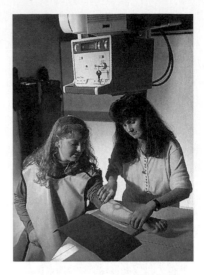

FIGURE 3.9 Medical use of X rays.
Radiologic technicians receive extensive training in the safe use of radiation for medical purposes. X rays will pass through soft tissues relatively easily but are stopped by dense tissues such as bone. This allows an X ray to be used to show if a bone is broken and the extent of damage if it is broken.

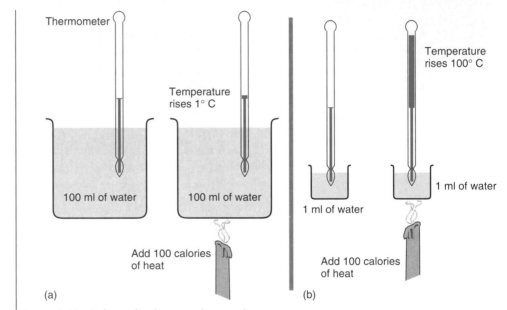

FIGURE 3.10 Relationship between heat and temperature.
Equal amounts of energy (one hundred calories of heat energy) are added to both of these beakers. However, the temperature in the large beaker (a) only increases by one degree. The same amount of heat results in a temperature increase of one hundred degrees in the small beaker (b). Why?

speeding up of the movement of the molecules. So, although there is a relationship between heat and temperature, the amount of heat in calories that an object has depends on the size of the object and its particular properties (figure 3.10).

Keeping the Human Body Warm

The human body usually maintains a temperature at which it functions most efficiently, about 37° C. This temperature is maintained by a balance between the rate of cellular metabolism (all the chemical reactions that take place in a cell), which generates heat, and radiation of heat from the surface of the skin. In addition, evaporation of fluid from the surface of the skin removes a great deal of heat from the body. During normal metabolism, the body is converting chemical-bond energy in food to different chemical bonds it can use to do its normal activities. As with all energy conversions, heat energy is also produced. Some of this heat will raise the temperature of the body. If the body temperature begins to drop, shivering begins. Shivering is a movement of muscles. As muscle cells move, their increased metabolism generates additional amounts of heat. In cold climates, it is very important to keep the temperature of the body near normal. Humans generally accomplish this by wearing special clothing, as well as ensuring that the body has enough food energy for conversion to heat energy when needed. Survival kits usually contain candy, which can provide quick energy.

Cooling the Human Body

Thus far, we have examined heat generation within the human body. Often the body may contain too much heat. Exposing more body surface for heat radiation and moving to an area with a greater difference between body temperature and environmental temperature will reduce the heat content. Increasing the quantity of sweat evaporation from the skin surface also reduces heat. The sweat absorbs large quantities of body heat as it evaporates. This is similar to changing liquid water into water vapor when we boil something. The amount of heat needed to cause this change from the liquid stage or phase to the gas phase is quite large. Young children frequently require quick heat removal when they have higher-than-normal temperatures. Because children can dehydrate quickly if they increase sweating, they might be placed in lukewarm baths. This will lower body temperature without removing excessive amount of fluids from the child's body.

Why do we take a person's temperature? Since the body's size and composition usually does not change in a short time, any change in temperature means that the body has either gained or lost heat. If the temperature is high, the body has usually increased its heat content as a result of increased cell metabolism. This increase in temperature is a symptom of abnormality. A low body temperature can also indicate abnormal body functioning.

PRESSURE

Gases have some properties relating to temperature and pressure that are not generally associated with liquids or solids. If a gas is kept in a closed container, it will exert pressure on the walls of the container. This **pressure** is due to the number of times that the molecules of gas collide with the inside wall of the container. If we increase the temperature of the gas in the container, the molecules will move faster, and they will collide more frequently with the walls of the container. Thus, there is an increase in pressure on the walls of the container. If we had an elastic container, like a balloon, this increased pressure would push out the walls of the container and increase its volume. If we put all these ideas together, we can see that the pressure is directly related to the temperature and inversely proportional to the volume. Stated as a formula, pressure is proportional to the temperature divided by the volume of the gas, or $P = T/V$. If you change any one of these terms, at least one of the others must change also. For instance, if the volume of the gas decreases (but the number of molecules remains the same), the pressure must increase or the temperature must decrease (figure 3.11).

ELECTRICITY IN LIFE

You might not think that electricity has much to do with life, but there are many electrical activities that occur inside the human body. The conduction of nerve impulses and muscular contraction are just two of them. Electrical energy is the result of uneven distribution of electrical charges. We know that the electrons of certain molecules can be detached from the original molecule and attached to a second molecule. Because the electron is negatively charged, the molecule that has lost an electron becomes positive; and the molecule that has gained an electron becomes negatively charged.

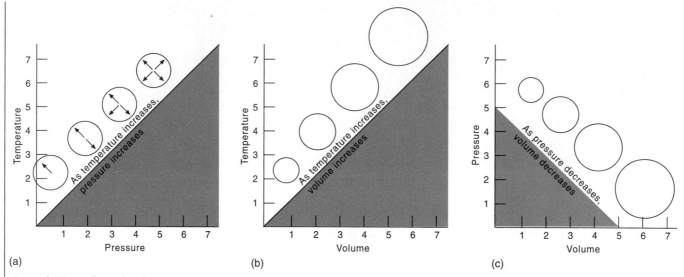

Figure 3.11 Relationship between pressure, temperature, and volume of a gas.
(a) As the temperature of a gas increases, the pressure of the gas (represented by the arrows in the balloons) must increase. (b) As the temperature of a gas increases, the volume of the gas (represented by the size of the balloons) must increase. (c) As the pressure of a gas decreases, the volume of the gas (represented by the size of the balloons) must increase.

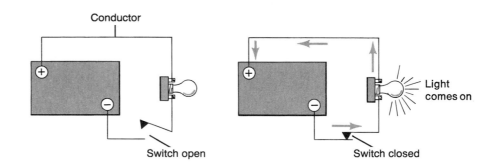

Figure 3.12 Storage battery.
A normal storage battery maintains unlike charged areas separate from one another. When a conductor connects the two poles, electrons are able to flow.

When two areas have unequal electrical charges, there will be a flow of electrons from the most negative area to the most positive area if a **conductor** of electrons connects the two areas. A battery consists of an arrangement that maintains a positive region separated from a negative region until the two poles of the battery are connected (figure 3.12).

Some materials are good conductors and others are very poor conductors of electricity. We make use of both on a routine basis. For example, we usually use metals to conduct electricity and are likely to use rubber, glass, or similar materials when we want to prevent the flow of electrons from one place to another. Those materials that prohibit the free movement of electrons are known as **insulators** or **nonconductors.**

Often when we are working with electricity, we use the term **grounding.** The ground (earth) is the ultimate receptor of displaced electrons. It is enormous compared to any battery or other electrical device likely to give shocks. Because electricity will follow the path of least resistance, and wires are better conductors than humans, electrons will flow through a ground wire (connected at some point by a pathway to the actual ground) rather than through a person. Therefore, a ground wire protects a person working with electrical devices.

INTERACTIONS OF MATTER AND ENERGY

A **force** is anything that has the potential to make an object move or alter its movement. All kinds of energy can be used to apply a force. Depending on the amount of energy a force has, it may not actually cause a movement. We frequently view energy in terms of forces or resistance to forces. If you try to move a patient from the bed to a chair, you may not be able to apply enough force to move them without help. You are spending energy and exerting a force against the patient, but the patient is resisting your force. As you sit reading this book, you are exerting force on whatever you are sitting on. The furniture is resisting the downward force.

The force exerted, and its action, are directly related to the amount of matter on which the

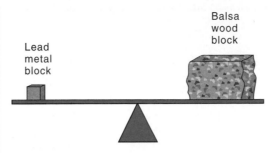

FIGURE 3.13 Density.

Since these two materials balance each other, they must have the same mass. It is obvious, however, that they do not have the same volume. Lead has a density of 11.3 g/ml and balsa wood has a density of 0.13 g/ml. Therefore, a volume of balsa 8.7 times as large as the volume of lead is required to obtain a balance.

force is applied. This is expressed as the weight of the matter. The **weight** of an object is the force that is pulling it toward the center of the earth (gravity). Let's examine this idea of force and matter a little further. The weight of an object changes depending on the force of gravity. Astronauts weigh much less on the moon than they do on the earth, but they still have the same resistance to forces. Mass is a term that relates weight to the energy required to move it. **Mass** is defined as resistance to force; i.e., how much matter there is in an object. The larger the mass, the larger the force necessary to move the mass.

If you have ever pushed a car, you know it is more difficult to push a van than a compact automobile. You might think this is due to the fact that the van is larger than the compact car. While it is true that the van is larger in volume, its mass is a different story. The van has a mass of 2155 kg and the compact has a mass of 1100 kg. It would be just as difficult to move the compact car if it was loaded with 1055 kg of bricks as it would be to move the van. The size of the two cars is different but if the compact is loaded with bricks, the masses are similar. The fact that the mass of a given volume of one material is different from the mass of a different material gives rise to the idea of density (figure 3.13). Density is equal to the mass per unit volume, or D = M/V.

The van has a mass of 2155 kg and a volume of 10 kl. Therefore, it has a density of 215 kg/kl. The empty compact has a mass of 1100 kg, a volume of 5 kl, and a density of 220 kg/kl. Even though both cars have almost the same density, the van has twice as much mass. If we load 1055 kg of bricks into the compact, it has the same mass as the van, 2155 kg. The compact, however, now has a density of 437 kg/kl.

Specific gravity is closely related to density. The specific gravity of a substance is its density compared to the density of water. One cubic centimeter of water (also equals one milliliter) weighs one gram. Water has a density of 1 gram/cubic centimeter. Anything with a higher density will sink in water, and anything with a lower density will float. Any substance with a specific gravity of less than 1.00 floats. If you mix water and gasoline, the gasoline (specific gravity of 0.75) floats to the top. In a mixture of water and mercury, the mercury (specific gravity of 13.6) sinks to the bottom.

One clinical test performed on urine is to measure its specific gravity. This determines how similar the urine is to pure water and how much dissolved materials it contains. A specific gravity test—along with other tests—can be very valuable information in diagnosing illnesses such as kidney diseases. People also vary in the specific gravity of their bodies. Some persons find it very easy to float in water while others find it impossible. This is directly related to their individual specific gravity, which in turn is a measure of their ratio of body fat to muscle and bone.

SUMMARY

Energy is the ability to do something. Energy of motion is kinetic energy, whereas energy of position is potential energy. The First Law of Thermodynamics states that there is a constant amount of energy in the universe. Energy can take a variety of forms, such as light, heat, and electricity. These forms of energy may be interconverted, but in that interconversion useful energy is lost and forms heat. The Second Law of Thermodynamics states that conversions from one form of energy to another result in the formation of heat. Energy of the electromagnetic spectrum including light, heat, radio waves, and X rays can be analyzed if we think of them as moving waves. When these energy waves hit an object, they can pass through the object or be refracted, reflected, or absorbed. Heat is a common form of energy that is extremely important to humans. Temperature is the measure of the amount of heat in an object. The larger amount of heat energy an object has, the faster the movement of molecules and the higher the temperature. Materials with little heat energy are likely to be solids. As heat energy is added, these solids will change to liquids and then to gases.

Electrical energy is the result of an uneven distribution of positive and negative charges. Electrical energy in the body is responsible for nerve impulse conduction and muscular activity. Other physical concepts include force, mass, density, weight, and specific gravity—all related to one another. A force tries to move something and the mass of an object tends to resist movement. All the other terms are used to compare force with mass.

QUESTIONS

1. Define potential energy and describe how it is different from kinetic energy.

2. What are the first and second laws of thermodynamics?

3. What happens to the frequency of a form of energy, such as light, as wavelength increases?

4. What is the difference between absorption, reflection, and refraction of energy?

5. What does temperature measure?

6. Explain why it is important to cool an infant by placing him or her in a lukewarm water bath.

7. List the units of measure of the metric system and the meanings of their prefixes.

8. What happens to the volume of a container of gas when the temperature increases? What happens when the pressure decreases?

9. What is the difference between mass and weight?

10. What is a decibel and what does it have to do with hearing loss?

absorption (ab-sorp'shun) Energy that enters an intercepting object and stops.

Angstrom (ang'strem) (Å) Unit of measurement of wavelengths of energy in the electromagnetic spectrum; one 100 millionth (10^{-8}) of a centimeter.

calorie (kal'o-re) The amount of heat necessary to raise the temperature of one gram of water one degree Celsius.

Celsius (sel'se-us) Scale of measuring temperature (abbreviated ° C).

conductor (kon-duk'tor) Connector of two areas that allows the flow of electrons.

cycles per second (si'kls) Numbers of waves of energy in regard to the electromagnetic spectrum.

electromagnetic spectrum (e-lek"tro-mag'net-ik spek'trum) Wavelike forms of energy such as radio waves, X rays, and light.

First Law of Thermodynamics (furst law uv ther"mo-di-nam'iks) Also known as the **Law of Conservation of Energy** states that the total amount of energy in the universe remains constant; it can neither be created nor destroyed but only transferred and transformed.

force (fōrs) Anything that has the potential to make an object move or alter its movement.

frequency (fre'kwen-se) The number of waves of energy produced per second.

grounding (grownd'ing) Connecting an area with the ground (earth), which then acts as the ultimate receptor of displaced electrons.

heat (hēt) A form of energy produced by the random motion of atoms and molecules.

insulators (in'su-la"tors) Material that prohibits the flow of electrons.

mass (mas) Resistance to forces.

nanometers (na"no-me'ters) A billionth of a meter.

nonconductors (non"kon-duk'tors) Material that prohibits the flow of electrons.

pressure (presh'ur) The force of the collisions of molecules on the surface of an area.

reflection (re-flek'shun) Energy that bounces off of the object it intersects.

refraction (re-frak'shun) Energy that passes through an object and leaves in a direction different from the direction that it entered.

Second Law of Thermodynamics (sek'ond law uv ther"mo-di-nam'iks) Basic principle that states that one form of energy can be converted to a second form of energy, but in doing so, a third form, heat, is also produced.

specific gravity (spĕ-sif'ik grav'ĭ-te) Density of a substance compared to the density of water.

temperature (tem'per-ah-tūr) The measure of molecular kinetic energy.

transparency (trans-par'en-sē) Property of material that allows the transmission of energy through it.

wavelength (wāv'length) Distance from one crest to the next crest of a wave of energy in the electromagnetic spectrum.

weight (wāt) The force of gravity on an object.

THE DYNAMIC HUMAN   Correlations to Chapter Three:

Respiratory System → Exploration → Boyle's Law

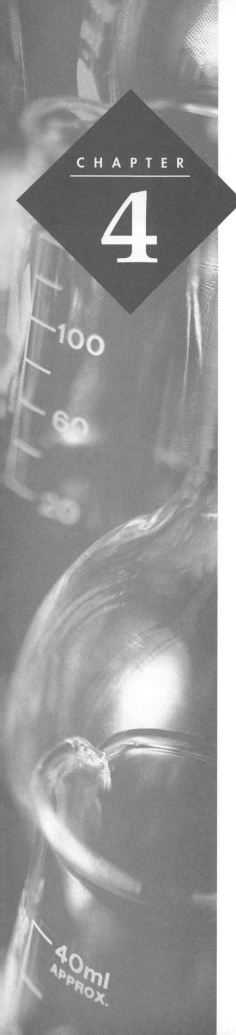

Organic Chemistry— The Chemistry of Life

CHAPTER OUTLINE

PURPOSE

The chemistry of living things is really the chemistry of the carbon atom and a few other atoms that can combine with carbon. In order to understand some aspects of the structure and function of living things, which will be covered later, you should first learn some basic organic chemistry.

CLINICAL VIEWPOINT

Among the vast number of proteins found in the body, one group stands out. *Immunoglobulins*, Ig, (immuno = resistant; globulin = globular protein) are commonly referred to as antibodies since they were once thought to be little bodies that defended against (anti-) infectious agents such as bacteria and viruses. There are five classes of these Y-shaped molecules, each identified by a particular letter of the Greek alphabet:

- IgM (*Mu*) is found in the blood serum and is very effective as a first line defense against bacterial blood infections.
- IgG (*Gamma*) is the most abundant immunoglobulin in body fluids, and is particularly effective in combating microorganisms and their toxins.
- IgA (*Alpha*) is found in the blood and secretions and serves as a defense against initial microbial invasion.
- IgE (*Epsilon*) is found in the blood and body fluids and is associated with certain types of allergies (hypersensitivities).
- IgD (*Delta*) is also in the blood; however, its function is not clear.

Each class can contain an infinite variety of unique protein molecules that are able to combine with specific agents recognized to be nonself, or dangerous to the body. An immunoglobulin is always a globular protein molecule manufactured by white blood cells known as B lymphoctyes (B cells) and plasma cells. The presence of nonself agents, called *immunogens*, is able to stimulate (*generate*) the production of this form of resistance (*immun*ity). When an immunoglobulin reacts with the immunogen, a sequence of events occurs that results in the destruction of the newly formed immunogen-immunoglobulin complex. In this way nonself and dangerous agents such as bacteria, viruses, toxic molecules, and cancer cells can be eliminated from the body. The production of protective immunoglobulins can occur as the result of vaccination. Several types of vaccinations are regularly given to infants and children to stimulate their bodies to become protected against infectious diseases. The DPT vaccination immunizes against diphtheria, pertussis (whooping cough), and tetanus; the MMR against measles, mumps, and rubella; and, against polio, either OPV (oral polio vaccine) or IPV (inactivated polio vaccine) is used.

LEARNING OBJECTIVES

- Recognize the difference between inorganic and organic molecules
- Understand the importance of structure in organic molecules
- Know the major functional groups found in organic molecules
- Describe the structure and function of the three major groups of organic molecules

MOLECULES CONTAINING CARBON

The principles and concepts discussed in chapter 2 apply to all types of matter—nonliving as well as living matter. Living systems are composed of various types of molecules. Most of the things we described in the previous chapter did not contain carbon atoms and so were classified as **inorganic molecules.** This chapter is mainly concerned with more complex structures, **organic molecules,** which contain carbon atoms arranged into rings or chains.

The original meaning of the terms *inorganic* and *organic* is related to the fact that organic materials were thought to be either alive or produced only by living things. Therefore, a very strong link exists between organic chemistry and the chemistry of living things, which is called **biochemistry,** or biological chemistry. Modern chemistry has considerably altered the original meaning of the terms *organic* and *inorganic,* since it is now possible to manufacture unique organic molecules that cannot be produced by living things. Many of the materials we use daily are the result of the organic chemist's art. Nylon, aspirin, polyurethane varnish, silicones, Plexiglas, food wrap, Teflon, and insecticides are just a few of the unique molecules that have been invented by organic chemists (figure 4.1).

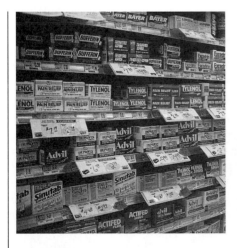

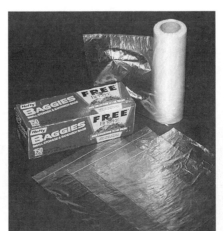

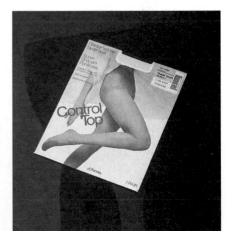

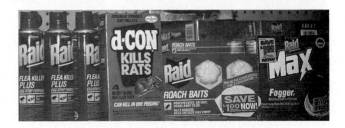

FIGURE **4.1** Some common synthetic organic materials. These items are examples of useful organic compounds invented by chemists.

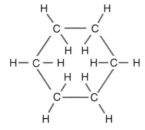

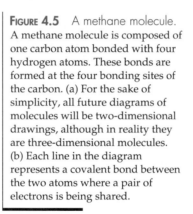

Figure 4.3 A ring or chain structure. The ring structure shown on the bottom is formed by joining the two ends of a chain of carbon atoms.

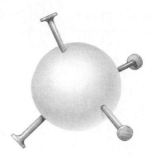

Figure 4.4 Bonding sites of a carbon atom. The arrangement of bonding sites around the carbon is similar to a ball with four equally spaced nails in it. Each of the four bondable electrons inhabits an area as far away from the other three as possible.

Figure 4.5 A methane molecule. A methane molecule is composed of one carbon atom bonded with four hydrogen atoms. These bonds are formed at the four bonding sites of the carbon. (a) For the sake of simplicity, all future diagrams of molecules will be two-dimensional drawings, although in reality they are three-dimensional molecules. (b) Each line in the diagram represents a covalent bond between the two atoms where a pair of electrons is being shared.

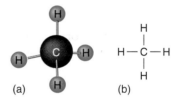

(a)   (b)

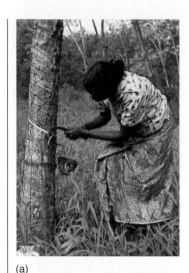

(a)

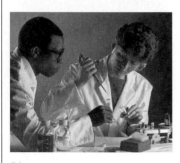

(b)

Figure 4.2 Natural and synthetic organic compounds. Some organic materials, such as rubber, were originally produced by plants but are now synthesized in industry. (a) The collection of latex from the rubber tree. (b) An organic chemist testing one of the steps in a manufacturing process.

Carbon—The Central Atom

In other instances, organic chemists have taken their lead from living organisms and have been able to produce organic molecules more efficiently, or in forms that are slightly different from the original natural molecule. Some examples of these are rubber, penicillin, some vitamins, insulin, and alcohol (figure 4.2).

All organic molecules, whether they are natural or synthetic, have certain common characteristics. The carbon atom, which is the central atom in all organic molecules, has some unusual properties. Carbon is unique in that it can combine with other carbon atoms to form long chains. In many cases, the ends of these chains may join together to form ring structures (figure 4.3). Only a few other atoms have this ability. What is really unusual is that these bonding sites are all located at equal distances from one another. If you were to take a rubber ball and stick four nails into it so that they were equally distributed around the ball, you would have a good idea of the geometry involved. These bonding sites are arranged this way because in the carbon atom there are four electrons in the second energy level. These four electrons in the L shell, or the $2s$, $2px$, $2py$, and $2pz$ orbitals, are all as far away from each other as possible (figure 4.4). Carbon atoms are usually involved in covalent bonds. Since carbon has four places where it can bond, the carbon atom can combine with four other atoms by forming four separate *single* covalent bonds with other atoms. This is the case with the methane molecule, which has four hydrogen atoms attached to a single carbon atom. Pure methane is a colorless and odorless gas that makes up 95% of natural gas (figure 4.5). The aroma of the

Box 4.1

Chemical Shorthand

Y ou have probably noticed that sketching the entire structural formula of a large organic molecule takes a great deal of time. If you know the structure of the major functional groups, you can use several shortcuts to more quickly describe chemical structures.

When multiple carbons with two hydrogens are bonded to each other in a chain, we sometimes write it as follows:

$$-\overset{\displaystyle H}{\underset{\displaystyle H}{C}}-\overset{\displaystyle H}{\underset{\displaystyle H}{C}}-\overset{\displaystyle H}{\underset{\displaystyle H}{C}}-\overset{\displaystyle H}{\underset{\displaystyle H}{C}}-\overset{\displaystyle H}{\underset{\displaystyle H}{C}}-\overset{\displaystyle H}{\underset{\displaystyle H}{C}}-\overset{\displaystyle H}{\underset{\displaystyle H}{C}}-\overset{\displaystyle H}{\underset{\displaystyle H}{C}}-\overset{\displaystyle H}{\underset{\displaystyle H}{C}}-\overset{\displaystyle H}{\underset{\displaystyle H}{C}}-\overset{\displaystyle H}{\underset{\displaystyle H}{C}}-\overset{\displaystyle H}{\underset{\displaystyle H}{C}}-$$

or we might write it this way:

$$-CH_2-CH_2-CH_2-CH_2-CH_2-CH_2-CH_2-CH_2-CH_2-CH_2-CH_2-CH_2-$$

or more simply, we may write it as follows: $(-CH_2-)_{12}$. If the twelve carbons were in a pair of two rings, we probably would not label the carbons or hydrogens unless we wished to focus on a particular group or point. We would probably draw the two six-carbon rings with only hydrogen attached as follows:

Or

Don't let these shortcuts throw you. You will soon find that you will be putting an —OH group onto a carbon skeleton and neglecting to show the bond between the oxygen and hydrogen, just like a professional.

natural gas is the result of mercaptan (and trimethyl disulfide) added to let consumers know when a leak occurs. Box 4.1 explains how chemists and biologists diagram the kind of bonds formed in organic molecules.

Some atoms may be bonded to a single atom more than once. This results in a slightly different arrangement of bonds around the carbon atom. An example of this type of bonding occurs when oxygen is attracted to a carbon. Oxygen has two bondable electrons—if it shares one of these with a carbon and then shares the other with the same carbon, it forms a *double bond.* A **double bond** is two covalent bonds formed between two atoms that share two pairs of electrons. Oxygen is not the only atom that can form double bonds, but double bonds are common between it and carbon. The double bond is denoted by two lines between the two atoms:

$$-\underset{\displaystyle |}{C}=O$$

Two carbon atoms might form double bonds between each other and then bond to other atoms at the remaining bonding sites. Figure 4.6 shows several compounds that contain double bonds. Some organic molecules contain *triple covalent bonds* such as the flammable gas acetylene, $H-C\equiv C-H$. Others like hydrogen cyanide, $H-C\equiv N$, have biological significance. This molecule inhibits production of energy and can result in death.

Although most atoms can be involved in the structure of an organic molecule, only a few are commonly found. Hydrogen (H) and oxygen (O) are almost always present. Nitrogen (N), sulfur (S), and phosphorus (P) are also very important in specific types of organic molecules.

An enormous variety of organic molecules is possible because carbon is able to bond at four different sites, form long chains, and combine with many other kinds of atoms. The types of atoms in the molecule are important in determining the properties of the molecule. The three-dimensional arrangement of the atoms within the molecule is also important. Since most inorganic molecules are small and involve few atoms, there is usually only one way in which a group of atoms can be arranged to form a molecule. There is only one arrangement for a single

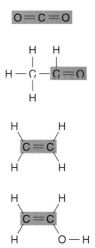

FIGURE 4.6 Double bonds. These diagrams show several molecules that contain double bonds. A double bond is formed when two atoms share two pairs of electrons with each other.

oxygen atom and two hydrogen atoms in a molecule of water. In a molecule of sulfuric acid, there is only one arrangement for the sulfur atom, the two hydrogen atoms, and the four oxygen atoms.

$$
\begin{array}{c}
O \\
\parallel \\
H-O-S-O-H \\
\parallel \\
O
\end{array}
$$

However, consider these two organic molecules:

$$
\begin{array}{ccccc}
H & & & H \\
| & & & | \\
H-C & -O- & C-H \\
| & & & | \\
H & & & H
\end{array}
$$

dimethyl
ether

and

$$
\begin{array}{cccc}
H & H \\
| & | \\
H-C- & C-O-H \\
| & | \\
H & H
\end{array}
$$

ethyl
alcohol

Both the dimethyl ether and the ethyl alcohol contain two carbon atoms, six hydrogen atoms, and one oxygen atom, but they are quite different in their arrangement of atoms and in the chemical properties of the molecules. While the first is an ether, the second is an alcohol. Since the ether and the alcohol have the same number and kinds of atoms, they are said to have the same empirical formula, which in this case is written C_2H_6O. An **empirical formula** simply indicates the number of each kind of atom within the molecule. When the arrangement of the atoms and their bonding within the molecule is indicated, we call this a **structural formula.** Figure 4.7 shows several structural formulas for the empirical formula $C_6H_{12}O_6$. Molecules that have the same empirical formula but different structural formulas are called **isomers.**

CARBON SKELETON AND FUNCTIONAL GROUPS

To help us understand organic molecules a little better, let's consider some of their similarities. All organic molecules have a **carbon skeleton,** which is composed of rings or chains of carbons. It is this carbon skeleton in the organic molecule that determines the overall shape of the molecule. The differences between various organic molecules depend on the length and arrangement of the carbon skeleton. In addition, the kinds of atoms that are bonded to this carbon skeleton determine the way the organic compound acts. Attached to the carbon skeleton are specific combinations of atoms called **functional groups.** These functional groups determine specific chemical properties. By learning to recognize some of the functional groups, it is possible to identify an organic molecule and to predict something about its activity. Figure 4.8 shows some of the functional groups that are important in biological activity. Remember that a functional group does not exist by itself; it must be a part of an organic molecule (*see* box 4.1).

COMMON ORGANIC MOLECULES

One way to make organic chemistry more manageable is to organize different kinds of compounds into groups on the basis of their similarity of structure or the chemical properties of the molecules. Frequently you will find that organic molecules are composed of subunits that are attached to each other. If you recognize

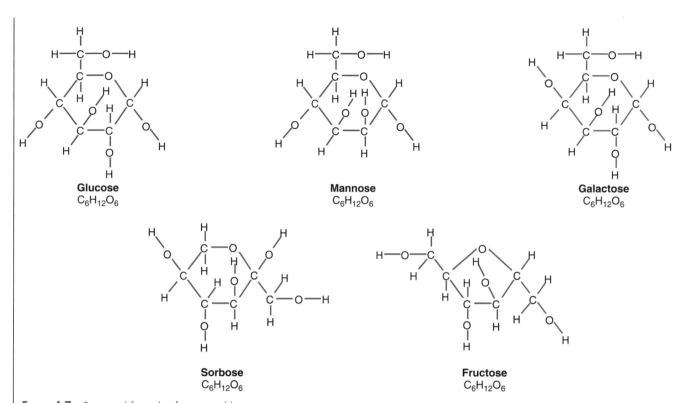

FIGURE 4.7 Structural formulas for several hexoses.

Several six-carbon sugars are represented here. Each has the same empirical formula, but they each have a different structural formula. They will also act differently from each other.

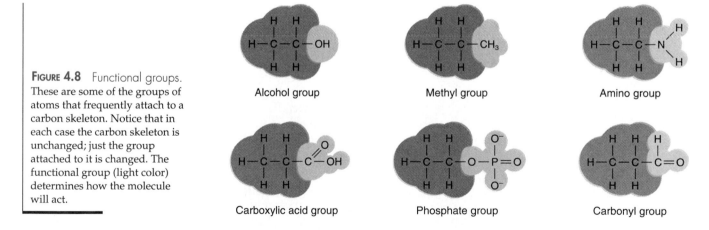

FIGURE 4.8 Functional groups. These are some of the groups of atoms that frequently attach to a carbon skeleton. Notice that in each case the carbon skeleton is unchanged; just the group attached to it is changed. The functional group (light color) determines how the molecule will act.

the subunit, then the whole organic molecule is much easier to identify. It is similar to distinguishing between a passenger train and a freight train by recognizing the individual cars unique to each.

When there are several subunits (*monomers; mono* = single; *mer* = segment or piece) bonded together, the molecule is referred to as a macromolecule or a *polymer* (*poly* = many; *mer* = segments). The word *monomer* means a single unit, while the term *polymer* means composed of many parts. The plastics industry has polymer chemistry as its foundation. The monomers in a polymer are usually combined by a **dehydration synthesis reaction** (*de* = remove; *hydro* = water; *synthesis* = combine). This reaction results in the synthesis or formation of a macromolecule when water is removed from between the two smaller component parts. For example, when a monomer with an "—OH group" attached to its carbon skeleton approaches

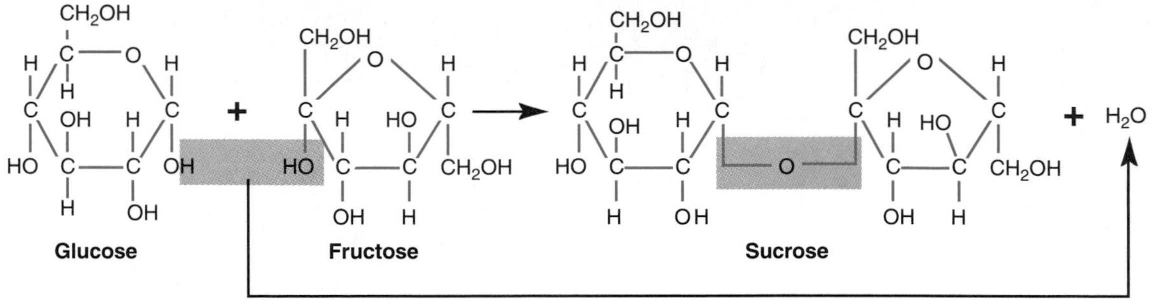

Figure 4.9 The dehydration synthesis reaction.
In the reaction illustrated here, the two —OH groups form water, and the oxygen that remains acts as an attachment site between the two larger sugar molecules. Many structural formulas appear to be complex at first glance, but if you look for the points where subunits are attached and dissect each subunit, they become much simpler to deal with.

another monomer with an available hydrogen, dehydration synthesis can occur. Figure 4.9 shows the removal of water from between two such subunits. Notice that in this case the structural formulas are used to help identify just what is occurring. However, the chemical equation also indicates the removal of the water. You can easily recognize a dehydration synthesis reaction because the reactant side of the equation shows numerous small molecules, while the product side lists fewer, larger products and water.

The reverse of a dehydration synthesis reaction is known as *hydrolysis* (*hydro* = water; *lyse* = to split or break). **Hydrolysis** is the process of splitting a larger organic molecule into two or more component parts by the addition of water. Digestion of food molecules in the stomach is an important example of hydrolysis.

Carbohydrates

One class of organic molecules, **carbohydrates,** is composed of carbon, hydrogen, and oxygen atoms linked together to form monomers called *simple sugars* or *monosaccharides* (*mono* = single, *saccharine* = sweet, sugar). The empirical formula for a simple sugar is easy to recognize because there are equal numbers of carbons and oxygens and twice as many hydrogens—for example, $C_3H_6O_3$ or $C_5H_{10}O_5$. We usually describe the kinds of simple sugars by the number of carbons in the molecule. The ending *-ose* indicates you are dealing with a carbohydrate. A tri*ose* has three carbons, a pent*ose* has five, and a hex*ose* has six. If you remember that the number of carbons equals the number of oxygen atoms and that the number of hydrogens is double that number, these names tell you the empirical formula for the simple sugar. Simple sugars, such as glucose, fructose, and galactose, provide the chemical energy necessary to keep organisms alive. These simple sugars combine with each other by dehydration synthesis to form **complex carbohydrates** (figure 4.9). When two simple sugars bond to each other, a *disaccharide* (*di-* = two) is formed; when three bond together, a *trisaccharide* (*tri-* = three) is formed (figure 4.10). Generally we call a complex carbohydrate that is larger than this a *polysaccharide* (many sugar units). In all cases, the complex carbohydrates are formed by the removal of water from between the sugars. Some common examples of polysaccharides are starch and glycogen. Cellulose is an important polysaccharide used in constructing the cell walls of plant cells. Humans cannot digest (*hydrolyze*) this complex carbohydrate, so we are not able to use it as an energy source. Plant cell walls add bulk or fiber to our diet, but no calories. Fiber is an important addition because it helps to control weight, reduce the risk of colon cancer, and control constipation and diarrhea.

Simple sugars can be used by the cell as components in other, more complex molecules. Sugar molecules are a part of other, larger molecules such as DNA, RNA, or ATP. ATP is important in energy transfer. It has a simple sugar (ribose) as part of its structural makeup. The building blocks of the genetic material (DNA) also have a sugar component (*see* figure 4.18).

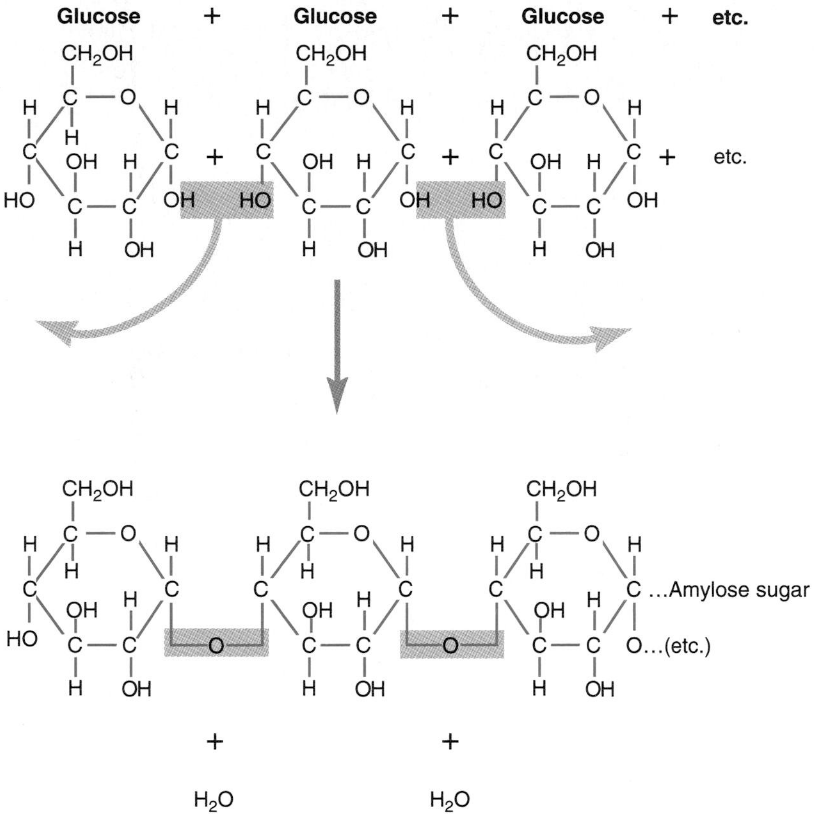

FIGURE 4.10 A trisaccharide.

Three simple sugars are attached to each other by the removal of two waters from between them. This is an example of a complex carbohydrate.

Lipids

We generally describe **lipids** as large organic molecules that do not easily dissolve in water. Just like carbohydrates, the lipids are composed of carbon, hydrogen, and oxygen. They do not, however, have the same ratio of carbon, hydrogen, and oxygen in their empirical formulas. Lipids generally have very small amounts of oxygen in comparison to the amounts of carbon and hydrogen. Fats, phospholipids, and steroids are all examples of lipids, but they are all quite different from each other in their structure.

Fats are important organic molecules that are used to provide energy. The building blocks of a fat are a glycerol molecule and fatty acids. The **glycerol** is a carbon skeleton that has three alcohol groups attached to it. Its chemical formula is $C_3H_5(OH)_3$.

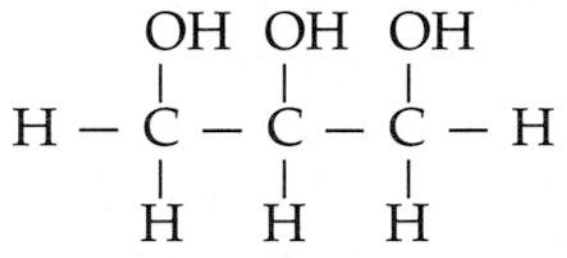

Glycerol

A **fatty acid** is a long-chain carbon skeleton that has a carboxylic acid functional group. If the carbon skeleton has as much hydrogen bonded to it as possible, we call it **saturated.** The saturated fatty acid shown is stearic acid, a component of solid meat fats such as mutton tallow. Notice that at every point in this structure the carbon has as much hydrogen as it can hold. Saturated fats are generally found in animal tissues—they tend to be solids at room temperatures. Some examples of saturated fats are butter, whale blubber, suet, lard, and fats associated with such meats as steak or pork chops.

Organic Chemistry—The Chemistry of Life   57

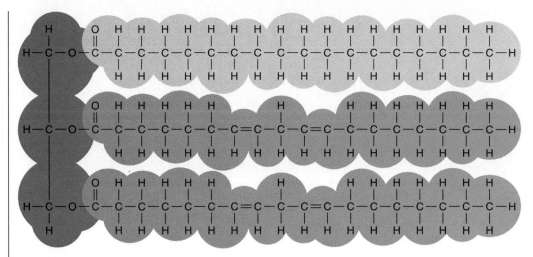

FIGURE 4.11 A fat molecule.

The arrangement of the three fatty acids attached to a glycerol molecule is typical of the formation of a fat. The structural formula of the fat appears to be very cluttered until you dissect the fatty acids from the glycerol; then it becomes much more manageable. This example of a triglyceride contains a glycerol molecule, two unsaturated fatty acids (linoleic acid), and a third saturated fatty acid (stearic acid).

stearic acid

If the carbons are double-bonded to each other at one or more points, the fatty acid is said to be **unsaturated.** The unsaturated fatty acid below is linoleic acid, a component of sunflower and safflower oils.

linoleic acid

Notice that there are two double bonds between the carbons and fewer hydrogens than in the saturated fatty acid. Unsaturated fats are frequently plant fats or oils—they are usually liquids at room temperature. Peanut oil, corn oil, and olive oil are considered unsaturated because they have double bonds between the carbons of the carbon skeleton. A polyunsaturated fatty acid is one that has a great number of double bonds in the carbon skeleton. When glycerol and three fatty acids are combined by three dehydration synthesis reactions, a fat is formed. Notice that dehydration synthesis is almost exactly the same as the reaction that causes simple sugars to bond together.

Fats are important molecules for storing energy. There is twice as much energy in a gram of fat as in a gram of sugar. This is important to an organism because fats can be stored in a relatively small space and still yield a high amount of energy. Fats in animals also provide protection from heat loss. Some animals have a layer of fat under the skin that serves as an insulating layer. The thick layer of blubber in whales, walruses, and seals prevents the loss of internal body heat to the cold, watery environment in which they live. This same layer of fat, together with the fat deposits around some internal organs—such as the kidneys and heart—serves as a cushion that protects these organs from physical damage. If a fat is formed from a glycerol molecule and three attached fatty acids, it is called a **triglyceride;** if two, a *diglyceride;* and if one, a *monoglyceride* (figure 4.11). Triglycerides account for about 95% of the fat stored in human tissue.

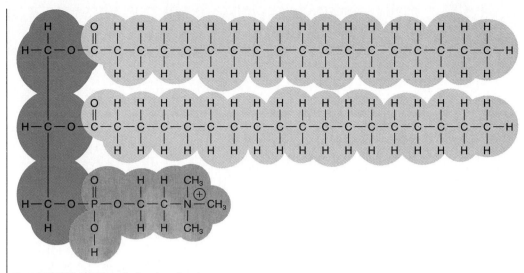

FIGURE 4.12 A phospholipid molecule.
This molecule is similar to a fat but has a phosphate group in its structure. The phosphate group is bonded to the glycerol by a dehydration synthesis reaction. This phospholipid contains glycerol, two fatty acids, and the phosphate-containing portion. Molecules like this are known as the lecithins.

Phospholipids are a class of water-insoluble molecules that resemble fats but contain a phosphate group (PO_4) in their structure (figure 4.12). One of the reasons phospholipids are important is that they are a major component of membranes in cells. Without these lipids in our membranes, the cell contents would not be able to be separated from the watery exterior environment. Some of the phospholipids are better known as *lecithins*. Lecithins are found in cell membranes and also help in the emulsification of fats. They help to separate large portions of fat into smaller units. This allows the fat to mix with other materials. Lecithins are added to many types of food for this purpose (chocolate bars, for example). Some people take lecithin as a nutritional supplement because they believe it leads to healthier hair and better reasoning ability. But once inside your intestines, lecithins are destroyed by enzymes, just like any other phospholipid (box 4.2).

Steroids, a third group of lipid molecules, are characterized by their arrangement of interlocking rings of carbon. They often serve as hormones that aid in regulating body processes. We have already mentioned one steroid molecule that you are probably familiar with: cholesterol. While serum cholesterol (the kind found in your blood associated with lipoproteins) has been implicated in many cases of atherosclerosis, this steroid is made by your body for use as a component of cell membranes. It is also used by your body to make bile acids. These products of your liver are channeled into your intestine to emulsify fats. Cholesterol is also necessary for the manufacture of vitamin D. Cholesterol molecules in the skin react with ultraviolet light to produce vitamin D, which assists in the proper development of bones and teeth. Figure 4.13 illustrates some of the steroid compounds that are typically manufactured by organisms.

A large number of steroid molecules are hormones. Some of them regulate reproductive processes such as egg and sperm production, while others regulate such things as salt concentration in the blood. Athletes have been known to use certain hormonelike steroids to increase their muscular bulk. The medical community is certain that use of these chemicals is potentially harmful, possibly resulting in liver disfunction, sex-characteristic changes, changes in blood chemistry, and even death.

Box 4.2 — Fat and Your Diet

When triglycerides are eaten in fat-containing foods, digestive enzymes hydrolyze them into monoglycerides and fatty acids. These molecules are absorbed by the intestinal tract and coated with protein to form *lipoprotein*, as shown in the accompanying diagram.

There are four types of lipoproteins in the body: (1) chylomicrons, (2) very-low-density-lipoproteins (VLDL), (3) low-density-lipoproteins (LDL), and (4) high-density-lipoproteins (HDL). Chylomicrons are very large particles formed in the intestine and are between 80% and 95% triglycerides in composition. As the chylomicrons circulate through the body, the triglycerides are removed by cells in order to make hormones, store energy, and build new cell parts. When most of the triglycerides have been removed, the remaining portions of the chylomicrons are harmlessly destroyed.

The VLDLs and LDLs are formed in the liver. VLDLs contain all types of lipid, protein, and 10%–15% cholesterol, while the LDLs are about 50% cholesterol. As with the chylomicrons, the body taps these molecules for their lipids. However, in some people, high levels of LDLs in the blood are associated with the disease *atherosclerosis* (hardening of the arteries). While in the blood, LDLs may stick to the insides of the vessels, forming deposits that restrict blood flow and contribute to high blood pressure, strokes, and heart attacks. Even though they are 30% cholesterol, a high level of HDLs (made in the intestine) in comparison to LDLs is associated with a lower risk of atherosclerosis. One way to reduce the risk of this disease is to lower your intake of LDLs. This can be done by reducing your consumption of saturated fats, since these are most easily converted by your body into LDLs and cholesterol.

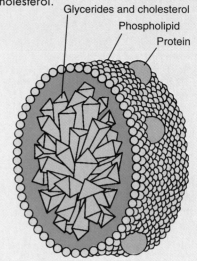

Glycerides and cholesterol
Phospholipid
Protein

Reprinted with permission, Best Foods, a division of CPC International, Inc.

FIGURE 4.13 Steroids.
(a) Cholesterol is produced by the human body and is found in your cells' membranes. (b) Vitamin D$_2$ is important to the normal growth of teeth and bones. (c) Cholic acid is a bile salt produced by the liver and used to break down fats. (d) Cortisol controls the metabolism of food and helps to control inflammation. Testosterone (e) and estradiol (f) are male and female sex hormones. (g) Progesterone is a female sex hormone produced by the ovaries and placenta.

(a) Cholesterol

(b) Vitamin D$_2$

(c) Cholic acid

(d) Cortisol

(e) Testosterone

(f) Estradiol

(g) Progesterone

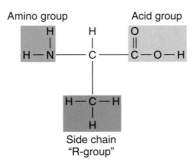

FIGURE 4.14 The structure of an amino acid.

An amino acid is composed of a short carbon skeleton with three functional groups attached: an amino group, a carboxylic acid group (acid group), and an additional variable group ("R-group"). It is the variable group that determines which specific amino acid is constructed.

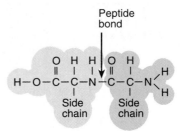

FIGURE 4.15 A peptide bond.

The bond that results from a dehydration synthesis reaction between two amino acids is called a peptide bond. This bond forms as a result of the removal of the hydrogen and hydroxyl groups. In the formation of this bond, the nitrogen is bonded directly to the carbon.

Proteins

Proteins are polymers made up of monomers known as *amino acids*. An **amino acid** is a short carbon skeleton that contains an amino group (a nitrogen and two hydrogens) on one end of the skeleton and a carboxylic acid group at the other end (figure 4.14). In addition, the carbon skeleton may have one of several different side chains on it. There are about twenty common amino acids that are important to cells. All are identical except for their side chains (box 4.3).

The amino acids can bond together by dehydration synthesis reactions. When two amino acids form a bond by removal of water, the nitrogen of the amino group of one is bonded to the carbon of the acid group of another. This bond is termed a **peptide bond** (figure 4.15).

Any amino acid can form a peptide bond with any other amino acid. They fit together in a specific way, with the amino group of one bonding to the acid group of the next. You can imagine that by using twenty different amino acids as building blocks, you can construct millions of different combinations. Each of these combinations is termed a **polypeptide chain.** A specific polypeptide is composed of a specific sequence of amino acids bonded end to end. This is called its *primary structure.* A listing of the amino acids in their proper order within a particular polypeptide constitutes its primary structure. The specific sequence of amino acids in a polypeptide is controlled by the genetic information of an organism.

The string of amino acids in a polypeptide is likely to twist into a particular shape: a coil or a pleated sheet. These forms are referred to as the *secondary structure* of polypeptides. For example, some proteins (e.g., hair) take the form of a *helix:* a shape like that of a coiled telephone cord. The helical shape is maintained by hydrogen bonds formed between different amino acid side chains at different locations in the polypeptide. Remember from chapter 2 that hydrogen bonds do not form molecules but result in the orientation of one part of a molecule to another part of a molecule. Other polypeptides form hydrogen bonds that cause them to make several flat folds that resemble a pleated skirt.

It is also possible for a single polypeptide to contain one or more coils and pleated sheets along its length. As a result, these different portions of the molecule can interact to form an even more complex three-dimensional structure. This occurs when the coils and pleated sheets twist and combine with each other. The complex three-dimensional structure formed in this manner is the polypeptide's *tertiary* (third degree) *structure.* A good example of tertiary structure can be seen when a coiled phone cord becomes so twisted that it folds around and back on itself in several places. The oxygen-holding protein found in muscle cells, myoglobin, displays tertiary structure: it is composed of a single (153 amino acids), helical molecule folded back and bonded to itself in several places.

Frequently, several different polypeptides, each with its own tertiary structure, twist around each other and chemically combine. The larger, three-dimensional

Box 4.3

Structure of Amino Acids

All of the individual amino acids drawn here have the amino group to the left, the carboxylic acid group to the right, and the side chain shaded in below. The side chain is usually symbolized as an "R-group." The various R-groups determine the particular amino acid and its activity. You do not need to memorize the structures of these different amino acids.

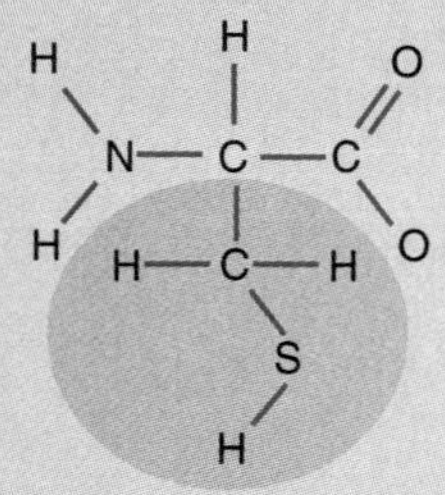

Cysteine

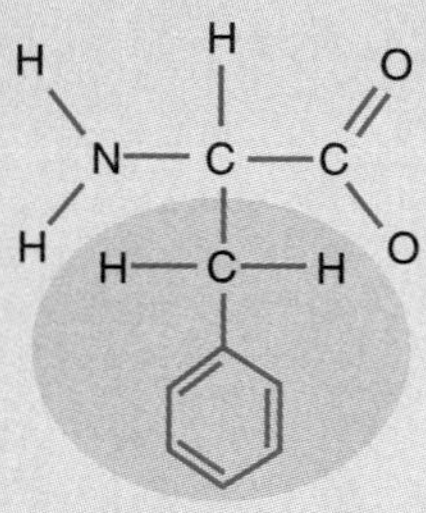

Phenylalanine

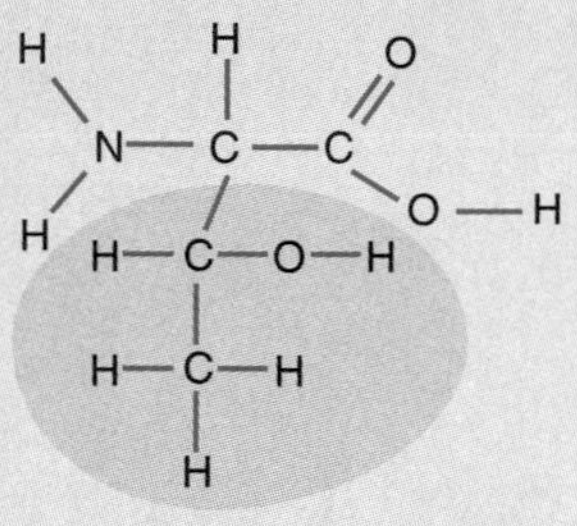

Threonine

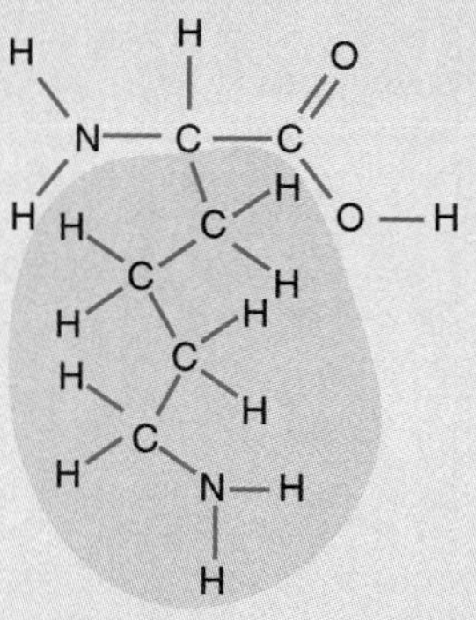

Lysine

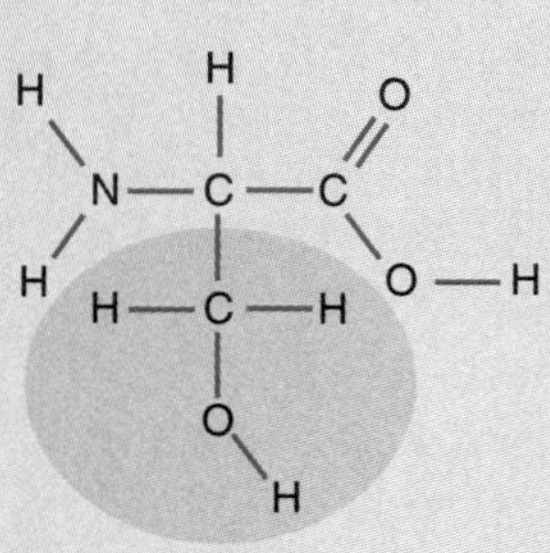

Serine

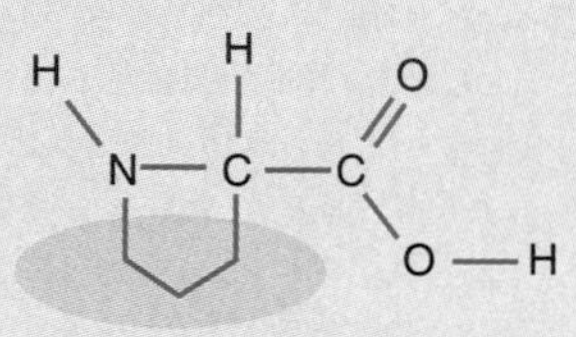

Proline

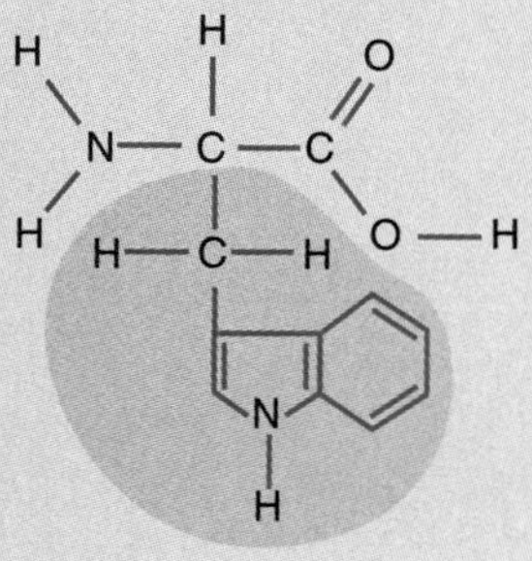

Tryptophan

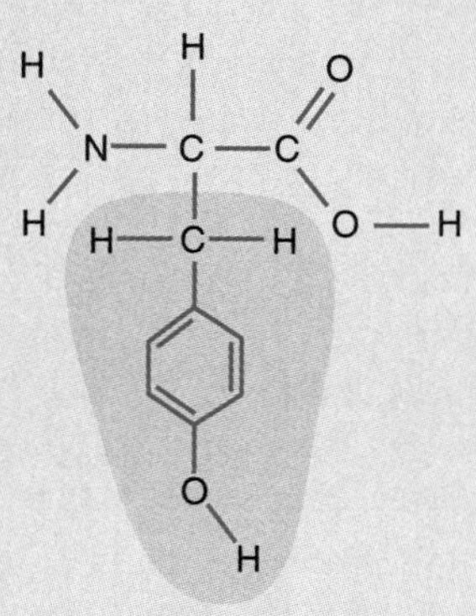

Tyrosine

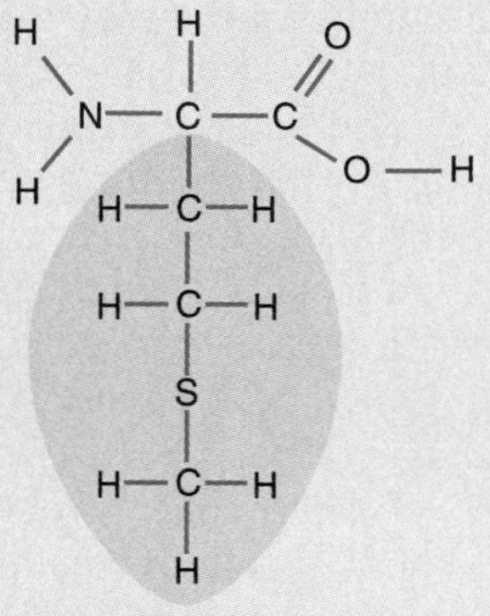

Methionine

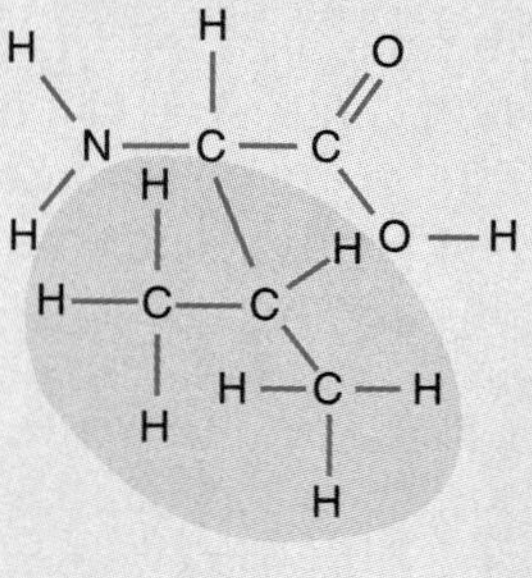

Valine

structure formed by these interacting polypeptides is referred to as the protein's *quaternary* (fourth degree) *structure*. The individual polypeptide chains are bonded to each other by the interactions of certain side chains, which can form disulfide bonds (figure 4.16). Quaternary structure is displayed by the protein molecules called *antibodies,* which are involved in fighting diseases such as mumps and chicken pox. The protein portion of the hemoglobin molecule (globin) also demonstrates quaternary structure.

Individual polypeptide chains or groups of chains forming a particular configuration are proteins. The structure of a protein is closely related to its function. We will consider two aspects of the structure of proteins: the sequence of amino acids within the protein and the overall three-dimensional shape of the molecule. Any changes in the arrangement of amino acids within a protein can have far-reaching

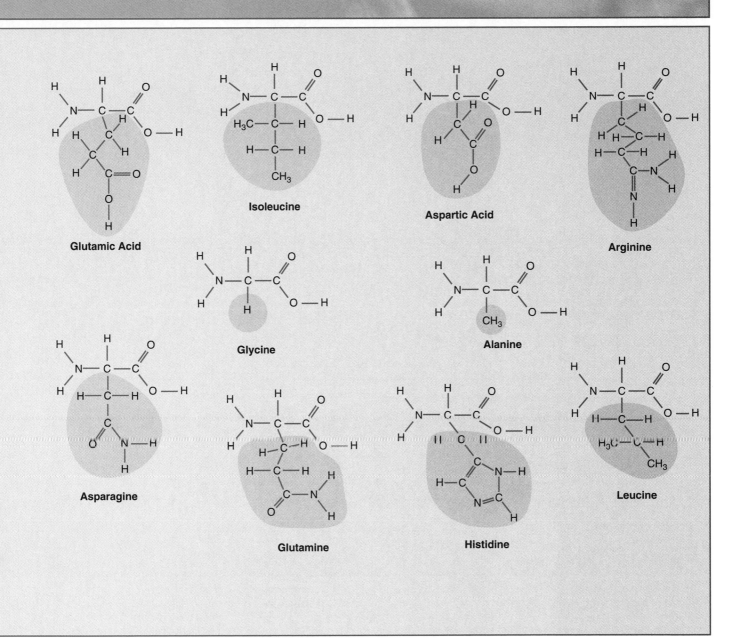

Glutamic Acid

Isoleucine

Aspartic Acid

Arginine

Glycine

Alanine

Asparagine

Glutamine

Histidine

Leucine

effects on its function. For example, normal hemoglobin found in red blood cells consists of two kinds of polypeptide chains called the alpha and beta chains. The beta chain is 146 amino acids long. If just one of these amino acids is replaced by a different one, the hemoglobin molecule may not function properly. A classic example of this results in a condition known as *sickle-cell anemia*. In this case, the sixth amino acid in the beta chain, which is normally glutamic acid, is replaced by valine. This minor change causes the hemoglobin to fold differently, and the red blood cells that contain this altered hemoglobin assume a sickle shape when the body is deprived of an adequate supply of oxygen.

When a particular sequence of amino acids forms a polypeptide, the stage is set for that particular arrangement to bond with another polypeptide in a certain way. Think of a telephone cord that has curled up and formed a helix (its secondary

Organic Chemistry—The Chemistry of Life   **63**

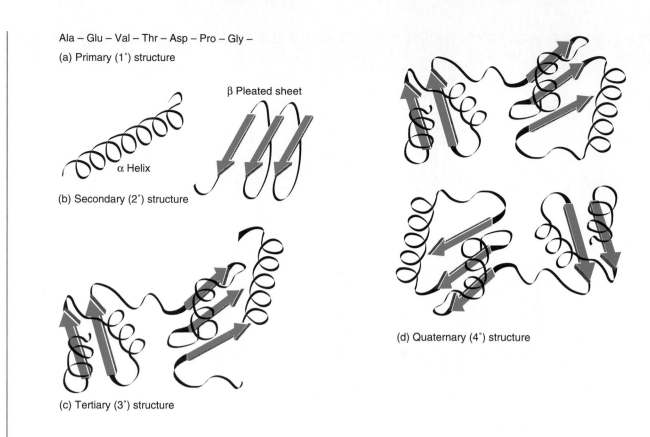

Ala – Glu – Val – Thr – Asp – Pro – Gly –

(a) Primary (1°) structure

β Pleated sheet

α Helix

(b) Secondary (2°) structure

(c) Tertiary (3°) structure

(d) Quaternary (4°) structure

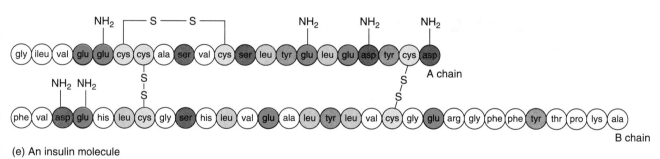

(e) An insulin molecule

FIGURE 4.16 Levels of protein structure and an insulin molecule.
(a) The primary (first degree) structure of a molecule is a list of its component amino acids in the order in which they occur. (b) This figure illustrates the secondary (second degree) structure of protein molecules or how the molecule may coil or fold. (c) Tertiary (third degree) structure is formed when molecules with folds and coils fold on themselves to make an even more complex structure. (d) Quaternary (fourth degree) structure is displayed when two separate molecules (each with their own tertiary structure) combine into one large macromolecule. (e) The protein insulin is composed of two polypeptide chains bonded together at specific points by reactions between the side chains of particular amino acids. The side chains of one interact with the side chains of the other and form a particular three-dimensional shape. The bonds that form between the polypeptide chains are called disulfide bonds.

structure). Now imagine that at several irregular intervals along that cord, you have attached magnets. You can see that the magnets at the various points along the cord will attract each other, and the curled cord will form a particular three-dimensional shape. You can more closely approximate the complex structure of a protein (its tertiary structure) if you imagine several curled cords, each with magnets attached at several points. Now imagine these magnets as bonding the individual cords together. The globs or ropes of telephone cords approximate the quaternary structure of a protein. This shape can be compared to the shape of a key. In order for a key to do its job effectively, it has to have particular bumps and grooves on its surface. Similarly, if a particular protein is to do its job effectively, it must have a particular shape. The protein's shape can be altered by changing the order of the amino acids

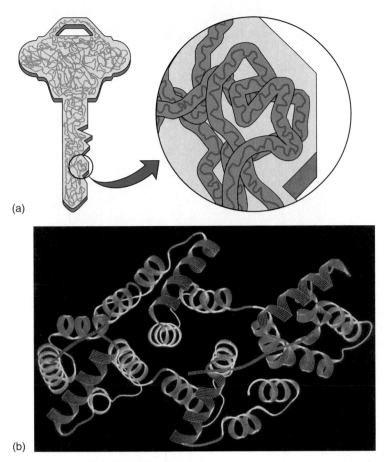

(a)

(b)

Figure 4.17 The three-dimensional shape of proteins.

(a) The specific arrangement of amino acids results in side chains that are available to bond with other side chains. The results are specific three-dimensional proteins that have a specific surface geometry. We frequently compare this three-dimensional shape to the three-dimensional shape of a specific key. (b) This is an x-ray diffraction of a protein called annexin. This molecule is located just inside cell membranes and is involved in the transport of materials through the membrane.

that cause different cross linkages to form. Changing environmental conditions also influences the shape of the protein. Figure 4.17 shows the importance of the three-dimensional shape of the protein. Energy in the form of heat or light may break the hydrogen bonds within protein molecules. When this occurs, the chemical and physical properties of the protein are changed and the protein is said to be **denatured.** A common example of this occurs when the gelatinous, clear portion of an egg is cooked and the protein changes to a white solid. Some medications are proteins and must be protected from denaturation so as not to lose their effectiveness. Insulin is an example. For protection, such medications may be stored in brown-colored bottles or kept under refrigeration.

The thousands of kinds of proteins can be placed into two categories. Some proteins are important for maintaining the shape of cells and organisms—they are usually referred to as **structural proteins.** The proteins that make up the cell membrane, muscle cells, tendons, and blood cells are examples of structural proteins. The other kinds of proteins, **regulator proteins,** help determine what activities will occur in the organism. These regulator proteins include enzymes and some hormones. These molecules help control the chemical activities of cells and organisms. Enzymes are important, and they are dealt with in detail in chapter 5. Some examples of enzymes are the digestive enzymes in the intestine and the mouth. Two hormones that are regulator proteins are insulin and oxytocin. Insulin is produced by the pancreas and

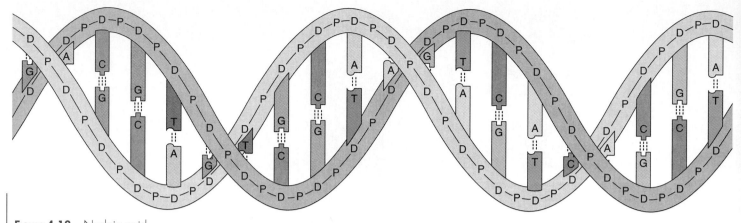

Figure 4.18 Nucleic acid.
Deoxyribonucleic acid (DNA) is an organic molecule composed of four nucleotides. Each nucleotide is composed of a sugar, deoxyribose (D); an inorganic acid, phosphoric acid (P); and one of four nitrogen-containing bases: adenine (A), cytosine (C), guanine (G), or thymine (T).

controls the amount of glucose in the blood. If insulin production is too low, or if the molecule is improperly constructed, glucose molecules are not removed from the bloodstream at a fast enough rate. The excess sugar is then eliminated in the urine. Other symptoms of excess sugar in the blood include excessive thirst, and even loss of consciousness. The disease caused by improperly functioning insulin is known as *diabetes.* Oxytocin, a second protein-type hormone, stimulates the contraction of the uterus during childbirth. It is also an example of an organic molecule that has been produced artificially and is used by physicians to induce labor.

Nucleic Acids

The last group of organic molecules that we will consider are the *nucleic acids.* **Nucleic acids** are complex molecules that store and transfer information within a cell. They are constructed of fundamental monomers known as **nucleotides.** Each nucleic acid is a polymer composed of nucleotides bonded together. There are eight different nucleotides, but each is constructed of a phosphate group, a sugar, and an organic nitrogenous base.

The two kinds of sugar that can be part of the nucleotide are ribose and deoxyribose. These are five-carbon simple sugars. The phosphate group is attached to the sugar and the nitrogenous base is attached to another part of the sugar. There are five common organic molecules containing nitrogen that are likely to be part of the nucleotide structure. The nitrogen-containing bases are adenine, guanine, cytosine, thymine, and uracil.

The nucleotides can then connect to form long chains by dehydration synthesis reactions. The long chains of nucleotides are of two types—RNA, ribonucleic acid, and DNA, deoxyribonucleic acid. The RNA forms a single polymer, whereas the DNA is generally composed of two matching polymers twisted together and held by hydrogen bonds (figure 4.18). These two types of molecules contain the information needed for the formation of particular sequences of amino acids; they determine what kinds of proteins an organism can manufacture. The mechanism of storing and using this information is the topic of chapter 8. Nucleotides are also components of molecules used to transfer chemical-bond energy. One, ATP and its role in metabolism, will be discussed in chapter 7.

Table 4.1 A Summary of the Types of Organic Molecules Found in Living Things

TYPE OF ORGANIC MOLECULE	BASIC SUBUNIT	FUNCTION	EXAMPLES
Carbohydrates	Simple sugar	Provide energy Provide support	Glucose Cellulose
Lipids			
1. Fats	Glycerol and fatty acids	Provide energy Provide insulation Serve as shock absorber	Lard Olive oil Linseed oil Tallow
2. Steroids	A complex ring structure	Often serve as hormones that control the body processes	Testosterone Vitamin D Cholesterol
3. Phospholipids	Glycerol, fatty acids, and phosphorus compounds	Form a major component of the structure of the cell membrane	Cell membrane
Proteins	Amino acid	Maintain the shape of cells and parts of organisms	Cell membrane Hair Muscle
		As enzymes, regulate the rates of cell reactions	Ptyalin in the mouth
		As hormones, effect physiological activity, such as growth or metabolism	Insulin
Nucleic acids	Nucleotide	Store and transfer genetic information that controls the cell	DNA RNA

SUMMARY

The chemistry of living things involves a variety of large and complex molecules. This chemistry is based on the carbon atom and the fact that carbon atoms can connect to form long chains or rings. This results in a vast array of molecules. The structure of each molecule is related to its function. Changes in the structure may result in abnormal functions, which we call disease. Some of the most common types of organic molecules found in living things are carbohydrates, lipids, proteins, and nucleic acids. Table 4.1 summarizes the major types of biologically important organic molecules and their roles in living things.

QUESTIONS

1. Diagram an example of each of the following: amino acid, simple sugar, glycerol, and fatty acid.
2. Give an example of each of the following classes of organic molecules: carbohydrate, protein, lipid, and nucleic acids.
3. What is the structural difference between a saturated fat and an unsaturated fat?
4. Describe three different kinds of lipids.
5. What are the differences among the primary, secondary, tertiary, and quaternary structures of proteins?
6. What two characteristics of the carbon atom make it unique?
7. What is the difference between inorganic and organic molecules?
8. What is meant by HDL, LDL, VLDL, and chylomicron? Where are they found? What relationship do they have to disease?
9. Describe five functional groups.
10. List three monomers and the polymers that can be constructed from them.

CHAPTER GLOSSARY

amino acid (ah-mēn'o ǎ'sid) A short carbon skeleton that contains an amino group, a carboxylic acid group, and one of various side groups.

biochemistry (bi-o-kem'iss-tre) The chemistry of living things, often called biological chemistry.

carbohydrate (kar-bo-hi'drāt) One class of organic molecules composed of carbon, hydrogen, and oxygen in a ratio of 1:2:1 in most monosaccharides. The basic building block of a carbohydrate is a simple sugar (= monosaccharide).

carbon skeleton (kar'bon skel'uh-ton) Central portion of an organic molecule composed of rings or chains of carbon atoms.

complex carbohydrates (kom'pleks kar-bo-hi'drāts) Macromolecules composed of simple sugars combined by dehydration synthesis to form a polymer.

dehydration synthesis reaction (de-hi-dra'shun sin'thuh-sis re-ak'shun) A reaction that results in the formation of a macromolecule when water is removed from between the two smaller component parts.

denature (de-na'chur) Irreversible change of the chemical and physical properties of a protein.

double bond (dubl bond) A pair of covalent bonds between two atoms formed when they share two pairs of electrons.

empirical formula (em-pēr'ĭ-kal for'miu-lah) Chemical shorthand that indicates the number of each kind of atom within a molecule.

fat (fat) A class of water-insoluble macromolecules composed of a glycerol and three fatty acids.

fatty acid (fat-te ǎ'sid) One of the building blocks of a fat, composed of a long-chain carbon skeleton with a carboxylic acid functional group.

functional groups (fung'shun-al grūps) Specific combinations of atoms attached to the carbon skeleton that determine specific chemical properties.

glycerol (glis'er-ol) One of the building blocks of a fat, composed of a carbon skeleton that has three alcohol groups (OH) attached to it.

hydrolysis (hi-drol'ĭ-sis) A process that occurs when a large molecule is broken down into smaller parts by the addition of water.

inorganic molecules (in-or-gan'ik mol'uh-kiuls) Molecules that do not contain carbon atoms in rings or chains.

isomers (i'so-meers) Molecules that have the same empirical formula but different structural formulas.

lipids (lĭ'pids) Large organic molecules that do not easily dissolve in water; classes include fats, phospholipids, and steroids.

nucleic acids (nu'kle-ik ǎ'sids) Complex molecules that store and transfer information within a cell. They are constructed of fundamental monomers known as nucleotides.

nucleotide (nu"kle-o-tīd') A fundamental subunit of nucleic acid constructed of a phosphate group, a sugar, and an organic nitrogenous base.

organic molecules (or-gan'ik mol'uh-kiuls) Complex molecules whose basic building blocks are carbon atoms in chains or rings.

peptide bond (pep'tīd bond) A covalent bond between amino acids in a protein.

phospholipid (fos"fo-lĭ'pid) A class of water-insoluble molecules that resemble fats but contain a phosphate group (PO_4) in their structure.

polypeptide chain (pŏ"le-pep'tīd chān) A macromolecule composed of a specific sequence of amino acids.

protein (pro'te-in) Macromolecules made up of one or more polypeptides attached to each other by bonds.

regulator proteins (reg'yu-la-tor pro'te-ins) Proteins that influence the activities that occur in an organism—for example, enzymes and some hormones.

saturated (sat'yu-ra-ted) Carbon skeleton of a fatty acid that contains no double bonds between carbons.

steroid (stēr'oid) One of the three kinds of lipid molecules characterized by their arrangement of interlocking rings of carbon.

structural formula (struk'chu-ral for'miu-lah) An illustration that shows the arrangement of the atoms and their bonding within a molecule.

structural proteins (struk'chu-ral pro'te-ins) Proteins that are important for holding cells and organisms together, such as the proteins that make up the cell membrane, muscles, tendons, and blood.

triglyceride (tri-glis'er-ide) A form of lipid composed of a glycerol molecule that has three attached fatty acids.

unsaturated (un-sat'yu-ra-ted) A carbon skeleton of a fatty acid containing carbons that are double-bonded to each other at one or more points.

 THE DYNAMIC HUMAN   Correlations to Chapter Four:

Cardiovascular System → Clinical Concepts → Myocardial Infarction

Endocrine System → Clinical Concepts → Diabetes

Immune and Lymphatic Systems → Clinical Concepts → Vaccinations

Respiratory System → Exploration → Oxygen Transport

Cell Structure and Function

CHAPTER OUTLINE

PURPOSE

The cell is the simplest structure capable of existing as an individual living unit. Within this unit, certain chemical reactions are required for maintaining life. These reactions do not occur at random, but are associated with specific parts of the many kinds of cells. This chapter deals with certain cellular structures found within most types of cells and discusses their functions.

CLINICAL VIEWPOINT

The cells in the human immune system respond to the presence of foreign proteins (antigens) found on organisms such as parasites, viruses, fungi, and bacteria. It has generally been thought that only the presence of antigens would trigger growth and changes in the cells of the immune system. When so stimulated by an antigen, the T-cells in the immune system produce new cells. The growth of these new T-cells destroys the antigens in the body.

Immunologists have discovered a hormone, interleukin-2 (Il-2), that allows for communication between the individual cells of the immune system. (It has been demonstrated that cells in the immune system produce antigens and interleukin-2.) This hormone stimulates the rapid growth of cells in the immune system. Since this rapid proliferation of cells in the immune system increases the number of cells, there is an increased production of antibodies, which more rapidly eliminates the invading organism.

Interleukin-2 can be injected into the body, causing an increase in production of T-cells. When this is done in conjunction with a vaccination, it increases the effectiveness of the vaccination. Interleukin-2 has also been shown to be a form of immunotherapy in the treating of certain types of cancer.

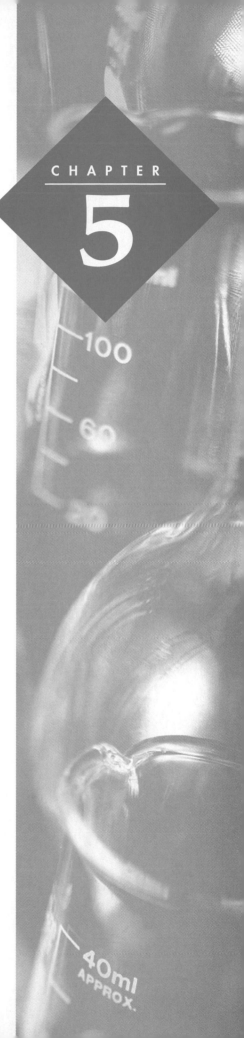

- Recognize the historical perspective of the development of the cell theory
- Describe the molecular structure of a membrane and relate this structure to the process whereby a cell accumulates and releases materials
- Describe the processes whereby a cell accumulates some materials and releases others to the environment, and the conditions controlling these various processes
- Identify the cytoplasmic organelles in most eukaryotic cells
- Associate the organelle structure with its major function in eukaryotic cells
- Identify the nuclear components of a cell and associate the functions with the nuclear structures

THE CELL THEORY

 The concept of a cell is one of the most important ideas in biology because it applies to all living things. It did not emerge all at once, but has been developed and modified over many years. It is still being modified today.

Several individuals made key contributions to the cell concept. Anton van Leeuwenhoek (1632–1723) was one of the first to make use of a **microscope** to examine biological specimens (box 5.1). When van Leeuwenhoek discovered that he could see things moving in pond water using his microscope, his curiosity stimulated him to look at a variety of other things. He studied blood, semen, feces, pepper, and tartar, for example. He was the first to see individual cells and recognize them as living units, but he did not call them cells. The name he gave to these "little animals" that he saw moving around in the pond water was *animalcules.*

The first person to use the term *cell* was Robert Hooke (1635–1703) of England, who was also interested in how things looked when magnified. He chose to study thin slices of cork, the tissue from the bark of a cork oak tree. He saw a mass of cubicles fitting neatly together, which reminded him of the barren rooms in a monastery. Hence, he called them by the same name, *cells.* As it is currently used, the term **cell** refers to the basic structural unit that makes up all living things. When Hooke looked at cork, the tiny boxes he saw were, in fact, only the cell walls that surrounded the living portions of plant cells. We now know that plant cell walls are composed of the complex carbohydrate cellulose, which provides strength and protection to the living contents of the cell. The cell wall appears to be a rigid, solid layer of material, but in reality it is composed of many interwoven strands of cellulose molecules. Its structure allows certain very large molecules to pass through it readily, but it acts as a screen to other molecules.

Hooke's use of the term *cell* in 1666 in his publication *Micrographia* was only the beginning, for it took nearly two hundred years before it was generally recognized that all living things were made of cells and that these cells could reproduce themselves. In 1838, Mathias Jakob Schleiden stated that all plants were made up of smaller cellular units. In 1839, Theodor Schwann published the idea that all animals were composed of cells.

Soon after the term cell caught on, it was recognized that its vitally important portion was inside the cell wall. This living material was termed **protoplasm,** which means *first-formed substance.* The use of the term *protoplasm* allowed the living portion of the cell to be distinguished from the nonliving cell wall. Very soon microscopists were able to distinguish two different regions of protoplasm. One type of protoplasm was more viscous and darker than the other. This region, called the **nucleus,** or core, appeared as a central body within the more fluid material surrounding it. **Cytoplasm** (*cyto* = cell, *plasm* = first-formed substance) is the name given to the more fluid portion of the protoplasm (figure 5.1). While the term protoplasm is seldom used today, the term cytoplasm is very common in the vocabulary of cell biologists.

The development of better light microscopes and, ultimately the electron microscope, revealed that protoplasm contains many structures called **organelles**

Box 5.1   The Microscope

In order to view very small objects we use a magnifying glass as a way of extending observational powers. A magnifying glass is a lens that bends light in such a way that the object appears larger than it really is. Such a lens might magnify objects ten or even fifty times. Anton van Leeuwenhoek (1632–1723), a Dutch drape and clothing maker, was one of the first individuals to carefully study magnified cells. He made very detailed sketches of the things he viewed with his simple microscopes and communicated his findings to Robert Hooke and the Royal Society of London. His work stimulated further investigation of magnification techniques and description of cell structure. These first microscopes were developed in the early 1600s.

Compound microscopes, developed soon after the simple microscopes, are able to increase magnification by bending light through a series of lenses. One lens, the *objective lens*, magnifies a specimen that is further magnified by the second lens, known as the *ocular lens*. With the modern technology of producing lenses, the use of specific light waves, and the immersion of the objective lens in oil to collect more of the available light, objects can be magnified one hundred to fifteen hundred times. Microscopes typically available for student use are compound light microscopes.

The major restriction of magnification with a light microscope is the ability of the viewer to distinguish two very close objects as two distinct things. The ability to separate two objects is termed *resolution* or *resolving power*. Some people have extremely good eyesight and are able to look at letters on a page and recognize that they are separate objects, while other persons see the individual letters as being "blurred together." Their eyes have different resolving powers. We can enhance the resolving power of the human eye by using lenses as in eyeglasses or microscopes. All lens systems, whether in the eye or in microscopes, have a limited resolving power.

If two structures in a cell are very close to each other, you may not be able to distinguish that there are actually two structures rather than one. The limits of resolution of a light microscope are related to the wavelengths of the light being transmitted through the specimen. If you could see ultraviolet light waves, which have shorter wavelengths, it would be possible to resolve more individual structures.

An electron microscope makes use of this principle: the moving electrons have much shorter wavelengths than visible light. Thus, they are able to magnify 200,000 times and still resolve individual structures. The difficulty is, of course, that you are unable to see electrons with your eyes. Therefore, in order to use the electron microscope, the electrons strike a photographic film or television monitor, and this "picture" shows the individual structures. Heavy metals scattered on the structures to be viewed with the electron microscope increase the contrast between areas where there are structures that interfere with the transmission of the electrons and areas where the electrons are transmitted easily. The techniques for preparing the material to be viewed—slicing the specimen very thinly and focusing the electron beam on the specimen—make electron microscopy an art as well as a science.

(*elle* = little). It has been determined that these organelles perform particular functions in each cell. The job that an organelle does is related to its structure. Each organelle is dynamic in its operation, changing shape and size as it works. Organelles move throughout the cell, and some even self-duplicate.

To date, most biologists recognize two major cell types, *prokaryotes* and *eukaryotes*. **Prokaryotic cells** are structurally more simple since they do not have as great a variety of organelles in comparison to eukaryotes. Most single-celled organisms we commonly refer to as bacteria are prokaryotic cells. Other bacteria display significantly different traits that have caused biologists to believe that they are more ancient than prokaryotes. This has resulted in some biologists creating a new category for this cell type, the *archaebacteria*. All other living things are based on the **eukaryotic cell** plan. Members of the kingdoms Protista, Mycetae, Plantae, and Animalia are all comprised of eukaryotic cells.

CELL MEMBRANES

One feature common to all cells, and many of the organelles they contain, is a thin layer of material called *membrane*. Membrane can be folded, molded, and twisted into many different structures, shapes, and forms. The particular arrangement of membrane within an organelle is related to the functions it is capable of performing. This is similar to the way a piece of fabric can be fashioned into a pair of pants, a shirt, sheets, pillowcases, or a rag doll. All cellular membranes have a fundamental molecular structure that allows them to be fashioned into a variety of different organelles, each with a very specific function.

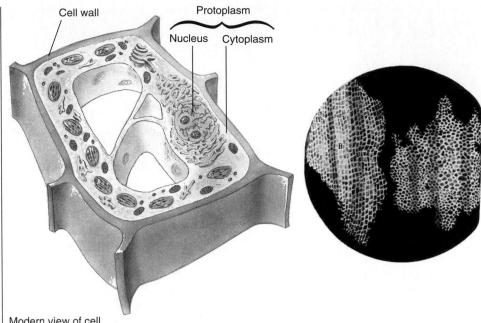

Cell wall

Protoplasm

Nucleus   Cytoplasm

Modern view of cell

FIGURE 5.1 Cells—basic structure of life.
The cell concept has changed considerably over the last 300 years. Robert Hooke's idea of a cell was based on his observation of slices of cork. One of the first subcellular differentiations was to divide the protoplasm into cytoplasm and nucleus. We know now that cells are composed of many kinds of subcellular particles.

Cellular membranes are thin sheets composed primarily of phospholipids and proteins. The current hypothesis of how membranes are constructed is known as the **fluid-mosaic model,** which proposes that the various molecules in the membrane are able to flow and move about, but that the membrane maintains its form because of the physical interaction of its molecules with surrounding water molecules. The phospholipid molecules of the membrane have one end (the glycerol portion) that is soluble in water and is therefore called **hydrophilic** (water-loving). The other end that is not water soluble, called **hydrophobic** (water-hating), is comprised of fatty acid. We commonly represent this molecule like a balloon with two strings. The inflated balloon represents the glycerol and phosphate, while the strings represent the two fatty acids. Consequently, when phospholipid molecules are placed in water, they form a double-layered sheet, with the water-soluble (hydrophilic) portions of the molecules facing away from each other. This is commonly referred to as a phospholipid bilayer. If phospholipid molecules are shaken in a glass of water, the molecules will automatically form double-layered membranes. It is important to understand that the membrane formed is not rigid or stiff but resembles a heavy olive oil in consistency. The component phospholipids are in constant motion as they move with the surrounding water molecules and slide past one another.

The protein component of cellular membranes can be found on either surface of the membrane or in the membrane, among the phospholipid molecules. Many of the protein molecules are capable of moving from one side to the other. These proteins can help with the chemical activities of the protoplasm. Still others aid in the movement of molecules across the membrane by forming channels through which substances may travel or by acting as transport molecules (figure 5.2). In addition to phospholipids and proteins, some protein molecules found on the outside surfaces of cellular membranes have carbohydrates or fats attached to them. These combination molecules are important in determining the "sidedness"

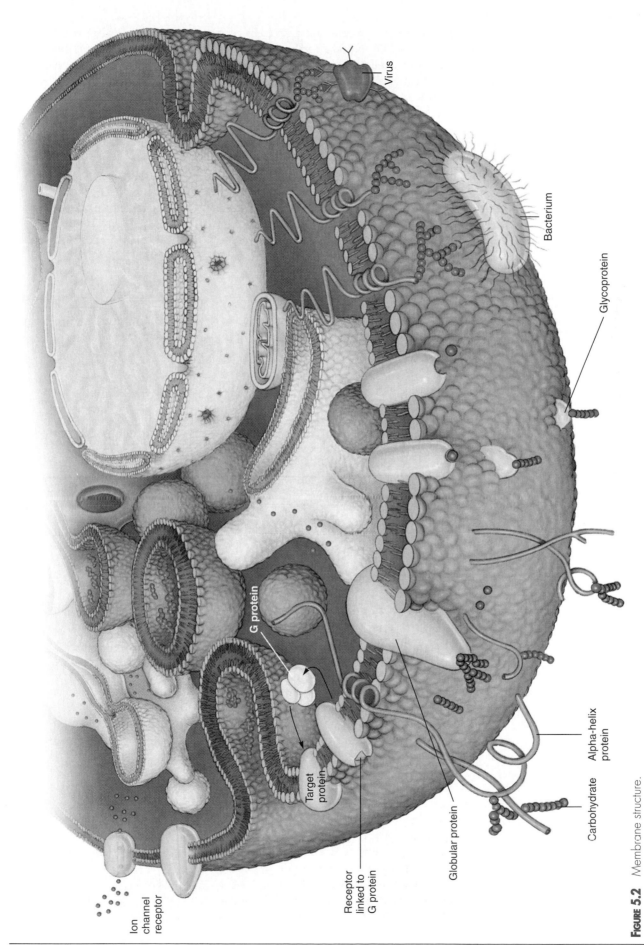

FIGURE 5.2 *Membrane structure.*

Membranes in cells are composed of protein and phospholipids. Two layers of phospholipid are oriented so that the hydrophobic fatty ends extend toward each other and the hydrophilic glycerol portions are on the outside. The phosphate-containing chain of the phospholipid is coiled near the glycerol portion. Buried within the phospholipid layer and/or floating on it are the globular proteins. Some of these proteins accumulate materials from outside the cell; others act as sites of chemical activity. Carbohydrates are often attached to one surface of the membrane.

Virus

Bacterium

Glycoprotein

Alpha-helix protein

Carbohydrate

Globular protein

G protein

Target protein

Receptor linked to G protein

Ion channel receptor

(inside-outside) of the membrane and also help organisms recognize differences between types of cells. Your body can recognize disease-causing organisms because their surface proteins are different from those of its own cellular membranes. Some of these molecules also serve as attachment sites for specific chemicals, bacteria, protozoa, white blood cells, and viruses. Many dangerous agents that cannot stick to the surface of a cell cannot cause harm. It is for this reason that cell biologists explore the exact structure and function of these molecules. They are also attempting to identify molecules that can interfere with the binding of such agents as viruses and bacteria in the hope of controlling infections.

Other molecules that are found in cell membranes are cholesterol and carbohydrates. Cholesterol is found in the middle of the membrane, in the hydrophobic region, because cholesterol is not water-soluble. It appears to play a role in stabilizing the membrane and keeping it flexible. Carbohydrates are usually found on the outside of the membrane, where they are bound to proteins or lipids. They appear to play a role in cell-to-cell interactions and are involved in binding with regulatory molecules.

GETTING THROUGH MEMBRANES

If a cell is to stay alive, it must meet the characteristics of life outlined in chapter 1. This includes taking nutrients in, and eliminating wastes and other by-products of metabolism. There are several mechanisms that allow cells to carry out the processes characteristic of life including *diffusion, osmosis, dialysis, facilitated diffusion, active transport,* and *phagocytosis.*

Diffusion

There is a natural tendency in gases and liquids for molecules of different types to completely mix with each other. This is because they are moving constantly. Their movement is random and is due to the kinetic energy found in the individual molecules. Consider two types of molecules. As the molecules of one type move about, they tend to scatter from a central location. The other type of molecule also tends to disperse. The result of this random motion is that the two types of molecules are eventually mixed with each other. Remember that the motion of the molecules is completely random. They do not move because of conscious thought— they move because of their kinetic energy. If you follow the paths of molecules from a sugar cube placed in a glass of water, you would find that some of the sugar molecules would move away from the cube, while others would move in the opposite direction. (Recall that when discussing a solution, the material in which you dissolve a substance is called the *solvent.* The material being dissolved is called the *solute.*) However, there would be more sugar molecules moving away from the original cube because there were more to start with. We generally are not interested in the individual movement, but rather the overall movement. This overall movement is termed **net movement.** It is the movement in one direction minus the movement in the opposite direction. The direction of greatest movement (net movement) is determined by the relative concentration of the molecules. **Diffusion** is the resultant movement; it is defined as the net movement of a kind of molecule from a place where that molecule is in higher concentration to a place where that molecule is more scarce. When a kind of molecule is completely dispersed, and movement is equal in all directions, we say that the system has reached a state of **dynamic equilibrium.** There is no longer a net movement because movement in one direction equals movement in the other. It is dynamic, however, because the system still has energy, and the molecules are still moving.

Because the cell membrane is composed of phospholipid and protein molecules that are in constant motion, temporary openings are formed that allow small molecules to cross from one side of the membrane to the other. Molecules close to the membrane are in constant motion as well. They are able to move into and out of a cell by passing through these openings in the membrane.

FIGURE 5.3 The concentration gradient.
Gradual changes in concentrations of molecules over distance are called concentration gradients. This bar shows a color gradient with full color at one end and no color at the other end. A concentration gradient is necessary for diffusion to occur. Diffusion results in net movement of molecules from an area of higher concentration to an area of lower concentration.

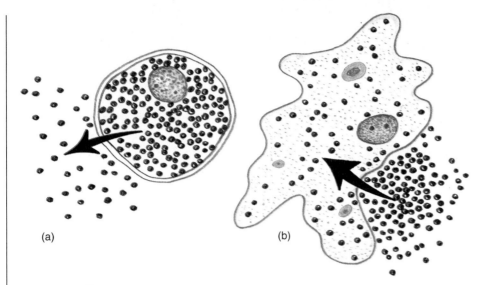

(a)   (b)

FIGURE 5.4 Diffusion.
As a result of molecular motion, molecules move from areas where they are concentrated to areas where they are less concentrated. This figure shows (a) molecules leaving a cell by diffusion and (b) molecules entering a cell by diffusion. The direction is controlled by concentration, and the energy necessary is supplied by the kinetic energy of the molecules themselves.

The rate of diffusion is related to the kinetic energy and size of the molecules. Since diffusion only occurs when molecules are unevenly distributed, the relative concentration of the molecules is important in determining how fast diffusion occurs. The difference in concentration of the molecules is known as a **concentration gradient** or **diffusion gradient.** When the molecules are equally distributed, no such gradient exists (figure 5.3).

Diffusion can take place only as long as there are no barriers to the free movement of molecules. In the case of a cell, the membrane permits some molecules to pass through, while others are not allowed to pass or only allowed to pass more slowly. *This permeability is based on size, ionic charge, and solubility of the molecules involved.* The membrane does not, however, distinguish direction of movement of molecules; therefore, the membrane does not influence the direction of diffusion. The direction of diffusion is determined by the relative concentration of specific molecules on the two sides of the membrane, and the energy that causes diffusion to occur is supplied by the kinetic energy of the molecules themselves (figure 5.4).

Diffusion is an important means by which materials are exchanged between a cell and its environment. Since the movement of the molecules is random, the cell has little control over the process; thus, diffusion is considered a passive process; i.e., chemical bond energy does not have to be expended. For example, animals are constantly using oxygen in various chemical reactions. Consequently,

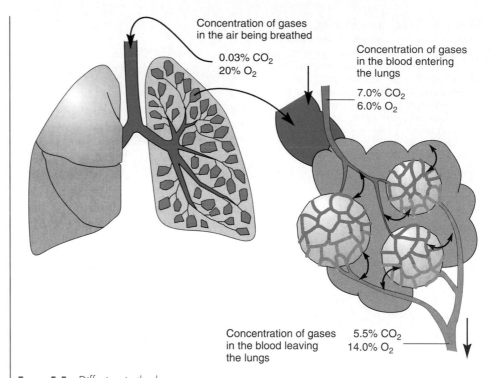

Concentration of gases
in the air being breathed

0.03% CO_2
20% O_2

Concentration of gases
in the blood entering
the lungs

7.0% CO_2
6.0% O_2

Concentration of gases
in the blood leaving
the lungs

5.5% CO_2
14.0% O_2

FIGURE 5.5 Diffusion in the lungs.
As blood enters the lungs, it has a higher concentration of carbon dioxide and a lower concentration
of oxygen than the air in the lungs. The concentration gradient of oxygen is such that the oxygen
diffuses from the lungs into the blood, and the concentration gradient of the carbon dioxide is such
that it diffuses from the blood into the lungs. These two different diffusions happen simultaneously,
and the direction of diffusion is controlled by the relative concentrations of each kind of molecule in
the blood and in the lungs.

the oxygen concentration in cells always remains low. The cells then contain a
lower concentration of oxygen in comparison to the oxygen level outside of the
cell. This creates a diffusion gradient, and the oxygen molecules diffuse from the
outside of the cell to the inside of the cell.

In humans, many of the cells are buried deep within the body; if it were not
for their circulatory systems, there would be little opportunity for cells to exchange gases directly with their surroundings. The circulatory system is a
transportation system within a body composed of blood vessels of various
sizes. These vessels carry many different molecules from one place to another.
Oxygen may diffuse into blood through the membranes of the lungs or other
moist surfaces of a human's body. The circulatory system then transports the
oxygen-rich blood throughout the body. The oxygen automatically diffuses
into cells that are low in oxygen. The opposite is true of carbon dioxide. Human
cells constantly produce carbon dioxide, and so there is always a high concentration of it within the cells. These molecules diffuse from the cells into the
blood, where the concentration of carbon dioxide is lower. The blood is
pumped to the moist surfaces (lungs, oral cavity, etc.), and the carbon dioxide
again diffuses into the surrounding environment, which has a lower concentration of this gas. In a similar manner, many other types of molecules constantly
enter and leave cells (figure 5.5).

Dialysis and Osmosis

Another characteristic of all membranes is that they are **selectively permeable.** Selective permeability means that a membrane will allow certain molecules to pass across it and will prevent others from doing so. Molecules that are able to dissolve in phospholipids, such as vitamins A and D, can pass through the membrane rather easily; however, many molecules cannot pass through at all. In certain cases, the membrane differentiates (selects) on the basis of molecular size; that is, the membrane allows small molecules, such as water, to pass through and prevents the passage of larger molecules. The membrane may also regulate the passage of ions. If a particular portion of the membrane has a large number of positive ions on its surface, positively charged ions in the environment will be repelled and prevented from crossing the membrane.

We make use of diffusion across a selectively permeable membrane when we use a dialysis machine to remove wastes from the blood. If a kidney is unable to function normally, blood from a patient is diverted to a series of tubes composed of selectively permeable membrane. The toxins that have concentrated in the blood diffuse into the surrounding fluids in the dialysis machine, and the cleansed blood is returned to the patient. Thus, the machine functions in place of the kidney.

Water is a molecule that easily diffuses through cell membranes. The net movement (diffusion) of water molecules through a selectively permeable membrane is known as **osmosis.** In any osmotic situation, there must be a selectively permeable membrane separating two solutions. For example, a solution of 90% water and 10% sugar separated by a selectively permeable membrane from a different sugar solution, such as one of 80% water and 20% sugar, demonstrates osmosis. The membrane allows water molecules to pass freely but prevents the larger sugar molecules from crossing. There is a higher concentration of water molecules in one solution (compared to the concentration of water molecules in the other), so more of the water molecules move from the solution with 90% water to the other solution with 80% water. Be sure that you recognize that osmosis is really diffusion in which the diffusing substance is water (the solvent), and that the regions of different concentrations are separated by a membrane that is more permeable to water.

A proper amount of water is required if a cell is to function efficiently. Too much water in a cell may dilute the cell contents and interfere with the chemical reactions necessary to keep the cell alive. Too little water in the cell may result in a buildup of poisonous waste products. As with the diffusion of other molecules, osmosis is a passive process because the cell has no control over the diffusion of water molecules. This means that the cell can remain in balance with an environment only if that environment does not cause the cell to lose or gain too much water.

If a cell contains a concentration of water and dissolved materials that is equal to that of its surroundings, the cell is said to be **isotonic** to its surroundings. Cells within the human body must have a concentration of water and dissolved materials within the cells that is equal to the concentration outside the cells. For example, blood plasma is 91.5% water and 8.5% dissolved materials. Red blood cells are isotonic when they have the same percentage of water and dissolved materials as the plasma. Many products are isotonic. For example, over-the-counter eyewashes are labeled *isotonic,* as are many medically important solutions. *Physiological saline* solution is isotonic, as are other intravenous (IV) solutions (0.9% dissolved salts).

However, if cells or tissues are going to survive in an environment that has a different concentration of water, they must expend energy to maintain this difference. Red blood cells having a lower concentration of water (higher concentration of dissolved materials, solutes) than their surroundings tend to gain water by osmosis very rapidly. They are said to be **hypertonic** to their surroundings

Table 5.1 The Effects of Osmosis on Different Cell Types

CELL TYPE	WHAT HAPPENS WHEN CELL IS PLACED IN HYPOTONIC SOLUTION	WHAT HAPPENS WHEN CELL IS PLACED IN HYPERTONIC SOLUTION
With cell wall; ex., bacteria, fungi	Swells; does not burst due to presence of protective cell wall. Cells will become *swollen* (*turgid*) under these conditions.	Shrinks; cell membrane pulls away from inside of cell wall and forms compressed mass of protoplasm, a process known as *plasmolysis*. Cells will shrink under these conditions. Placing cells in salt water causes certain types of bacterial cells to tear their cell membranes away from the cell wall and results in their death.
Without cell wall; ex., human	Swells and may burst, a process called *hemolysis*. Red blood cells will *hemolyze* under these conditions.	Shrinks into compact mass, a process known as *crenation*.

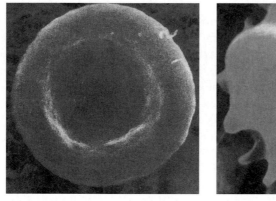
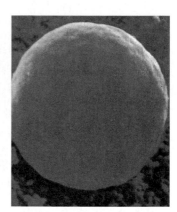

(a) Isotonic   (b) Cell in hypertonic solution   (c) Cell in hypotonic solution

Figure 5.6 Osmotic influences on cells.
The cells in these three photographs were subjected to three different environments. (a) The cell is isotonic to its surroundings. The water concentration inside the red blood cell and the water concentration in the environment are in balance with each other, so movement of water into the cell equals movement of water out of the cell, and the cell has its normal shape. (b) The cell is in a hypertonic solution. Water has diffused from the cell to the environment because a higher concentration of water was in the cell, and the cell has shrunk. (c) A cell has accumulated water from the environment because a higher concentration of water was outside the cell than in its protoplasm. The cell is in a hypotonic solution so it has swollen.

and the surroundings are **hypotonic.** These two terms are always used to compare two different solutions. The hypertonic solution is the one with more solutes (dissolved material) and less solvent (water); the hypotonic solution has less solutes (dissolved material) and more solvent (water). It may help to remember that the water goes where the salt is (table 5.1).

Organisms whose cells gain water by osmosis must expend energy to eliminate any excess if they are to keep from swelling and bursting (figure 5.6).

Under normal conditions, when we drink small amounts of water the cells of the brain will swell a little, and signals are sent to the kidneys to rid the body of excess water. By contrast, marathon runners may drink large quantities of water in a very short time following a race. This rapid addition of water to the body may cause abnormal swelling of brain cells because the excess water cannot be gotten rid of rapidly enough. If this happens, the person may lose consciousness, or even die, because the brain cells have swollen too much.

So far, we have considered only those situations in which the cell has no control over the movement of molecules. Cells cannot rely solely on diffusion and osmosis, because many of the molecules they require either cannot pass through the membrane or occur in relatively low concentrations in the cell's surroundings.

Controlled Methods of Transporting Molecules

Some molecules move across the membrane by combining with specific carrier proteins. When the rate of diffusion of a substance is increased in the presence of a carrier, we call this **facilitated diffusion.** Since this is diffusion, the net direction of movement is in accordance with the concentration gradient. Therefore, this is considered a passive transport method, although it can only occur in living organisms with the necessary carrier proteins. One example of facilitated diffusion is the movement of glucose molecules across the membranes of certain cells. In order for the glucose molecules to pass into these cells, specific proteins are required to carry them across the membrane. The action of the carrier does not require an input of energy other than the kinetic energy of the molecules (figure 5.7).

When molecules are moved across the membrane from an area of *low* concentration to an area of *high* concentration, the cell must be expending energy. The process of using a carrier protein to move molecules up a concentration gradient is called **active transport** (figure 5.8). Active transport is very specific: only certain molecules or ions are able to be moved in this way, and they must be carried by specific proteins in the membrane. The action of the carrier requires an input of energy other than the kinetic energy of the molecules; therefore, this process is termed *active* transport. For example, some ions, such as sodium and potassium, are actively pumped across cell membranes. Sodium ions are pumped out of cells up a concentration gradient. Potassium ions are pumped into cells up a concentration gradient.

In addition to active transport, materials can be transported into a cell by *endocytosis* and out by *exocytosis.* **Phagocytosis** (*phag* = to eat; *cyto* = cell; *-osis* = condition of) is another name for one kind of endocytosis, which is the process that cells use to wrap membrane around a particle (usually food) and engulf it (figure 5.9). This is the process leukocytes (white blood cells) in your body use to surround invading bacteria, viruses, and other foreign materials. Because of this, these kinds of cells are called *phagocytes.* When phagocytosis occurs, the material to be engulfed touches the surface of the phagocyte and causes a portion of the outer cell membrane to be indented. The indented cell membrane is pinched off inside the cell to form a sac containing the engulfed material. This sac, composed of a single membrane, is called a **vacuole.** Once inside the cell, the membrane of the vacuole is broken down, releasing its contents inside the cell, or it may combine with another vacuole containing destructive enzymes.

Phagocytosis is used by many types of cells to acquire large amounts of material from their environment. However, if the cell is not surrounding a large quantity of material, but is merely engulfing some molecules dissolved in water, the process is termed **pinocytosis.** In this form of endocytosis, the sacs that are formed are very small in comparison to those formed during phagocytosis. Because of this size difference, they are called **vesicles.** In fact, an electron microscope is needed to see them.

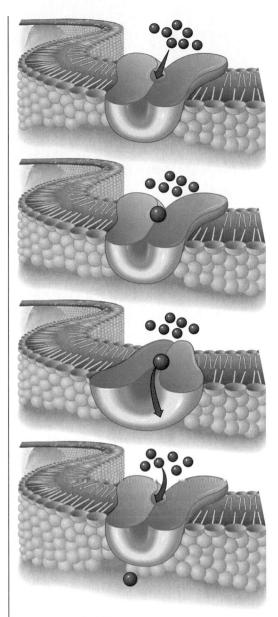

FIGURE 5.7 Facilitated diffusion.

This method of transporting materials across membranes is a diffusion process; i.e., a movement of molecules from a high to a low concentration. However, the process is helped (facilitated) by a particular membrane protein. No chemical bond energy in the form of ATP is required for this process. The molecules being moved through the membrane attach to a specific transport carrier protein in the membrane. This causes a change in its shape that propels the molecule or ion through to the other side.

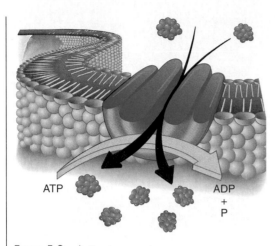

FIGURE 5.8 Active transport.
One possible method whereby active transport could cause materials to accumulate in a cell is illustrated here. Notice that the concentration gradient is such that if simple diffusion were operating, the molecules would leave the cell. The action of the carrier protein requires an active input of energy other than the kinetic energy of the molecules—therefore, this process is termed *active* transport.

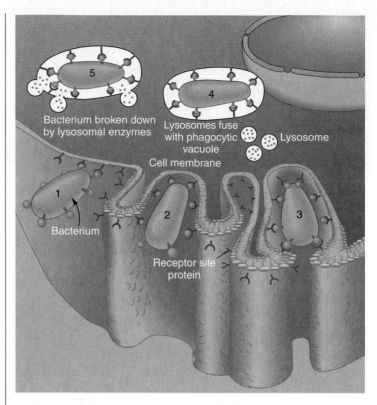

FIGURE 5.9 [▣] Phagocytosis.
This cell is engulfing a large amount of material at one time and surrounding it with a membrane. A lysosome adds its digestive enzymes to aid in the breakdown. Finally, the digested material is able to be absorbed from the vacuole into the cytoplasm of the cell.

The processes of phagocytosis and pinocytosis differ from active transport in that the cell surrounds large amounts of material with a membrane rather than taking the material in through the membrane, molecule by molecule. The movement of materials into the cell by either phagocytosis or pinocytosis is referred to as *endocytosis*. The transport of material from the cell by the reverse process is called *exocytosis*.

Cell Size

The size of a cell is directly related to its level of activity and the rate of movement of molecules across cell membranes. In order to stay alive, a cell must have a constant supply of nutrients, oxygen, and other molecules. It must also be able to get rid of carbon dioxide and other waste products that are harmful to it. The larger a cell becomes, the more difficult it is to satisfy these requirements; consequently most cells are very small. There are a few exceptions to this general rule, but they are easily explained. Egg cells, like the yolk of a hen's egg, are very large cells. However, the only part of an egg cell that is metabolically active is a small spot near its surface. The central portion of the egg is simply inactive, stored food called *yolk*.

All cells are highly organized living units that require a constant exchange of food, gases, and waste products through the cell membrane. The membrane is the surface area (outer face) of the cell. The living material is the volume (amount of space) within the cell. There is a mathematical relationship between the surface area and volume of a cell referred to as the *surface-to-volume ratio*. As cells grow, the amount of surface area increases by the square (X^2) but volume increases by the cube (X^3). They do not increase at the same rate. The surface area increases at a slower rate than the volume. Thus, the surface area-to-volume ratio changes as the cell grows. As a cell gets larger, cells have a problem with transporting materials across the plasma membrane. For example, diffusion of molecules is quite rapid over a short distance, but becomes slower over a longer distance. If a cell were to get too large, the center of the cell would die because diffusion would not be rapid enough to allow for the exchange of materials. When the surface area is not large enough to permit sufficient exchange between the cell volume and the outside environment, cell growth stops.

Now that you have some background concerning the structure and the function of membranes, let's turn our attention to the way cells use the membranes to build specific structural components of their protoplasm. The outer boundary of the cell is termed the **cell membrane** or **plasma membrane.** It is associated with a great variety of metabolic activities, including the uptake and release of molecules, the sensing of stimuli in the environment, the recognition of other cell types, and attachment to other cells and nonliving objects. In addition to the cell membrane, there are many other organelles composed of membranes. Each of these membranous organelles has a unique shape or structure that is associated with particular functions. One of the most common organelles found in cells is the endoplasmic reticulum.

The Endoplasmic Reticulum

The **endoplasmic reticulum, ER,** is a set of folded membranes and tubes throughout the cell. This system of membranes provides a large surface upon which chemical activities take place. Since the ER has an enormous surface area, many chemical reactions can be carried out in an extremely small space. Picture the vast surface area of a piece of newspaper crumpled into a tight little ball. The surface contains hundreds of thousands of tidbits of information in an orderly arrangement, yet it is packed into a very small volume. Proteins on the surface of the ER are actively involved in controlling and encouraging chemical activities—whether they are reactions involving growth and development of the cell or those resulting in the accumulation of molecules from the environment. The arrangement of the proteins allows them to control the sequences of metabolic activities so that chemical reactions can be carried out very rapidly and accurately.

Upon close examination using an electron microscope, it becomes apparent that there are two different types of ER—*rough* and *smooth.* The rough ER appears rough because it has ribosomes attached to its surface. *Ribosomes* are nonmembranous organelles that are associated with the synthesis of proteins from amino acids. Therefore, cells with an extensive amount of rough ER—for example, your pancreas cells—are capable of synthesizing large quantities of proteins. Smooth ER lacks attached ribosomes but is the site of many other important cellular chemical activities, including fat metabolism and detoxification reactions that are involved in the destruction of toxic substances such as alcohol and drugs. Your liver cells contain extensive smooth ER.

In addition, the spaces between the folded membranes serve as canals for the movement of molecules within the cell. Some researchers suggest that this system of membranes allows for rapid distribution of molecules within a cell (figure 5.10). The rough and smooth ER may also be connected to one another and to the nuclear membrane.

The Golgi Apparatus

Another organelle composed of membrane is the **Golgi apparatus.** Even though this organelle is also composed of membrane, the way in which it is structured

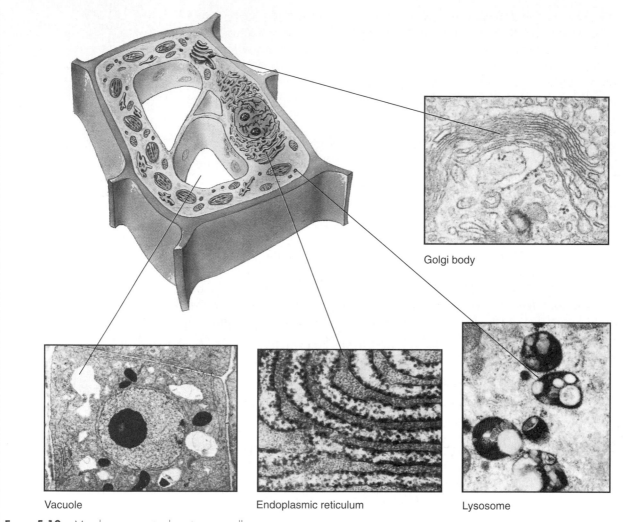

Golgi body

Vacuole

Endoplasmic reticulum

Lysosome

FIGURE 5.10 Membranous cytoplasmic organelles.

Certain structures in the cytoplasm are constructed of membranes. Membranes are composed of protein and phospholipids. The four structures here—the endoplasmic reticulum, the Golgi body, vacuoles, and lysosomes—are constructed of simple membranes.

enables it to perform jobs different from those performed by the ER. The typical Golgi is composed of from five to twenty flattened, smooth, membranous sacs, which resemble a stack of pancakes. The Golgi apparatus is the site of the synthesis and packaging of certain molecules produced in the cell. It is also the place where particular chemicals are concentrated prior to their release from the cell or distribution within the cell. Some Golgi vesicles are used to transport such molecules as mucus, carbohydrates, glycoproteins, insulin, and enzymes to the outside of the cell. The molecules are concentrated inside the Golgi, and tiny vesicles are pinched, or budded, off the outside surfaces of the Golgi sacs. The vesicles move to and merge with the endoplasmic reticulum or cell membrane. In so doing, the contents are placed in the ER where they can be utilized or transported from the cell.

An important group of molecules that is necessary to the cell are the hydrolytic enzymes. This group of enzymes is capable of destroying carbohydrates, nucleic acids, proteins, and lipids. Since cells contain large amounts of these molecules, these enzymes must be controlled in order to prevent the destruction of the cell. The Golgi is the site where these enzymes are converted from their inactive to their active forms and packaged in membranous sacs. These vesicles are pinched off from the outside surfaces of the Golgi sacs and given the special name **lysosomes,** meaning bursting body. The lysosomes are used by cells in four major ways:

1. When a cell is damaged, the membranes of the lysosomes break and the enzymes are released. These enzymes then begin to break down the contents of the damaged cell so that the component parts can be used by surrounding cells.

2. Lysosomes also play a part in the normal development of an organism. For example, as a tadpole slowly changes into a frog, the cells of the tail are destroyed by the action of lysosomes. In humans, the developing embryo has paddle-shaped hands or feet. At a prescribed point in the development, the cells between the bones of the fingers or toes release the enzymes that have been stored in the lysosomes. As these cells begin to disintegrate, individual fingers or toes begin to take shape. Occasionally this process does not take place, and the infant is born with "webbed fingers or toes." This developmental defect, called *syndactylism*, may be surgically corrected soon after birth (figure 5.11).

3. In many kinds of cells, the lysosomes are known to combine with food vacuoles. When this occurs, the enzymes of the lysosome break down the food particles into smaller and smaller molecular units. This process is common in one-celled organisms such as *Paramecium*.

4. Lysosomes are also used in the destruction of engulfed, disease-causing microorganisms such as bacteria, viruses, and fungi. As these invaders are taken into the cell by phagocytosis, lysosomes fuse with the phagocytic vacuole. When this occurs, the hydrolytic enzymes of the lysosome move into the vacuole to destroy the microorganisms.

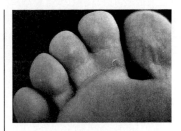

Figure 5.11 Syndactylism. This person displays the trait known as syndactylism (*syn* = connected, *dactyl* = finger or toe). In most people, enzymes break down the connecting tissue, allowing the toes to separate.

The many kinds of vacuoles and vesicles contained in cells are frequently described by their function. Thus, food vacuoles hold food, and water vacuoles store water. Specialized water vacuoles called *contractile vacuoles* are able to forcefully expel excess water that has accumulated in the cytoplasm as a result of osmosis. The contractile vacuole is a necessary organelle in cells that live in fresh water. The water constantly diffuses into the cell, since the environment contains a higher concentration than inside the cell and therefore must be actively pumped out. The special containers that hold the contents resulting from pinocytosis are called *pinocytic vesicles*. In all cases, these simple containers are constructed of a surrounding membrane.

The Nuclear Membrane

The nucleus is a place in the cell—not a solid mass. Just as a room is a place created by the walls, floor, and ceiling, the nucleus is a place in a cell created by the **nuclear membrane.** This membrane separates the *nucleoplasm*, liquid material in the nucleus, from the cytoplasm. Because they are separated, the cytoplasm and nucleoplasm can maintain a different chemical composition. If the membrane was not formed around the genetic material, the organelle we call the *nucleus* would not exist. The nuclear membrane is formed from many flattened sacs fashioned into a hollow sphere around the genetic material, DNA. It has large openings, called nuclear pores, that allow relatively large molecules to pass. The pores serve to select what types of molecules are allowed to pass.

Energy Converters

All of the membranous organelles described are able to be interconverted from one form to another (figure 5.12). For example, phagocytosis results in the formation of vacuolar membrane from cell membrane that fuses with lysosomal

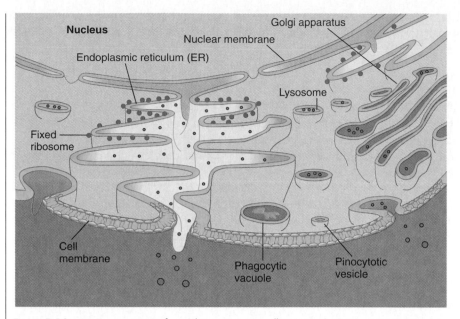

FIGURE 5.12 Interconversion of membranous organelles.
Eukaryotic cells contain a variety of organelles composed of phospholipids and proteins. Each has a unique shape and function. Many of these organelles are interconverted from one to another as they perform their essential functions. Cell membranes can become vacuolar membrane or endoplasmic reticulum, which can become vesicular membrane, which in turn can become Golgi or nuclear membrane. However, mitochondria cannot exchange membrane parts with other membranous organelles.

membrane, which in turn came from Golgi membrane. However, there are other organelles composed of membranes that are chemically different and incapable of interconversion. These organelles are associated with energy conversion reactions in the cell, *mitochondria* (figure 5.13).

The **mitochondrion** is an organelle resembling a small bag with a larger bag inside that is folded back on itself. These inner folded surfaces are known as the **cristae.** Located on the surface of the cristae are particular proteins and enzymes involved in *aerobic cellular respiration.* **Aerobic cellular respiration** is the series of reactions involved in the release of usable energy from food molecules, which requires the participation of oxygen molecules. Enzymes that speed the breakdown of simple nutrients are arranged in a sequence on the mitochondrial membrane. The average human cell contains upwards of ten thousand mitochondria. Cells that are involved in activities that require large amounts of energy such as muscle cells contain many more mitochondria. When properly stained, they can be seen with the compound light microscope. When cells are functioning aerobically, the mitochondria swell with activity. But when this activity diminishes, they shrink and appear as threadlike structures.

Mitochondria are different from other kinds of membranous structures in several ways. First, their membranes are chemically different from those of other membranous organelles; second, they are composed of double layers of membrane—an inner and an outer membrane; third, both of these structures have ribosomes and DNA that are similar to those of bacteria; and fourth, they have a certain degree of independence from the rest of the cell—they have a limited ability to reproduce themselves but must rely on nuclear DNA for assistance. The function of mitochondria will be discussed in chapter 7.

All of the organelles just described are composed of membranes. Many of these membranes are modified for particular functions. Each membrane is composed of the double phospholipid layer with protein molecules associated with it.

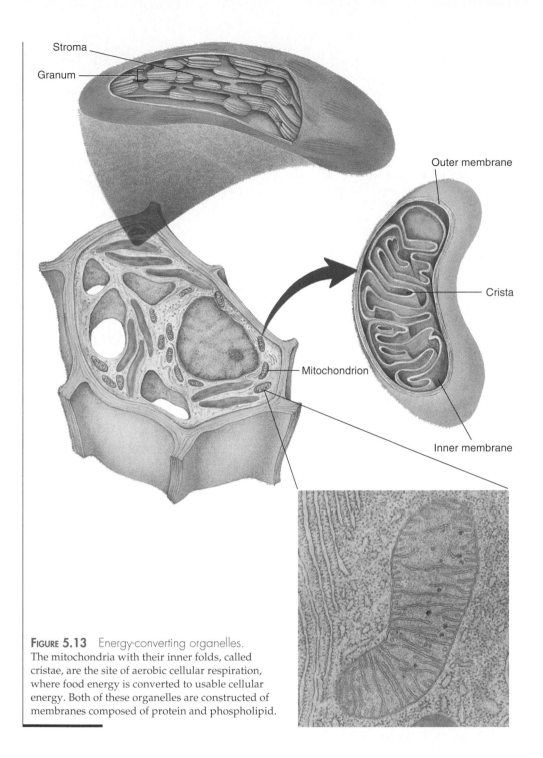

Stroma

Granum

Outer membrane

Crista

Mitochondrion

Inner membrane

Figure 5.13 Energy-converting organelles. The mitochondria with their inner folds, called cristae, are the site of aerobic cellular respiration, where food energy is converted to usable cellular energy. Both of these organelles are constructed of membranes composed of protein and phospholipid.

Suspended in the cytoplasm and associated with the membranous organelles are various kinds of structures that are not composed of phospholipids and proteins arranged in sheets.

NONMEMBRANOUS ORGANELLES

Ribosomes

In the cytoplasm are many very small structures called **ribosomes** that are composed of ribonucleic acid (RNA) and protein. Ribosomes function in the manufacture of protein. Each ribosome is composed of two oddly shaped subunits—a large one and a small one. The larger of the two subunits is composed of a specific type of RNA associated with several kinds of protein molecules. The smaller

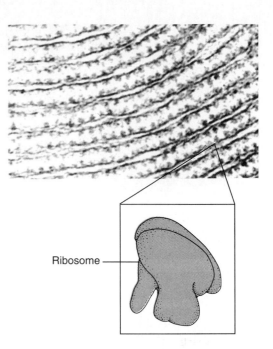

FIGURE 5.14 Ribosomes.
Each ribosome is constructed of two subunits of protein and ribonucleic acid. These globular organelles are associated with the construction of protein molecules from individual amino acids. They are sometimes located individually in the cytoplasm where protein is being assembled, or they may be attached to endoplasmic reticulum (ER). They are so obvious on the ER when using electron micrograph techniques that when they are present, we label this ER as rough ER.

Ribosome

is composed of RNA with fewer protein molecules than the large one. These globular organelles are involved in the assembly of proteins from amino acids—they are frequently associated with the endoplasmic reticulum to form rough ER. Areas of rough ER have been demonstrated to be active sites of protein production. Cells actively producing nonprotein materials, such as lipids, are likely to contain more smooth ER than rough ER. Many ribosomes are also found floating freely in the cytoplasm (figure 5.14), wherever proteins are being assembled. Cells (ex., of the liver) that are actively producing protein have great numbers of free and attached ribosomes. The details of how ribosomes function in protein synthesis are discussed in chapter 8.

Microtubules and Microfilaments

Another type of nonmembranous organelle, the **microtubules,** consist of small, hollow tubes composed of protein called *tubulin.* They function throughout the cytoplasm, where they provide structural support and enable movement. The microtubules are dynamic structures that are capable of being lengthened or shortened by the addition or subtraction of tubulin units (figure 5.15). As a result, there seems to be a constant shifting of microtubular material within a cell. Many of the structures with which microtubules are associated are able to move or grow. Microtubules participate in the movement of chromosomes during nuclear division, in the movement of flagella and cilia, and in the positioning of cellulose molecules during cell-wall synthesis. Important structures composed of microtubules are the *centrioles.*

Microfilaments are long, fiberlike contractile strands made of protein found in cells. Some are involved in the contraction of cells, while others serve as a cellular framework. It appears that microtubules and microfilaments are often interconnected to form a kind of cellular skeleton that allows the cell to have shape. However, this is not a rigid structural support, because both microtubules and microfilaments are involved in movement and may be assembled and disassembled. When a white blood cell or *Amoeba* moves by crawling or amoeboid motion, the filaments just under the cell membrane are being rearranged. This is much like what happens when an umbrella is opened or closed. When its metal frame changes position, the nylon or plastic cover changes shape and position. Figure 5.16 shows how these different elements might be used to form a cellular skeleton.

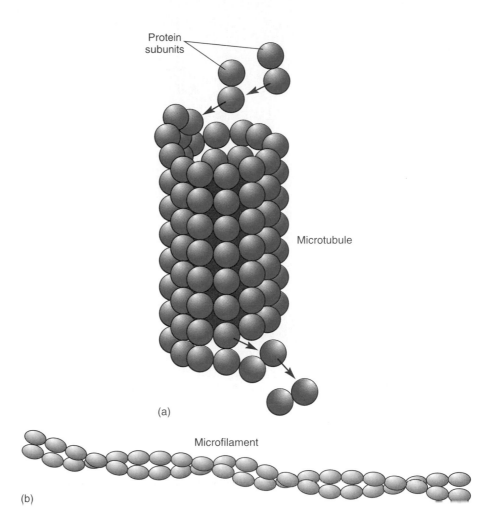

FIGURE 5.15 Microtubules and microfilaments.

(a) Microtubules are hollow tubes constructed of proteins. The dynamic nature of the microtubule is useful in the construction of certain organelles in a cell, such as centrioles and cilia or flagella.

(b) Microfilaments are composed of the contractile protein, actin. This is the same contractile protein found in human muscle cells.

Protein subunits

Microtubule

(a)

Microfilament

(b)

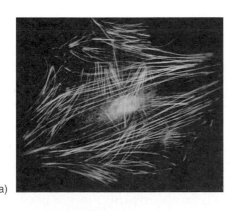

(a)

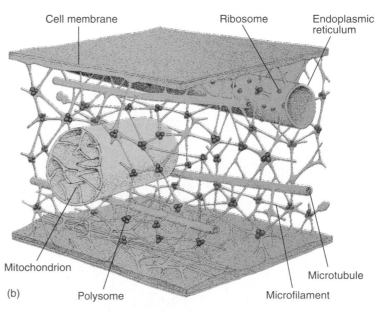

FIGURE 5.16 The cytoskeleton.

A complex array of microfilaments and microtubules provides a structure for the cell. The cellular skeleton is not a rigid structure but changes as the microfilaments and microtubules assemble and disassemble. (a) Elements of the cytoskeleton have been labeled with a fluorescent dye to make them visible. (b) How the various parts of the cytoskeleton are interconnected.

(b) From "The Ground Substance of the Living Cell" by Keith Porter and Jonathan Tucker. Copyright © 1981 by Scientific American, Inc. All rights reserved.

Cell membrane

Ribosome

Endoplasmic reticulum

Mitochondrion

Polysome

(b)

Microtubule

Microfilament

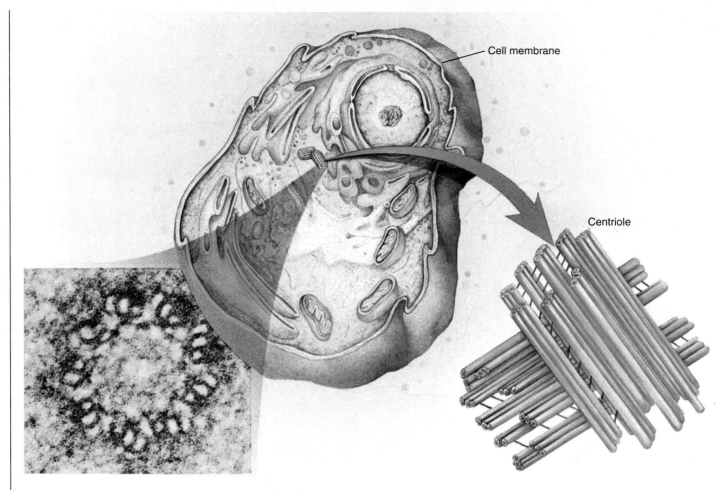

Cell membrane

Centriole

FIGURE 5.17 The centriole.

These two sets of short microtubules are located just outside the nuclear membrane in many types of cells. The micrograph shows an end view of one of these sets. Magnification is about 160,000 times.

Centrioles

An arrangement of two sets of microtubules at right angles to each other makes up a structure known as the **centriole.** The centrioles of many cells are located in a region known as the *centrosome,* or a structure called a *basal body.* The centrosome is usually located close to the nuclear membrane, while basal bodies are at the bases of cilia and flagella. It appears that the centriole acts as the overall director of microtubule activities. Each set is composed of nine groups of short microtubules arranged in a cylinder (figure 5.17). The centriole functions in cell division and is referred to again in chapter 9. One curious fact about centrioles is that they are present in most animal cells but not in many types of plant cells.

Cilia and Flagella

Many cells have microscopic, hairlike structures projecting from their surfaces; these are **cilia** or **flagella** (figure 5.18). In general, we call them *flagella* if they are long and few in number, and *cilia* if they are short and more numerous. They are similar in structure, and each functions to move the cell through its environment or to move the environment past the cell. They are constructed of a cylinder of nine sets of microtubules similar to those in the centriole, but they have an additional two microtubules in the center. These long strands of microtubules project from the cell surface and are covered by cell membrane. When cilia and

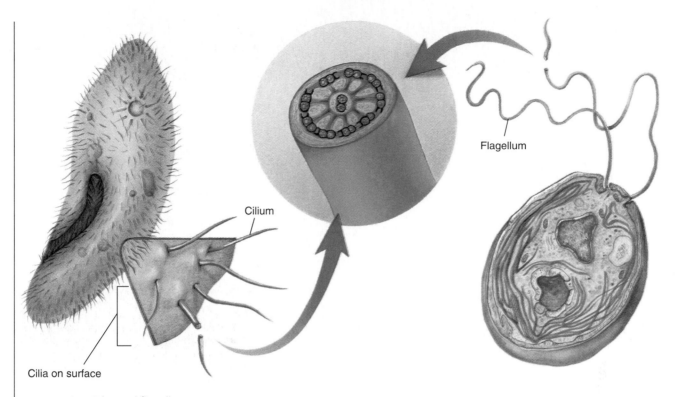

Figure 5.18 Cilia and flagella.

These two structures function like oars or propellers that move the cell through its environment or move the environment past the cell. Cilia and flagella are constructed of groups of microtubules. Flagella are longer than cilia.

flagella are sliced crosswise, their cut ends show what is referred to as the *9 + 2 arrangement* of microtubules. The cell has the ability to control the action of these microtubular structures, enabling them to be moved in a variety of different ways. Cilia are found on the cells of many of the tubes in the respiratory system and in the oviduct. In the respiratory system, the cilia move in a coordinated manner and move dust and other foreign material out of the lungs. In the oviduct, the coordinated movement of the cilia moves the egg toward the uterus.

Inclusions

Inclusions are collections of materials that do not have as well-defined a structure as the organelles we have discussed so far. They might be concentrations of stored materials, such as starch grains, sulfur, or oil droplets, or they might be a collection of miscellaneous materials known as **granules.** Unlike organelles, which are essential to the survival of a cell, the inclusions are generally only temporary sites for the storage of nutrients and wastes.

Some inclusion materials may be harmful to other cells. For example, rhubarb leaf cells contain an inclusion composed of an organic acid—oxalic acid. Needle-shaped crystals of calcium oxalate can cause injury to the kidneys of an organism that eats rhubarb leaves. The sour taste of this particular compound aids in the survival of the rhubarb plant by discouraging animals from eating it. Similarly, certain bacteria store crystals of a substance in their inclusions that is known to be harmful to insects. Spraying plants with these bacteria is a biological method of controlling the population of the insect pests, while not interfering with the plant or with humans.

In the past, cell structures such as ribosomes, centrioles, and mitochondria were also called *granules,* since their structure and function were not clearly known. As scientists learn more about unidentified particles in the cells, they too will be named and more fully described.

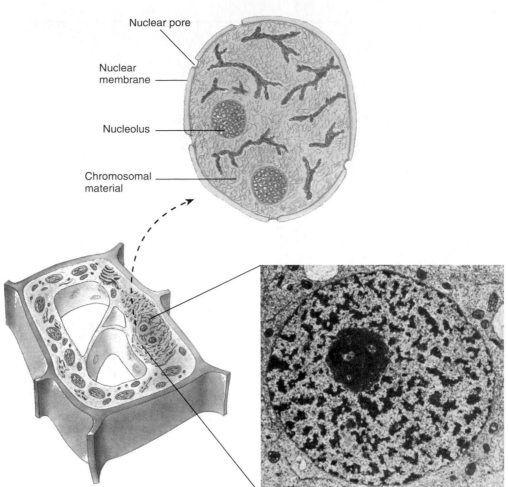

Nuclear pore

Nuclear membrane

Nucleolus

Chromosomal material

FIGURE 5.19 The nucleus. One of the two major regions of protoplasm, the nucleus has its own complex structure. It is bounded by a double membrane that separates it from the cytoplasm. Inside the nucleus are the nucleoli, chromosomes or chromatin material composed of DNA, and the liquid matrix (nucleoplasm). Magnification is about 20,000 times.

NUCLEAR COMPONENTS

As stated at the beginning of this chapter, one of the first structures to be identified in cells was the nucleus. The nucleus was referred to as the cell center. If the nucleus is removed from a cell, the cell can only live a short time. For example, human red blood cells begin life in bone marrow, where they have nuclei. Before they are released into the bloodstream to serve as oxygen and carbon dioxide carriers, they lose their nuclei. As a consequence, red blood cells are only able to function for about 120 days before they disintegrate.

When nuclear structures were first identified, it was noted that certain dyes stained some parts more than others. The parts that stained more heavily were called **chromatin,** which means colored material. Chromatin is composed of long molecules of deoxyribonucleic acid (DNA) in association with proteins. These DNA molecules contain the genetic information for the cell, the blueprints for its construction and maintenance. Chromatin is loosely organized DNA in the nucleus. When the chromatin is tightly coiled into shorter, denser structures, we call them **chromosomes** (*chromo* = color; *some* = body). Chromatin and chromosomes are really the same molecules but differ in structural arrangement. In addition to chromosomes, the nucleus may also contain one, two, or several *nucleoli*. A **nucleolus** is the site of ribosome manufacture. Nucleoli are composed of specific granules and fibers in association with the cell's DNA used in the manufacture of ribosomes. These regions, together with the completed or partially completed ribosomes, are called nucleoli.

The final component of the nucleus is its liquid matrix called the **nucleoplasm.** It is a mixture composed of water and the molecules used in the construction of ribosomes, nucleic acids, and other nuclear material (figure 5.19).

Prokaryotic cells Characterized by few membranous organelles; nuclear material not separated from the cytoplasm by a membrane	Eukaryotic cells Cells larger than prokaryotic cells; nucleus with a membrane separating it from the cytoplasm; many complex organelles composed of many structures including membranes			
Kingdom Prokaryotae	Kingdom Protista	Kingdom Mycetae	Kingdom Plantae	Kingdom Animalia
Unicellular organisms	Unicellular organisms; some in colonies; both photosynthetic and heterotrophic nutrition	Multicellular organisms or loose colonial arrangement of cells; organism is a row or filament of cells; decay fungi and parasites	Multicellular organisms; cells supported by a rigid cell wall of cellulose; some cells have chloroplasts; complex arrangement into tissues	Multicellular organisms with division of labor into complex tissues; no cell wall present; acquire food from the environment
Examples: bacteria and cyanobacteria	Examples: protozoans such as *Amoeba* and *Paramecium* and algae such as *Chlamydomonas* and *Euglena*	Examples: *Penicillium*, morels, button mushrooms, galls, and rusts	Examples: moss, ferns, cone-bearing trees, and flowering plants	Examples: worms, insects, starfish, frogs, reptiles, birds, and mammals

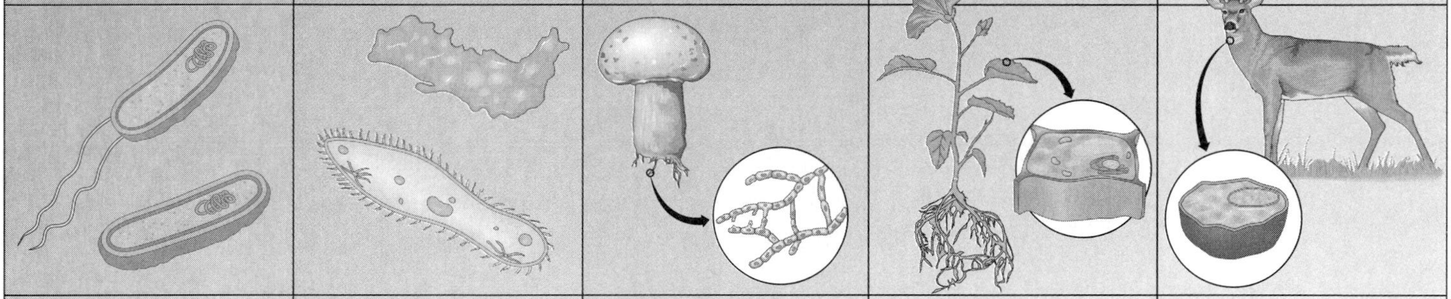

FIGURE 5.20 Comparison of cell types.
The five types of cells illustrated here indicate the major patterns of construction found in all living things. Note the similarities of all five and the subtle differences among them.

Not all of the cellular organelles we have just described are located in every cell. Some cells typically have combinations of organelles that differ from others. For example, some cells have a nuclear membrane, mitochondria, ER, and Golgi, while others have mitochondria, *centrioles*, Golgi, ER, and a nuclear membrane. Other cells are even more simple and lack the complex membranous organelles described in this chapter. Because of this fact, biologists have been able to classify cells into two major types: *prokaryotic* and *eukaryotic* (figure 5.20).

MAJOR CELL TYPES

The Prokaryotic Cell Structure

Prokaryotic cells do not have a typical nucleus bound by a nuclear membrane, nor do they contain mitochondria, Golgi, or extensive networks of ER. However, prokaryotic cells contain DNA and enzymes and are able to reproduce and engage in metabolism. They perform all of the basic functions of living things with fewer and more simple organelles. All the prokaryotic cells are commonly called bacteria and some cause tuberculosis, strep throat, gonorrhea, and acne. Other prokaryotic cells (bacteria) are responsible for the decay and decomposition of dead organisms. Some bacteria have a type of green photosynthetic pigment and carry on photosynthesis.

One significant difference between prokaryotic and eukaryotic cells is in the chemical makeup of their ribosomes. The ribosomes of prokaryotic cells contain different proteins than those found in eukaryotic cells. Prokaryotic ribosomes are also smaller. This discovery was important to medicine because many cells that cause common diseases are prokaryotic (bacteria). As soon as differences in the

Table 5.2 Antibiotics Classified by the Area They Disrupt

CELL-WALL SYNTHESIS	CELL-MEMBRANE FUNCTION	PROTEIN SYNTHESIS		NUCLEIC-ACID FUNCTION	METABOLIC PATHWAYS
Bacitracin	Amphotericin B	Chloramphenicol	Erythromycin	Griseofulvin	Isoniazid
Cephalosporins	Benzalkonium chloride	Dihydrostreptomycin	Clindamycin	Idoxuridine	Para-aminosalicyclic acid
Cycloserine	Colistin	Aminoglycosides	Lincomycin	Rifampicin	Sulfonamides
Penicillins	Nystatin	Neomycin	Methacycline		
Ristocetin	Polymyxins	Paromomycin	Oleandomycin		
Vancomycin		Puromycin	Oxytetracycline		
		Streptomycin	Tetracycline		
		Trobicin	Nitrofurans		
		Chlortetracycline			

ribosomes were noted, researchers began to look for ways in which to interfere with the prokaryotic ribosome's function but *not* interfere with the ribosomes of eukaryotic cells. **Antibiotics,** such as streptomycin, are the result of this research. This drug combines with prokaryotic ribosomes and causes the death of the prokaryote by preventing the production of proteins essential to its survival. Since eukaryotic ribosomes differ from prokaryotic ribosomes, streptomycin does not interfere with the normal function of ribosomes in human cells.

Antibiotics work by inhibiting one of five main areas of microbial cell metabolism. They may disrupt: (1) cell-wall synthesis, (2) cell-membrane function, (3) protein synthesis, (4) nucleic-acid function, and (5) select metabolic pathways (table 5.2).

The Eukaryotic Cell Structure

Eukaryotic cells contain a true nucleus and most of the membranous organelles described earlier. Eukaryotic organisms can be further divided into several categories based on the specific combination of organelles they contain. The cells of plants, fungi, protozoa and algae, and animals are all eukaryotic. The most obvious characteristic that sets the plants and algae apart from other organisms is their green color, which indicates that the cells contain chlorophyll. Chlorophyll is necessary for the process of photosynthesis—the conversion of light energy into chemical-bond energy in food molecules. These cells, then, are different from the other cells in that they contain chloroplasts in the cytoplasm. Another distinguishing characteristic of plants and algae is the presence of cellulose in their cell walls.

The group of organisms that have a cell wall but lack chlorophyll in chloroplasts is collectively known as *fungi.* They were previously thought to be either plants that had lost their ability to make their own food or animals that had developed cell walls. Organisms that belong in this category of eukaryotic cells include yeasts, molds, mushrooms, and fungi that cause such human diseases as athlete's foot, jungle rot, and ringworm. Now we have come to recognize this group as different enough from plants and animals to place them in a separate kingdom.

Eukaryotic organisms that lack cell walls and cannot photosynthesize are placed in separate groups. Organisms that consist of only one cell are called protozoans—examples are *Amoeba* and *Paramecium.* They have all the cellular organelles described in this chapter except the chloroplast; therefore, protozoans must consume food as do the fungi and the multicellular animals. An amoeba, *Entamoeba histolytica,* (*ent* = inside; *amoeba* = amoeba; *histo* = tissue; *lytic* = burst) is responsible for amoebic dysentery.

While the differences in these groups of organisms may seem to set them worlds apart, their similarity in cellular structure is one of the central themes that

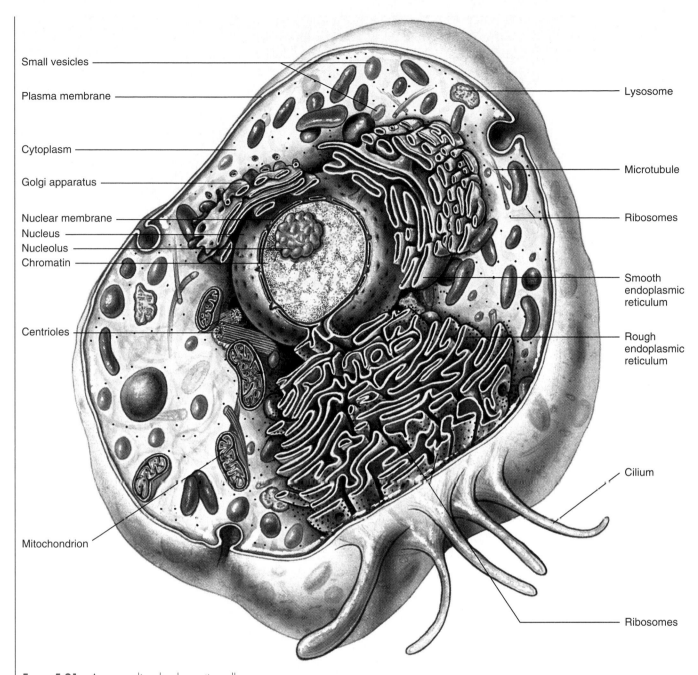

Small vesicles

Plasma membrane

Cytoplasm

Golgi apparatus

Nuclear membrane

Nucleus

Nucleolus

Chromatin

Centrioles

Mitochondrion

Lysosome

Microtubule

Ribosomes

Smooth endoplasmic reticulum

Rough endoplasmic reticulum

Cilium

Ribosomes

FIGURE 5.21 A generalized eukaryotic cell.

The major organelles of a typical animal cell are shown here. Use this illustration to identify structures when you are reviewing table 5.2.

From John W. Hole, Jr., *Human Anatomy and Physiology*, 6th ed. Copyright © 1993 Wm. C. Brown Communications, Inc. Reprinted by permission of Times Mirror Higher Education Group, Inc., Dubuque, Iowa. All Rights Reserved. Reprinted by permission.

unifies the field of biology (figure 5.21). One can obtain a better understanding of how cells operate in general by studying specific examples. Since the organelles have the same general structure and function regardless of the kind of cell in which they are found, we can learn more about how mitochondria function in plants by studying how mitochondria function in animals. There is a commonality among all living things with regard to their cellular structure and function. Table 5.3 compares the structure and function of cellular organelles.

Table 5.3 Comparison of the Structure and Function of the Cellular Organelles

ORGANELLE	TYPE OF CELL	STRUCTURE	FUNCTION
Plasma membrane	Prokaryotic Eukaryotic	Typical membrane structure; phospholipid and protein present	Controls passage of some materials to and from the environment of the cell
Granules	Prokaryotic Eukaryotic	Variable	May have a variety of functions
Chromatin material	Prokaryotic Eukaryotic	Composed of DNA and protein in eukaryotes, but just DNA in prokaryotes	Contains the hereditary information that the cell uses in its day-to-day life and passes it on to the next generation of cells
Ribosome	Prokaryotic Eukaryotic	Protein and RNA structure	Site of protein synthesis
Microtubules and microfilaments	Eukaryotic	Hollow tubes composed of protein	Provide structural support and allow for movement
Nuclear membrane	Eukaryotic	Typical membrane structure	Separates the nucleus from the cytoplasm
Nucleolus	Eukaryotic	Group of RNA molecules and DNA located in the nucleus	Site of ribosome manufacture and storage
Endoplasmic reticulum	Eukaryotic	Folds of membrane forming sheets and canals	Surface for chemical reactions and intracellular transport system
Golgi apparatus	Eukaryotic	Membranous stacks	Associated with the production of secretions and enzyme activation
Vacuoles	Eukaryotic	Membranous sacs	Containers of materials
Lysosome	Eukaryotic	Membranous container	Isolates very strong enzymes from the rest of the cell
Mitochondria	Eukaryotic	Large membrane folded inside of a smaller membrane	Associated with the release of energy from food; site of cellular respiration
Centriole	Eukaryotic	Microtubular	Associated with cell division
Contractile vacuole	Eukaryotic	Membranous container	Expels excess water
Cilia and flagella	Eukaryotic	9 + 2 tubulin in eukaryotes; different structure in prokaryotes	Movement

SUMMARY

The concept of the cell has developed over a number of years. It passed through a stage where only two regions, the cytoplasm and the nucleus, could be identified. At present, numerous organelles are recognized as essential components of both prokaryotic and eukaryotic cell types. The structure and function of some of these organelles are compared in table 5.3. This table also indicates whether the organelle is unique to prokaryotic or eukaryotic cells or if it is found in both.

The cell is the common unit of life. We study individual cells and their structure to understand how they function as individual living organisms and as parts of many-celled beings. Knowing how prokaryotic and eukaryotic cell types resemble or differ from each other helps physicians control some organisms dangerous to humans.

1. Make a list of the membranous organelles of a eukaryotic cell and describe the function of each.

2. Describe how the concept of the cell has changed over the past two hundred years.

3. What three methods allow the exchange of molecules between cells and their surroundings?

4. How do diffusion, facilitated diffusion, osmosis, and active transport differ?

5. What are the differences between a lysosome and mitochondrion?

6. Diagram a cell and show where proteins, nucleic acids, carbohydrates, and lipids are located.

7. Make a list of the nonmembranous organelles of the cell and describe their functions.

8. Define the following terms: cytoplasm, cristae, chromatin, and chromosome.

9. Why does putting salt on meat preserve it from spoilage by bacteria?

10. What is the function of lysosomes?

CHAPTER GLOSSARY

active transport (ak-tiv trans-port) Use of a carrier molecule to move molecules across a cell membrane in a direction opposite that of the concentration gradient. The carrier requires an input of energy other than the kinetic energy of the molecules.

aerobic cellular respiration (a-ro′bik sel′yu-lar res″pi-ra′shun) A series of reactions in the mitochondria involved in the release of usable energy from food molecules by combining them with oxygen molecules.

antibiotics (an-te-bi-ot′iks) Drugs that selectively kill or inhibit the growth of a particular cell type.

cell (sel) The basic structural unit that makes up all living things.

cellular membranes (sel′u-lar mem′brāns) Thin sheets of material composed of phospholipids and proteins. Some of the proteins have attached carbohydrates or fats.

centriole (sen′tre-ōl) Two sets of nine short microtubules, each arranged in a cylinder.

chromatin (kro′mah-tin) Areas or structures within the nucleus of a cell composed of long molecules of deoxyribonucleic acid (DNA) in association with proteins.

chromosomes (kro′mo-sōmz) Structures visible in the nucleus that consist of DNA and protein.

cilia (sil′e-ah) Numerous short, hairlike structures projecting from the cell surface that enable locomotion.

concentration gradient (kon″sen-tra′shun gra″de-ent) The gradual change in the number of molecules per unit of volume over distance.

cristae (kris′te) Folded surfaces of the inner membranes of mitochondria.

cytoplasm (si″to-plazm) The more fluid portion of the protoplasm that surrounds the nucleus.

diffusion (dĭ″fiu′zhun) Net movement of a kind of molecule from an area of higher concentration to an area of lesser concentration.

diffusion gradient (dĭ″fiu′zhun gra″de-ent) The difference in the concentration of diffusing molecules over distance.

dynamic equilibrium (di-nam′ik e″kwĭ-lib′re-um) A state of balance reached when molecules are completely dispersed and their movement is equal in all directions.

endoplasmic reticulum (ER) (en″do-plaz′mik re-tĭk′yu-lum) Folded membranes and tubes throughout the eukaryotic cell that provide a large surface upon which chemical activities take place.

eukaryotic cells (yu′ka-re-ah″tik sels) One of the two major types of cells; characterized by cells that have a true nucleus, as in plants, fungi, protists, and animals.

facilitated diffusion (fah-sil′-ĭ-ta″ted dĭ″fiu′zhun) Diffusion assisted by carrier molecules.

flagella (flah-jel′luh) Long, hairlike structures projecting from the cell surface that enable locomotion.

fluid-mosaic model (flu′id mo-za′ik mod′l) The concept that the cell membrane is composed primarily of protein and phospholipid molecules that are able to shift and flow past one another.

Golgi apparatus (gōl′je ap″pah-rat′us) A stack of flattened, smooth, membranous sacs; the site of synthesis and packaging of certain molecules in eukaryotic cells.

granules (gran′yūls) Materials whose structure is not as well defined as that of other organelles.

hydrophilic (hi′dro-fil′ik) Readily absorbing or dissolving in water.

hydrophobic (hi′dro-fo′bik) Tending not to combine with, or incapable of dissolving in, water.

hypertonic (hi-pur-tŏn′ik) A comparative term describing one of two solutions. The hypertonic solution is the one with the higher amount of dissolved material.

hypotonic (hi′po-tŏn′ik) A comparative term describing one of two solutions. The hypotonic solution is the one with the lower amount of dissolved material.

inclusions (in-klu′zhuns) A general term referring to materials inside a cell that are usually not readily identifiable; stored materials.

isotonic (i′so-tŏn′ik) A term used to describe two solutions that have the same concentration of dissolved material.

lysosome (li′so-sōm) A specialized organelle that holds a mixture of hydrolytic enzymes.

microfilaments (mi″kro-fil′ah-ments) Long, fiberlike structures made of actin protein and found in cells, often in close association with the microtubules; provide structural support and enable movement.

microscope (mi′kro-skōp) An instrument used to make an object appear larger than it appears to the naked eye.

microtubules (mi′kro-tū″byūls) Small, hollow tubes of protein that function throughout the cytoplasm to provide structural support and enable movement.

mitochondrion (mi-to-kahn′dre-on) A membranous organelle resembling a small bag with a larger bag inside that is folded back on itself; serves as the site of aerobic cellular respiration.

net movement (net muv′ment) Movement in one direction minus the movement in the other.

nuclear membrane (nu′kle-ar mem′brān) The structure surrounding the nucleus that separates the nucleoplasm from the cytoplasm.

nucleolus (plural, **nucleoli**) (nu″kle-o′lus) Nuclear structures composed of completed or partially completed ribosomes and the specific parts of chromosomes that contain the information for their construction.

nucleoplasm (nu′kle-o-plazm) The liquid matrix of the nucleus composed of a mixture of water and the molecules used in the construction of the rest of the nuclear structures.

nucleus (nu′kle-us) The central body that contains the information system for the cell.

organelles (or-gan-elz′) Cellular structures that perform specific functions in the cell. The function of an organelle is directly related to its structure.

osmosis (os-mo′sis) The net movement of water molecules through a selectively permeable membrane.

phagocytosis (fă″jo-si-to′sis) The process by which the cell wraps around a particle and engulfs it.

pinocytosis (pĭ″no-si-to′sis) The process by which a cell engulfs some molecules dissolved in water.

plasma membrane (plaz′muh mem′brān) The outer-boundary membrane of the cell; also known as the cell membrane.

prokaryotic cells (pro′ka-re-ot″ik sels) One of the two major types of cells. They do not have a typical nucleus bound by a nuclear membrane and lack many of the other membranous cellular organelles; for example, bacteria.

protoplasm (pro′to-plazm) The living portion of a cell as distinguished from the nonliving cell wall.

ribosomes (ri′bo-sōmz) Small structures composed of two protein and ribonucleic acid subunits involved in the assembly of proteins from amino acids.

selectively permeable (sĕ-lek′tiv-le per′me-ah-b′l) The property of a membrane that allows certain molecules to pass through it but interferes with the passage of others.

vacuole (vak′yu-ōl) A large sac within the cytoplasm of a cell, composed of a single membrane.

vesicles (vĕ′sĭ-kuls) Small, intracellular, membrane-bound sacs in which various substances are stored.

THE DYNAMIC HUMAN   Correlations to Chapter Five:

Respiratory System ➤ Exploration ➤ Gas Exchange

Enzymes

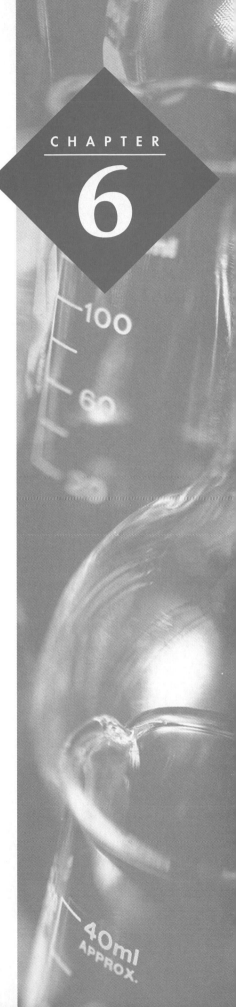

CHAPTER OUTLINE

PURPOSE

Living cells require various chemical reactions to conduct their vital functions. To prevent the malfunction and death of the cell, these reactions must be rapid and controlled. The problem is starting reactions and controlling their rate. Regulation of the rates of the many reactions in cells is the task of enzymes.

CLINICAL VIEWPOINT

Medical professionals primarily concerned with the effect of alcohol on humans assumed that only the liver was able to neutralize alcohol. But, a recent article in the *New England Journal of Medicine* reported the discovery of a stomach enzyme that also neutralizes alcohol.

   Normally this enzyme reduces the alcohol level in the stomach by 20%. This in turn reduces the amount of alcohol entering the bloodstream and being transported to the brain.

   However, large amounts of alcohol interfere with the enzyme. It was found that while male alcoholics lost some of their ability to digest alcohol in the stomach, females experienced a complete loss of the enzyme. The report stated, "For them (women), drinking alcohol has the same effect as injecting it intravenously."

LEARNING OBJECTIVES

- Explain the need for enzymes in the maintenance of living things
- Describe what happens when an enzyme and substrate combine
- Relate the three-dimensional structure of an enzyme to its ability to catalyze a reaction
- Explain the role of coenzymes and vitamins in enzyme operation
- Describe the influences of environmental factors such as temperature, pH, and concentration on turnover number
- Define the mechanisms of enzyme competition and inhibition
- Explain the methods used by cells to control and regulate their biochemical activities

All living things require a source of energy and building materials in order to grow and reproduce. Energy may be in the form of visible light, or it may be derived from energy-containing covalent bonds found in nutrients. **Nutrients** are molecules required by organisms for growth, reproduction, and/or repair—they serve as a source of energy and molecular building materials. The formation, breakdown, and rearrangement of molecules to provide organisms with essential energy and building blocks are known as *biochemical reactions.* These reactions occur when atoms or molecules come together and form new, more stable relationships. This results in the formation of new molecules and a change in the energy distribution among the reactants and end products (box 6.1). Most chemical reactions require an input of energy to get them started. This is referred to as **activation energy.** This energy is used to make the reactants unstable and more likely to react (figure 6.1).

If organisms are to survive, they must gain sizable amounts of energy and building materials in a very short time. Experience tells us that the sucrose in candy bars contains the potential energy needed to keep us active, as well as building materials to help us grow (sometimes to excess!). Yet, it could be millions of years before a candy bar is broken down by random chemical processes, releasing its energy and building materials. Of course, living things cannot wait that long. To sustain life, biochemical reactions must occur at extremely rapid rates. One way to increase the rate of any chemical reaction and make its energy and component parts available to a cell is to increase the temperature of the reactants. In general, the hotter the reactants, the faster they will react. However, this method of increasing reaction rates has a major drawback when it comes to living things. The organism will die because cellular proteins are denatured before the temperature reaches the point required to sustain the biochemical reactions necessary for life. This is of practical concern to people who are experiencing a fever. Should the fever stay too high for too long, major disruptions of cellular biochemical processes could be fatal.

However, there is a way of increasing the rate of chemical reactions without increasing the temperature. This involves using substances called *catalysts.* A **catalyst** is a chemical that speeds the reaction but is not used up in the reaction. It is able to be recovered unchanged when the reaction is complete. Catalysts function by lowering the amount of activation energy needed to start the reaction. A cell

Box 6.1 Enzyme Theory

Chemists use two different theories to explain how chemical reactions occur and how enzymes might speed these reactions. One theory suggests that reactants collide with one another as a result of their natural kinetic energy. However, not all collisions result in changes in the chemical bonds of the reactants. Those collisions that do bring about changes in the chemical bonds are called *effective collisions.* It is not enough that the two molecules touch or bump into each other; they

must both have the correct orientation to each other so that specific chemical bonds come to lie next to one another. You must orient the pieces so that the proper side of one piece will fit into the appropriate part of the other. It is believed that enzymes help the two reacting molecules to "line up" so that more effective collisions occur more frequently.

In the collision theory, it is necessary for the two reactants to make enough contact with each other so that eventu-

ally some of the collisions will be effective. The energy needed to start a reaction is used to increase the probability of an effective collision. The higher the temperature, the faster the molecules move and the more frequently the reactants will contact each other with the proper orientation. Because of their shape, enzymes probably increase the likelihood that the chemical bond energy involved in the reaction will be altered, increasing the chance that the reaction will take place.

manufactures specific proteins that act as catalysts. A protein molecule that acts as a catalyst to speed the rate of a reaction is called an **enzyme.** Enzymes can be used over and over again until they are worn out, broken. The production of these protein catalysts is under the direct control of an organism's genetic material (DNA). The instructions for the manufacture of all enzymes are found in the genes of the cell. Organisms make their own enzymes. How the genetic information is used to direct the synthesis of these specific protein molecules is discussed in chapter 7.

As the instructions for the production of an enzyme are read from the genetic material, a specific sequence of amino acids is linked together at the ribosomes. Once bonded, the chain of amino acids folds and twists to form a globular molecule. It is the nature of its three-dimensional shape that allows this enzyme to combine with a reactant and lower the activation energy. Each enzyme has a very specific three-dimensional shape which, in turn, is very specific to the kind of reactant with which it can combine. The enzyme physically fits with the reactant. The molecule to which the enzyme attaches itself (the reactant) is known as the **substrate.** When the enzyme attaches itself to the substrate molecule, a new, temporary molecule—the **enzyme-substrate complex**—is formed (figure 6.2). When the substrate is combined with the enzyme, its bonds are less stable and more likely to be altered and form new bonds. The enzyme is specific because it has a particular shape that can combine only with specific parts of certain substrate molecules.

You might think of an enzyme as a tool that makes a job easier and faster. For example, the use of an open-end crescent wrench can make the job of removing or attaching a nut and bolt go much faster than that same job done by hand. In order

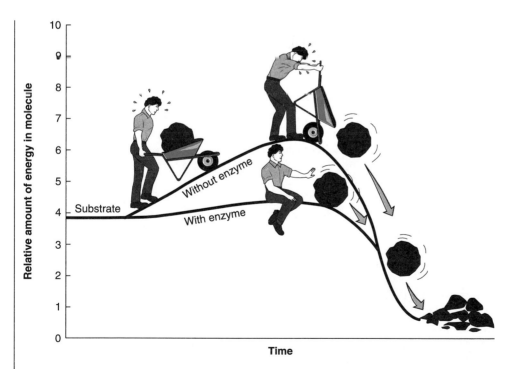

FIGURE 6.1 The lowering of activation energy.
Enzymes operate by lowering the amount of energy needed to get a reaction going—the activation energy. When this energy is lowered, the nature of the bonds is changed so they are more easily broken. While the cartoon shows the breakdown of a single reactant into many end products (as in a hydrolysis reaction), the lowering of activation energy can also result in bonds being broken so that new bonds may be formed in the construction of a single, larger end product from several reactants (as in a synthesis reaction).

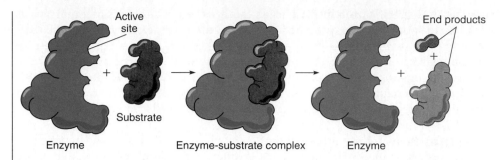

FIGURE 6.2 Enzyme-substrate complex formation.

During an enzyme-controlled reaction, the enzyme and substrate come together to form a new molecule—the enzyme-substrate complex molecule. This molecule exists for only a very short time. During that time, activation energy is lowered and bonds are changed. The result is the formation of a new molecule or molecules called the end products of the reaction. Notice that the enzyme comes out of the reaction intact and ready to be used again.

to accomplish this job, the proper wrench must be used. Just any old tool (screwdriver or hammer) won't work! The enzyme must also physically attach itself to the substrate; therefore, there is a specific **binding site** or **attachment site** on the enzyme surface. Figure 6.3 illustrates the specificity of both wrench and enzyme. Note that the wrench and enzyme are recovered unchanged after they have been used. This means that the enzyme and wrench can be used again. Eventually, like wrenches, enzymes wear out and need to be replaced by synthesizing new ones, using the instructions provided by the cell's genes. Generally, only very small quantities of enzymes are necessary because they work so fast and can be reused.

Both enzymes and wrenches are specific in that they have a particular surface geometry or shape that matches the geometry of their respective substrates. Note that both the enzyme and wrench are flexible. The enzyme can bend or fold to fit the substrate just as the wrench, to a limited extent, can be "adjusted" to fit the nut. This is called the *induced fit hypothesis.* The fit is induced because the presence of the substrate causes the enzyme to "mold" or "adjust" itself to the substrate as the two come together. The place on the enzyme that causes a specific part of the substrate to change is called the **active site** of the enzyme, or the place on the enzyme surface where chemical bonds are formed or broken. (Note in the case illustrated in figure 6.3 that the "active site" is the same as the "binding site." This is typical of many enzymes.) This site is the place where the activation energy is lowered and the electrons are shifted to change the bonds. The active site may enable a positively charged surface to combine with the negative portion of a reactant. While the active site does mold itself to a substrate, enzymes do not have the ability to fit all substrates. Enzymes are specific to a certain substrate or group of very similar substrate molecules. One enzyme cannot speed the rate of all types of biochemical reactions. Rather, a special enzyme is required to control the rate of each type of chemical reaction occurring in an organism.

Because the enzyme is specific to both the substrate to which it can attach and the reaction that it can encourage, a unique name can be given to each enzyme. The first part of an enzyme's name is the name of the molecule to which it can become attached. The second part of the name indicates what type of reaction it facilitates. The third part of the name is "-ase," which is the ending that tells you it is an enzyme. For example, *DNA polymerase* is the name of the enzyme that attaches to the molecule DNA and is responsible for increasing its length through a polymerization reaction. However, a few enzymes (i.e., pepsin and trypsin) are still referred to by their original names. The enzyme responsible for the dehydration synthesis reactions among several glucose molecules to form glycogen is known as *glycogen synthetase.* The enzyme responsible for breaking

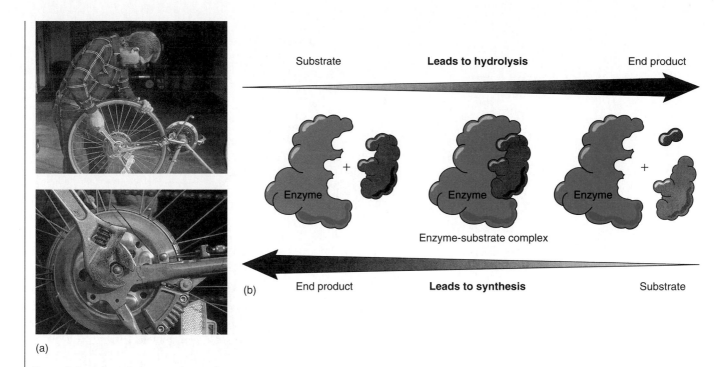

FIGURE 6.3 It fits, it's fast, and it works.
(a) While it could be done by hand, an open-end crescent wrench can be used to remove the wheel from this bicycle more efficiently. The wrench is adjusted and attached, temporarily forming a nut-bolt-wrench complex. Turning the wrench loosens the bonds holding the nut to the bolt and the two are separated. The use of the wrench makes the task much easier. Keep in mind that the same wrench that is used to disassemble the bicycle can be used to reassemble it. Enzymes function in the same way. (b) An enzyme will "adjust itself" as it attaches to its substrate, forming a temporary enzyme-substrate complex. The presence and position of the enzyme in relation to the substrate lowers the activation energy required to alter the bonds. Depending on the circumstances (what job needs to be done), the enzyme might be involved in synthesis (constructive) or hydrolysis (destructive) reactions.

the bond that attaches the amino group to the amino acid arginine is known as *arginine aminase.* When an enzyme is very common, we often shorten its formal name. The salivary enzyme involved in the digestion of starch should be *amylose* (starch) *hydrolase,* but it is generally known as *amylase.*

Certain enzymes use an additional molecule to enable them to function. This additional molecule is not a protein, but attaches to the enzyme and works with the protein catalyst to speed up a reaction. This enabling molecule is called a *coenzyme.* A **coenzyme** aids a reaction by removing one of the end products or by bringing in part of the substrate. Many coenzymes cannot be manufactured by organisms and must be obtained from their foods. Coenzymes are frequently constructed from minerals (ex., zinc, magnesium, or iron), vitamins, or nucleotides. You know that a constant small supply of vitamins in your diet is necessary for good health. The reason your cells require vitamins is to serve in the manufacture of certain coenzymes. A coenzyme can work with a variety of enzymes; therefore, you need extremely small quantities of vitamins. An example of enzyme-coenzyme cooperation is shown in figure 6.4. The metabolism of alcohol consists of a series of reactions resulting in its breakdown to carbon dioxide (CO_2), water (H_2O), and energy. During one of the reactions in this sequence, the enzyme alcohol dehydrogenase picks up hydrogen from alcohol and attaches it to NAD^+. In this reaction, NAD^+ (*n*icotinamide *a*denine *d*inucleotide, manufactured from the vitamin niacin) acts as a coenzyme because NAD^+ carries the hydrogen and electrons away from the reaction as the alcohol is broken down. The presence of the coenzyme NAD^+ is necessary for the enzyme to function properly.

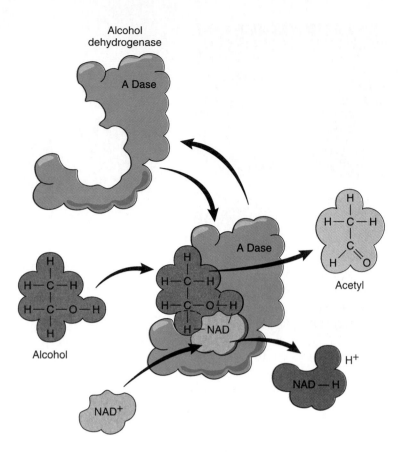

Alcohol
dehydrogenase

FIGURE 6.4 The role of coenzymes.
NAD is a coenzyme that works with the enzyme
alcohol dehydrogenase during the decomposition
of alcohol. The coenzyme carries the hydrogen
from the alcohol molecule after it is removed by
the enzyme. Notice that the hydrogen on the
alcohol is picked up by the NAD. The use of the
coenzyme NAD makes the enzyme function more
efficiently because one of the end products of this
reaction (hydrogen) is removed from the reaction
site. Because the hydrogen is no longer close to
the reacting molecules, the overall direction of the
reaction is toward the formation of acetyl. This
encourages more alcohol to be broken down.

ENVIRONMENTAL EFFECTS ON ENZYME ACTION

An enzyme forms a complex with one substrate molecule, encourages a reaction to occur, detaches itself, and then forms a complex with another molecule of the same substrate. The number of molecules of substrate that a single enzyme molecule can react with in a given time (e.g., reactions per minute) is called the **turnover number.** Sometimes the number of jobs an enzyme can perform during a particular time period is incredibly large—ranging between a thousand (10^3) and ten thousand trillion (10^{16}) times faster than uncatalyzed reactions per minute! Without the enzyme, perhaps only fifty or one hundred substrate molecules might be altered in the same time. With this in mind, let's identify the ideal conditions for an enzyme and consider how these conditions influence the turnover number.

An important environmental condition affecting enzyme-controlled reactions is temperature (figure 6.5), which has two effects on enzymes: (1) it can change the rate of molecular motion and (2) it can cause changes in the shape of an enzyme. As the temperature of an enzyme-substrate system increases, you would expect an increase in the amount of product molecules formed. This is true up to a point. The temperature at which the rate of formation of enzyme-substrate complex is fastest is termed the *optimum temperature. Optimum* means the best or most productive quantity or condition. In this case, the optimum temperature is the temperature at which the product is formed most rapidly.

As one lowers the temperature below the optimum, molecular motion slows, and the rate at which the enzyme-substrate complexes form decreases. Even though the enzyme is still able to operate, it does so very slowly. Therefore, it is possible to preserve foods for long periods by storing them in freezers or refrigerators.

When the temperature is raised above the optimum, some of the molecules of enzyme are changed in such a way that they can no longer form the enzyme-substrate complex; thus, the reaction is not encouraged. If the temperature continues to increase, more and more of the enzyme molecules will become inactive.

FIGURE 6.5 The effect of temperature on the turnover number.

As the temperature increases, the rate of the enzymatic reaction increases. The increasing temperature may increase the number of times an enzyme contacts and combines with a substrate molecule. Temperature may also influence the shape of the enzyme molecule, making it fit better with the substrate. At certain temperatures, the enzyme molecule is irreversibly changed so that it can no longer function as an enzyme. At that point, it has been denatured. Notice that the enzyme represented in this graph has an optimum (best) temperature range of between 30°C and 45°C.

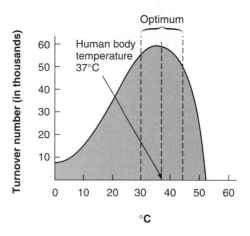

When heat is applied to an enzyme, it causes permanent changes in the three-dimensional shape of the molecule. The surface geometry of the enzyme molecule will not be recovered, even when the temperature is reduced. We can again use the wrench analogy. When a wrench is heated above a certain temperature, the metal begins to change shape. The shape of the wrench is changed permanently so that even if the temperature is reduced, the surface geometry of the end of the wrench is permanently lost. When this happens to an enzyme, we say that it has been *denatured*. A **denatured** enzyme is one whose protein structure has been permanently changed so that it has lost its original biochemical properties. Because enzymes are molecules and are not alive, they are not "killed," but denatured. Although egg white is not an enzyme, it is a protein and provides a common example of what happens when denaturation occurs as a result of heating. As heat is applied to the egg white, it is permanently changed (denatured).

Another environmental condition that influences enzyme action is pH. The three-dimensional structure of a protein leaves certain side chains exposed. These side chains may attract ions from the environment. Under the right conditions, a group of positively charged hydrogen ions may accumulate on certain parts of an enzyme. In an environment that lacked these hydrogen ions, this would not happen. Thus, variation in the most effective shape of the enzyme could be caused by a change in the number of hydrogen ions present in the solution. Because the environmental pH is so important in determining the shapes of protein molecules, there is an optimum pH for each specific enzyme. The enzyme will fit with the substrate only when it is at the proper pH. Many enzymes function best at the pH close to neutral (7.0). However, a number of enzymes perform best at pHs quite different from seven. Pepsin, an enzyme found in the stomach, works well at an acid pH of 1.5 to 2.2, while arginase, an enzyme in the liver, works well at a basic pH of 9.5 to 9.9 (figure 6.6).

In addition to temperature and pH, the concentration of enzymes, substrates, and products influences the rates of enzymatic reactions. Although the enzyme and the substrate are in contact with one another for only a short period of time, when there are huge numbers of substrate molecules it may happen that all the enzymes present are always occupied by substrate molecules. When this occurs, the rate of product formation cannot be increased unless the number of enzymes is increased. Cells can actually do this by synthesizing more enzymes. However, just because there are more enzyme molecules does not mean that any one enzyme molecule will be working any faster. The turnover number for each enzyme stays the same. As the enzyme concentration increases, the amount of product formed increases in a specified time. A greater number of enzymes are turning over substrates; they are not turning over substrates faster. Similarly, if enzyme numbers are decreased, the amount of product formed declines.

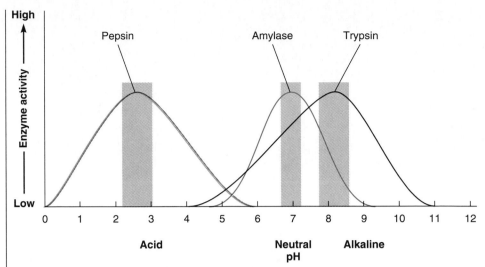

Figure 6.6 The effect of pH on the turnover number.
As the pH changes, the rate of the enzymatic reaction changes. The ions in solution alter the environment of the enzyme's active site and the overall shape of the enzyme. The enzymes illustrated here are amylase, pepsin, and trypsin. Amylase is found in saliva and is responsible for hydrolyzing starch to glucose. Pepsin is found in the stomach and hydrolyzes protein. Trypsin is produced in the pancreas and enters the small intestine, where it also hydrolyzes protein. Notice that each enzyme has its own pH range of activity, the optimum (shown in the color bars) being different for each.

We can also look at this from the point of view of the substrate. If substrate is in short supply, enzymes may have to wait for a substrate molecule to become available. Under these conditions, as the amount of substrate increases, the amount of product formed increases. The increase in product is the result of more substrates available to be changed. If there is a very large amount of substrate, even a small amount of enzyme can eventually change all the substrate to product; it will just take longer. Decreasing the amount of substrate results in reduced product formation because some enzymes will go for long periods without coming in contact with a substrate molecule.

CELLULAR CONTROLLING PROCESSES AND ENZYMES

In any cell there are thousands of kinds of enzymes. Each controls specific chemical reactions and is sensitive to changing environmental conditions such as pH and temperature. In order for a cell to stay alive in an ever-changing environment, its innumerable biochemical reactions must be controlled. **Control processes** are mechanisms that ensure that an organism will carry out all metabolic activities in the proper sequence (coordination) and at the proper rate (regulation). *Coordination* of enzymatic activities in a cell results when specific reactions occur in a given sequence; for example, $A \rightarrow B \rightarrow C \rightarrow D \rightarrow E$. This ensures that a particular nutrient will be converted to a particular end product that is necessary to the survival of the cell. Should a cell not be able to coordinate its reactions, essential products might be produced at the wrong time or never be produced at all, and the cell would die. *Regulation* of biochemical reactions refers to how a cell controls the amount of chemical product produced. The old expression "having too much of a good thing" applies to this situation. For example, if a cell manufactures too much lipid, the presence of those molecules could interfere with other life-sustaining reactions, resulting in the death of the cell. On the other hand, if a cell does not produce enough of an essential molecule, such as a digestive enzyme, it might also die. The cellular control process involves both enzymes and genes.

Keep in mind that any one substrate may be acted upon by several different enzymes. While these different enzymes may all combine with the same substrate, they do not all have the same chemical effect on the substrate, each converting the

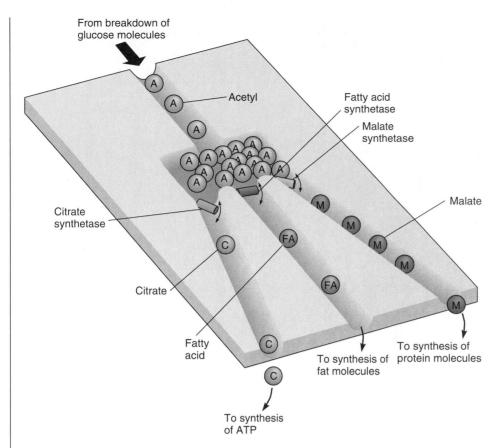

From breakdown of
glucose molecules

Acetyl

Fatty acid
synthetase

Malate
synthetase

Malate

Citrate
synthetase

Citrate

Fatty
acid

To synthesis of
fat molecules

To synthesis of
protein molecules

To synthesis
of ATP

Figure 6.7 *Enzymatic competition.*
Acetyl can serve as a substrate for a number of different reactions. Whether it becomes a fatty acid, malate, or citrate is determined by the enzymes present. Each of the three enzymes may be thought of as being in competition for the same substrate—the acetyl molecule. The cell can partially control which end product will be produced in the greatest quantity by producing greater numbers of one kind of enzyme and fewer of the other kind. If citrate synthetase is present in the highest quantity, more of the acetyl substrate will be acted upon by that enzyme and converted to citrate rather than to the other two end products, malate and fatty acids. The illustration represents the action of each enzyme as an "enzyme gate."

substrate to different end products. For example, acetyl is a substrate that can be acted upon by three different enzymes: citrate synthetase, fatty acid synthetase, and malate synthetase (figure 6.7). Which enzyme has the greatest success depends on the number of each type of enzyme available and the suitability of the environment for the enzyme's operation. The enzyme that is present in the greatest number, and/or is best suited to the job in the environment of the cell wins, and the amount of its end product becomes greatest. Whenever there are several different enzymes available to combine with a given substrate, **enzymatic competition** results. For example, the use a cell makes of the substrate molecule acetyl is directly controlled by the amount and kinds of enzymes it produces. The number and kinds of enzymes produced are regulated by the cell's genes. It is the job of chemical messengers to inform the genes as to whether specific enzyme-producing genes should be turned on or off or whether they should have their protein-producing activities increased or decreased. Such chemical messengers are called **gene-regulator proteins.** Gene-regulator proteins that decrease protein production are called *gene-repressor proteins,* while those that increase protein production are *gene-activator proteins.* Returning to our example, if the cell is in need of protein, the acetyl could be metabolized to

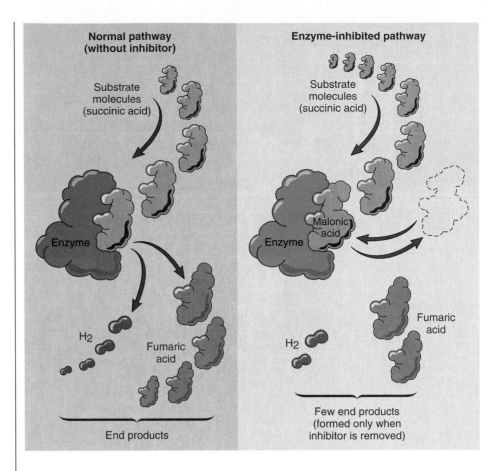

Normal pathway (without inhibitor)

Substrate molecules (succinic acid)

Enzyme

H₂

Fumaric acid

End products

Enzyme-inhibited pathway

Substrate molecules (succinic acid)

Malonic acid

Enzyme

H₂

Fumaric acid

Few end products (formed only when inhibitor is removed)

FIGURE 6.8 *Enzymatic inhibition.*
The left-hand side of the illustration shows the normal functioning of the enzyme. On the right-hand side, the enzyme is unable to function. This is because an inhibitor, malonic acid, is attached to the enzyme and prevents the enzyme from forming the normal complex with succinic acid. As long as malonic acid is present, the enzyme will be unable to function. If the malonic acid is removed, the enzyme will begin to function normally again. Its attachment to the inhibitor in this case is not permanent but has the effect of reducing the number of product molecules from per unit of time.

provide one of the building blocks for the construction of protein by turning up the production of the enzyme malate synthetase. If the cell requires energy to move or grow, more acetyl can be metabolized to release this energy by producing more citrate synthetase. When the enzyme fatty acid synthetase outcompetes the other two, the acetyl is used in fat production and storage.

Another method of controlling the synthesis of many molecules within a cell is called **negative-feedback inhibition.** This control process occurs within an enzyme-controlled reaction sequence. As the number of end products increases, some product molecules *feed back* to one of the previous reactions and have a *negative* effect on the enzyme controlling that reaction; i.e., they *inhibit* or prevent that enzyme from performing at its best. Since the end product can no longer be produced at the same rapid rate, its concentration falls. When there are too few end-product molecules to feed back and cease their inhibition, the enzyme resumes its previous optimum rate of operation, and the end-product concentration begins to increase. This also helps regulate the number of end products formed but does not involve the genes.

In addition, the operation of enzymes can be influenced by the presence of other molecules. An **inhibitor** is a molecule that attaches itself to an enzyme and interferes with its ability to form an enzyme-substrate complex (figure 6.8). One of the early kinds of pesticides used to spray fruit trees contained arsenic. The arsenic attached itself to insect enzymes and inhibited the normal growth and reproduction of insects. Organophosphates are pesticides that inhibit several enzymes necessary for the operation of the nervous system. When they are incorporated into nerve cells, they disrupt normal nerve transmission and cause the death of the affected organisms. In humans, death due to pesticides is usually caused by uncontrolled muscle contractions, resulting in breathing failure.

Some inhibitors have a shape that closely resembles the normal substrate of the enzyme. The enzyme is unable to distinguish the inhibitor from the normal substrate and so it combines with either or both. As long as the inhibitor is combined with an enzyme, the enzyme is ineffective in its normal role. Some of these enzyme-inhibitor complexes are permanent. An inhibitor removes a specific enzyme as a functioning part of the cell: the reaction that enzyme catalyzes no longer occurs, and none of the product is formed. This is termed **competitive inhibition** because the inhibitor molecule competes with the normal substrate for the active site of the enzyme.

We use enzyme inhibition to control disease. The sulfa drugs (sulfonamides) are used to control a variety of bacteria, such as the bacterium *Streptococcus pyogenes*, the cause of strep throat and scarlet fever. The drug resembles one of the bacterium's necessary substrates and so prevents some of the cell's enzymes from producing an essential cell component. As a result, the bacterial cell dies because its normal metabolism is not maintained.

SUMMARY

Enzymes are protein catalysts that speed up the rate of chemical reactions without any significant increase in the temperature. They do this by lowering activation energy. Enzymes have a very specific structure that matches the structure of particular substrate molecules. Actually, the substrate molecule comes in contact with only a specific part of the enzyme molecule—the attachment site. The active site of the enzyme is the place where the substrate molecule is changed. The enzyme-substrate complex reacts to form the end product. The protein nature of enzymes makes them sensitive to environmental conditions, such as temperature and pH, that change the structure of proteins. The number and kinds of enzymes are ultimately controlled by the genetic information of the cell. Other kinds of molecules, such as coenzymes, inhibitors, or competing enzymes, can influence specific enzymes. Changing conditions within the cell shift the enzymatic priorities of the cell by influencing the turnover number.

QUESTIONS

1. What is the difference between a catalyst and an enzyme?
2. Describe the sequence of events in an enzyme-controlled reaction.
3. How does changing temperature affect the rate of an enzyme-controlled reaction?
4. Would you expect a fat and a sugar molecule to be acted upon by the same enzyme? Why or why not?
5. What factors in the cell can speed up or slow down enzyme reactions?
6. What is the turnover number? Why is it important?
7. What is the relationship between vitamins and coenzymes?
8. What is enzyme competition, and why is it important to all cells?
9. What effect might a change in pH have on enzyme activity?
10. Where in a cell would you look for enzymes?

activation energy (ak″tī-va′shun en′ur-je) Energy required to start a reaction.

active site (ak′tiv sīt) The place on the enzyme that causes the substrate to change.

attachment site (uh-tatch′munt sīt) A specific point on the surface of the enzyme where it can physically attach itself to the substrate; also called **binding site.**

binding site (bīnding sīt) See **attachment site.**

catalyst (cat′uh-list) A chemical that speeds up a reaction but is not used up in the reaction.

coenzyme (ko-en′zīm) A molecule that works with an enzyme to enable the enzyme to function as a catalyst.

competitive inhibition (kum-pet′ĭ-tiv in″hĭ-bĭ′shun) The formation of a temporary enzyme-inhibitor complex that interferes with the normal formation of enzyme-substrate complexes, resulting in a decreased turnover.

control processes (kon-trol pro′ses-es) Mechanisms that ensure that an organism will carry out all metabolic activities in the proper sequence (coordination) and at the proper rate (regulation).

denature (de-nā′chur) To permanently change the protein structure of an enzyme so that it loses its ability to function.

enzymatic competition (en-zi-mă′tik com-pĕ-tī′shun) Competition among several different available enzymes to combine with a given substrate material.

enzyme (en′zīm) A specific protein that acts as a catalyst to speed the rate of a reaction.

enzyme-substrate complex (en′zīm-sub′strāt kom′pleks) A temporary molecule formed when an enzyme attaches itself to a substrate molecule.

gene-regulator proteins (jēn-reg′yu-la-tor pro′te-ins) Chemical messengers within a cell that inform the genes as to whether protein-producing genes should be turned on or off or whether they should have their protein-producing activities increased or decreased; for example, gene-repressor proteins and gene-activator proteins.

inhibitor (in-hib′ĭ-tor) A molecule that temporarily attaches itself to an enzyme, thereby interfering with the enzyme's ability to form an enzyme-substrate complex.

negative-feedback inhibition (neg′ă-tiv-fēd′băk in″hĭ-bĭ′shun) A metabolic control process that operates at the surfaces of enzymes. This process occurs when one of the end products of the pathway alters the three-dimensional shape of an essential enzyme in the pathway and interferes with its operation long enough to slow its action.

nutrients (nu′tre-ents) Molecules required by organisms for growth, reproduction, and/or repair.

substrate (sub′strāt) A reactant molecule with which the enzyme combines.

turnover number (turn′o-ver num′ber) The number of molecules of substrate that a single molecule of enzyme can react within a given time.

Biochemical Pathways

CHAPTER OUTLINE

PURPOSE

This chapter deals with how cells use chemical reactions to obtain and use energy, and how molecules can be altered and used as building materials. These chemical reactions are linked to one another in very specific ways. The series of changes a molecule undergoes from the beginning to the end of a particular chemical process is called a *biochemical pathway*.

There are hundreds of such pathways, all of which interlink, but we will deal only with those that form the core of all chemical reactions in a living cell—cellular respiration and some examples of alternative pathways.

CLINICAL VIEWPOINT

Anorexia nervosa is a nutritional deficiency disease characterized by severe, prolonged weight loss. An anorexic person's fear of becoming overweight is so intense that even though weight loss occurs, it does not lessen the fear of obesity. Anorexics continue to diet, even refusing to maintain the optimum body weight for their age, sex, and height. Anorexic individuals starve themselves to death. This nutritional deficiency disease is thought to stem from sociocultural factors. Our society's preoccupation with weight loss and the desirability of being thin strongly influence this disorder. Just turn on your television or radio, or look at newspapers, magazines, or billboards and you can see how our culture encourages people to be thin. Male and female models are thin. Muscle protein is considered to be healthy, and fat to be unhealthy. Unless you are thin, so the ads imply, you will never be popular, get a date, or even marry. In fact, you

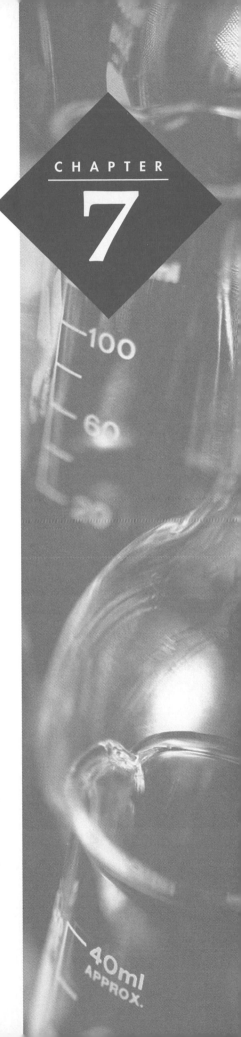

may die early. Are these prophecies self-fulfilling? Our culture's constant emphasis on being thin has influenced many people (primarily women) to lose too much weight and become anorexic. Here are some of the symptoms seen in persons with anorexia nervosa:

thin, dry brittle hair

degradation of fingernails

constipation

amenorrhea (lack of menstrual periods)

decreased heart rate

loss of body proteins

weaker heartbeat

calcium deficiency

osteoporosis

hypothermia (low body temperature)

hypotension (low blood pressure)

increased skin pigmentation

reduction in size of uterus

inflammatory bowel disease

slowed reflexes

fainting

weakened muscles

LEARNING OBJECTIVES

- Associate the major parts of aerobic respiration with the ultrastructure of the mitochondrion
- List the raw materials and products and describe the processes involved in the three major parts of aerobic respiration
- Describe the processes involved in the alternate pathways known as anaerobic respiration (fermentation)
- Follow a molecule through the steps of interconversion of fats, proteins, and carbohydrates
- List the six classes of nutrients
- Recognize the functions of the six types of nutrients
- Recognize the difference between a complete and incomplete protein
- Distinguish between calorie and kcalorie

ENERGY AND CELLS: CELLULAR RESPIRATION AND PHOTOSYNTHESIS

All living organisms require energy to sustain life. The source of this energy comes from the chemical bonds of molecules (figure 7.1). Burning wood is an example of a chemical reaction that results in the release of energy by breaking chemical bonds. The organic molecules of wood are broken and changed into the end products of ash, gases (ex., CO_2), water (H_2O), and energy (heat and light). Living organisms are capable of carrying out these same types of reactions but in a controlled manner. By controlling energy-releasing reactions, they are able to use the energy to power functions such as reproduction, movement, and growth. These reactions form a **biochemical pathway** when they are linked to each other. The products of one reaction are used as the reactants for another.

Organisms such as green plants, algae, and certain bacteria are capable of trapping sunlight energy and holding it in the chemical bonds of molecules such as carbohydrates. The process of converting sunlight energy to chemical-bond energy, **photosynthesis,** is a major biochemical pathway. Photosynthetic organisms

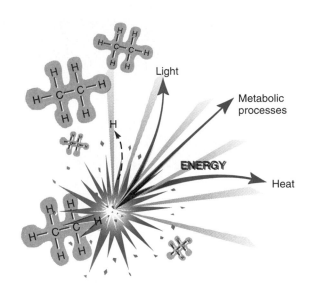

FIGURE 7.1 Life's energy: chemical bonds.

All living things utilize the energy contained in chemical bonds. As organisms decompose molecules, such as the organic molecule ethane shown in this illustration, the energy released may be used for metabolic processes such as growth and reproduction. Some organisms such as fireflies and certain bacteria are able to bioluminesce as some of this chemical bond energy is released as visible light. In all cases, there is a certain amount of heat freed from the breaking of chemical bonds.

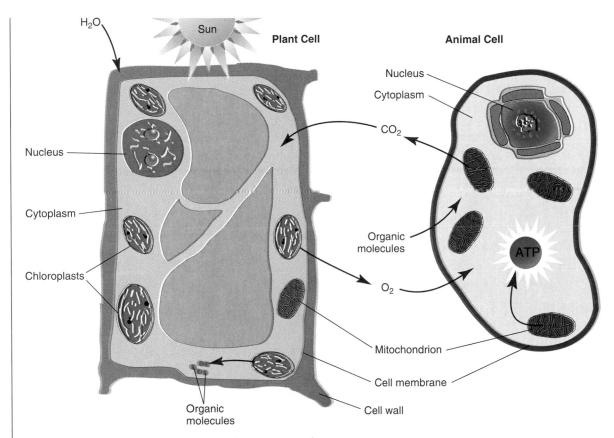

FIGURE 7.2 Biochemical pathways that involve energy transformation.

Photosynthesis and cellular respiration are a series of chemical reactions that control the flow of energy in many organisms. Organisms that contain photosynthetic machinery are capable of using light, water, and carbon dioxide to produce organic molecules such as sugars, proteins, lipids, and nucleic acids. The molecules, along with oxygen, may be used by other organisms such as animals to sustain their lives.

produce food molecules, such as carbohydrates, for themselves as well as for all the other organisms that feed on them. **Cellular respiration,** a second major biochemical pathway, is a chain of reactions during which cells release the chemical-bond energy and convert it into other usable forms (figure 7.2). All organisms must carry out cellular respiration if they are to survive. Whether organisms manufacture food or take it in from the environment, they all use chemical bond energy.

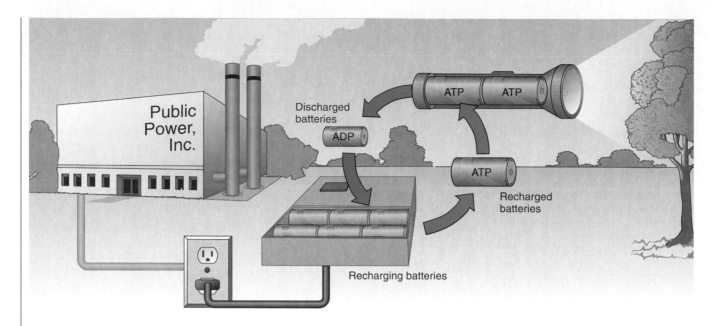

FIGURE 7.3 🔋 Just the right amount of power for the job.

When rechargeable batteries in a flashlight have been drained of their power, they can be recharged by placing them in a battery charger. This enables the right amount of power from a power plant to be packed into the batteries for reuse. Cells operate in much the same manner. When the cell's "batteries," ATP, have been drained while powering a job like muscle contraction, the discharged "batteries," ADP, can be recharged back to full ATP power.

GENERATING ENERGY IN A USEFUL FORM: ATP

Photosynthesis and cellular respiration consist of many steps. If the products of a reaction do not have the same amount of energy as the reactants, energy has either been released or added in the reaction. Some chemical reactions—like cellular respiration—may have a net release of energy, whereas others—like photosynthesis—require an input of energy.

To transfer the right amount of chemical-bond energy from energy-releasing to energy-requiring reactions, cells use the molecule ATP. **Adenosine *tri*phosphate (ATP)** is a handy source of the right amount of usable chemical-bond energy. Each ATP molecule used in the cell is like a rechargeable AAA battery used to power small toys and electronic equipment. Each contains just the right amount of energy to power the job. When the power has been drained, it can be recharged numerous times before it must be recycled. Recharging the AAA battery requires getting a small amount of energy from a source of high energy such as a hydroelectric power plant (figure 7.3). Energy from the electric plant is too powerful to directly run a small flashlight or portable tape recorder. If you plugged your recorder directly into the power plant, the recorder would be destroyed. However, the recharged AAA battery delivers just the right amount of energy at the right time and place. ATP functions in much the same manner. After the chemical-bond energy has been drained by breaking one of its bonds:

$$ATP \rightarrow ADP + P + Energy$$

A) used to power chemical reactions

B) lost as heat to the environment

the discharged molecule (ADP) is recharged by "plugging it in" to a high-powered energy source. This source may be (1) sunlight (photosynthesis) or (2) chemical-bond energy (released from cellular respiration from carbohydrates and fats):

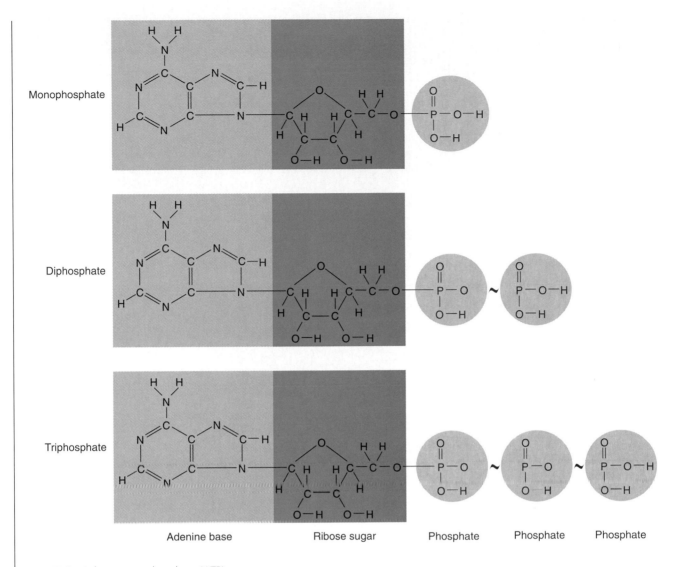

Monophosphate

Diphosphate

Triphosphate

Adenine base   Ribose sugar   Phosphate   Phosphate   Phosphate

FIGURE 7.4 Adenosine triphosphate (ATP).
A macromolecule of ATP consists of a molecule of adenine, a molecule of ribose, and three phosphate groups. The two end phosphate groups are bonded together by high-energy bonds. When these bonds are broken, they readily release their chemical-bond energy; therefore, they are known as high-energy bonds. These bonds are represented by the curved lines. The ATP molecule is considered to be an energy carrier.

A) Sunlight (photosynthesis)

$$ADP + P + Energy \rightarrow ATP$$

B) Chemical-bond energy (cellular respiration)

An ATP molecule is formed from adenine (nitrogenous base), ribose (sugar), and phosphates (figure 7.4). These three are chemically bonded to form AMP, *adenosine monophosphate* (one phosphate). When a second phosphate group is added to the AMP, a molecule of ADP (diphosphate) is formed. The ADP, with the addition of more energy, is able to bond to a third phosphate group and form ATP. The addition of phosphate to any molecule is called a *phosphorylation reaction*.

$$X + P + Energy \rightarrow XP$$

The covalent bond that attaches the second phosphate to the AMP molecule is easily broken to release energy for energy-requiring cell processes. Because the

Box 7.1

Oxidation-Reduction (Redox) Reactions in a Nutshell

The most important characteristic of **redox** (*reduction + oxidation*) reactions is that energy-containing electrons are transferred from one molecule to another. Such reactions enable cells to produce useful chemical-bond energy in the form of ATP (in cellular respiration), and to synthesize the energy-containing bonds of carbohydrates (in photosynthesis). Oxidation means the loss of electrons, and reduction means the gain of electrons. (Do not associate oxidation with oxygen; many different elements may enter into redox reactions. Do not associate reduction with weight loss. In this situation, to become reduced actually means to gain something.) Molecules that lose electrons (serve as electron donors) usually release this chemical-bond energy and are broken down into more simple molecules. Molecules that gain electrons (serve as electron acceptors) usually gain electron energy and are enlarged, forming a more complex molecule (box figure 7.1). Because electrons cannot exist apart from the atomic nucleus for a long period, both oxidation and reduction occur in a redox reaction; whenever an electron is donated, it is quickly gained by another molecule. A simple way to help identify a redox reaction is to use the mnemonic device, "LEO the lion says GER." LEO stands for "Loss of Electrons is Oxidation"; and GER stands for "Gain of Electrons is Reduction."

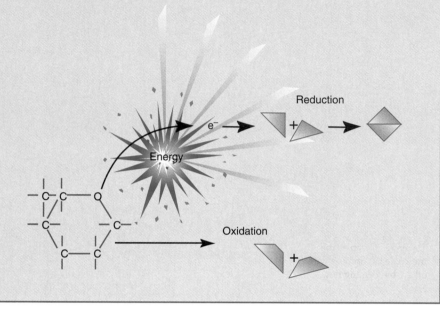

energy in this bond is so easy for a cell to use, it is called a **high-energy phosphate bond.** ATP has two high-energy phosphate bonds represented by curved solid lines. Both ADP and ATP, because they contain high-energy bonds, are very unstable molecules and readily lose their phosphates. When this occurs, the energy held in the high-energy bonds of the phosphate can be transferred to another molecule or released to the environment. Within a cell, enzymes speed this release of energy as ATP is broken down to ADP and P. ATP is used as the primary source of chemical-bond energy in cells.

UNDERSTANDING ENERGY TRANSFORMATION REACTIONS: OXIDATION-REDUCTION AND CELLULAR RESPIRATION

This equation summarizes the chemical reactions humans and many other organisms use to extract energy from the carbohydrate, glucose:

$$C_6H_{12}O_6 + 6\ O_2 + 6\ H_2O^* \rightarrow 6\ CO_2 + 12\ H_2O + \text{Energy (ATP + heat)}$$

This is known as aerobic cellular respiration, an oxidation-reduction reaction process. **Aerobic cellular respiration** is a specific series of chemical reactions involving the use of molecular oxygen (O_2) in which chemical-bond energy is released to the cell in the form of ATP. **Oxidation-reduction reactions** are electron transfer reactions in which the molecules losing electrons become oxidized and those gaining electrons become reduced (box 7.1). *Don't panic!* It is not difficult to understand if you think about it in simple terms.

---

*These H_2O molecules are added at various reaction points from the cytoplasm.

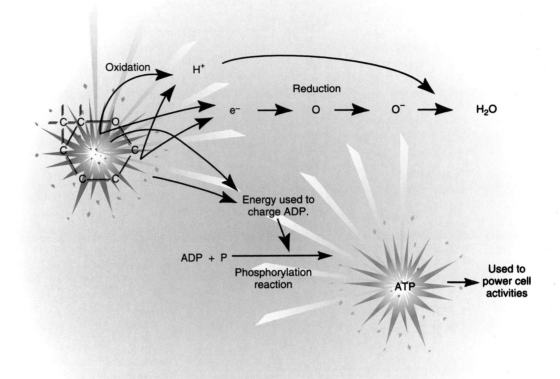

FIGURE 7.5 Oxidation-reduction (redox) reactions. During an oxidation-reduction reaction, a large molecule loses its electrons. This is the "oxidation" portion of the reaction. When the electrons are removed, the large molecule is unable to stay together and breaks into smaller units. The energy released during oxidation can be used to power cell activities such as the manufacture of sugars, fats, and nucleic acids. It may also be used to move molecules through cell membranes or contract muscle fibers. The reduction part of the reaction occurs when the electrons are picked up by another molecule. When they are acquired, it enables the molecule to combine with others by forming new bonds. Thus, during the reduction part of the reaction, new large molecules are formed.

Covalent bonds in the sugar glucose contain potential energy. Since this molecule contains more bonds than any of the other molecules listed in the equation, it contains the greatest amount of potential energy. That is, sugar contains more potential energy than oxygen, water, or carbon dioxide. (Which would you rather have for lunch?) The covalent bonds of glucose are formed by sharing pairs of fast-moving, energetic electrons. Of all the covalent bonds in glucose (H–O, H–C, C–C), those easiest to get at are on the outside of the molecule. If we could get the hydrogen electrons off glucose, their energy could be used to phosphorylate ADP molecules producing ATP. The ATP could be used to power the metabolic activities of the cell. The chemical reaction that results in the loss of electrons from this molecule is the *oxidation* part of this reaction. However, there are problems with removing the hydrogen electrons.

First, these high-energy electrons must be controlled since they could be dangerous. If they were allowed to fly about at random, they could combine with other molecules and cause cell death. They must be "handled" carefully! Once energy has been removed for ATP production, the electrons must be placed in a safe place. In *aerobic* cellular respiration, these electrons are attached to oxygen. Oxygen serves as the final resting place of the hydrogen electrons. When the electrons are added to oxygen, it becomes a negatively charged ion, $O^=$. This is the *reduction* portion of the reaction. Reduction occurs when electrons are gained by a molecule. *So, in the aerobic cellular respiration of glucose, glucose is oxidized and oxygen is reduced.* One cannot occur without the other (figure 7.5). If something is oxidized, something else must be reduced. A cell cannot simply lose its electrons; they have to go someplace!

Box 7.2

Mole Theory—It's Not What You Think!

In real life it is unreasonable to follow a chemical reaction on an atom-by-atom basis. Therefore, the formulas do not represent individual numbers of molecules but considerably larger amounts. The whole numbers that appear before the chemical formula in an equation describe how many *moles* of the compound are involved in the reaction. A *mole* is 6.023×10^{23} objects; i.e.,

602,300,000,000,000,000,000,000 items!

A mole of pencils would contain $6.023 ¥ 1023$ pencils. A mole of pop cans would be $6.023 ¥ 1023$ cans.

In a chemical reaction, this number of objects is equal to the atomic or molecular mass in grams. For example, a mole of hydrogen atoms (H) contains 6.023×10^{23} atoms of hydrogen. A mole of glucose contains 6.023×10^2 molecules of glucose. The number 6.023×10^{23} is known as Avogadro's number, after its discoverer. With respect to aerobic cellular respiration in humans,

$$C_6H_{12}O_6 + 6\ O_2 + 6\ H_2O \rightarrow 6\ CO_2 + 12\ H_2O +$$
$$36\ ATP + Heat$$

The number preceding each formula tells the number of moles of each substance. Therefore, we are really not talking about the number of individual molecules being respired, but the number of moles of each substance being respired! In this case there are:

$1 \times 6.023 \times 10^{23}$ molecules of $C_6H_{12}O_6$
$6 \times 6.023 \times 10^{23}$ molecules of O_2
$6 \times 6.023 \times 10^{23}$ molecules of H_2O
$6 \times 6.023 \times 10^{23}$ molecules of CO_2

being metabolized to produce 36 moles of ATP! How does this measure up on a scale? It amounts to:

180 grams of $C_6H_{12}O_6$ = molecular weight of $C_6H_{12}O_6$ × 1 mole = 0.5 cup
192 grams of O_2 = molecular weight of O_2 × 6 moles = 67 2-liter pop bottles of oxygen!
108 grams of H_2O (net) = molecular weight of H_2O × 6 moles = 0.45 cup
264 grams of CO_2 = molecular weight of CO_2 × 6 moles = 67 2-liter pop bottles

These are sizable amounts of food and water! How do these numbers compare to those noted on the nutrition labels of some of your snack foods?

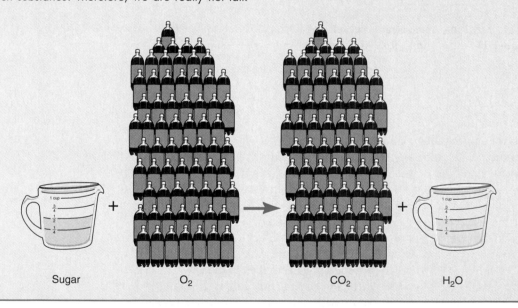

Sugar   + O_2 → CO_2 + H_2O

The second problem that occurs when electrons are removed from the glucose relates to what's left of the hydrogen atoms; i.e., the protons, (H⁺). As more and more electrons are removed from the glucose (oxidized) to power the phosphorylation of ADP (charge batteries), there is an increase in the hydrogen ion concentration. The pH of the cytoplasm decreases. This could also be fatal to the cell. However, this is controlled since these H⁺ ions can easily combine with the O⁼ ions to form molecules of harmless water, H_2O.

What happens to the remaining molecule of glucose? Once the hydrogens have all been stripped off, the remaining carbon and oxygen atoms are rearranged to form molecules of CO_2. The oxidation-reduction reaction is complete. All of the hydrogen originally a part of the glucose has been moved to the oxygen to form

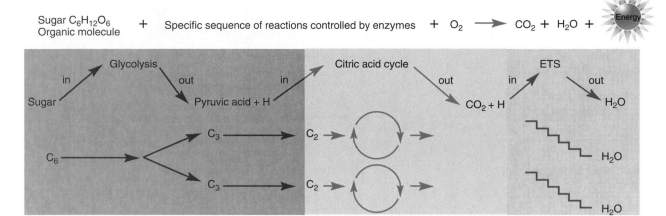

$$\text{Sugar } C_6H_{12}O_6 \text{ Organic molecule} + \text{Specific sequence of reactions controlled by enzymes} + O_2 \longrightarrow CO_2 + H_2O + \text{Energy}$$

FIGURE 7.6 Level 1 Aerobic cellular respiration.

This sequence of reactions in the aerobic oxidation of glucose is an overview of the energy-yielding reactions of a cell. The first top line presents the respiratory process in its most basic form. The next two lines expand on the generalized statement and illustrate how sugar (glucose) moves through a complex series of reactions to produce usable energy (ATP). Note that both CO_2 and H are products of the citric acid cycle, but only the H enters the ETS.

water. All of the remaining carbon and oxygen atoms of the original glucose are now in the form of CO_2. The total amount of energy released from this process is enough to generate 38 ATP molecules in prokaryotic (bacterial) cells and 36 ATPs in eukaryotic (human) cells (box 7.2).

> *The sections on aerobic cellular respiration are divided into levels from the most basic (level 1) to the more complex (level 3). Be sure to consult your instructor for the level that is required for your course of study.*

Level 1

In eukaryotic cells the process of releasing energy from food molecules begins in the cytoplasm and is completed in the mitochondrion. The mitochondrial enzymes allow for the step-by-step conversion of glucose into the smaller carbon dioxide and water molecules. The major parts of the cellular respiration process are:

1. **Glycolysis** (*glyco* = carbohydrate; *lys* = splitting; *sis* = the process of) breaks the 6-carbon sugar (glucose) into two smaller 3-carbon molecules of pyruvic acid; ATP is produced. Hydrogens and their electrons are sent to the electron-transport system (ETS) for processing.

2. The **Krebs cycle** removes the remaining hydrogen, electrons, and carbon from pyruvic acid. ATP is produced for cell use. The hydrogens and their electrons are sent to the ETS for processing.

3. The **electron-transport system (ETS)** converts the kinetic energy of hydrogen electrons to the high-energy phosphate bonds of ATP, while the hydrogen ions and electrons are bonded with oxygen to form water (figure 7.6).

Level 2

Glycolysis takes place in the cytoplasm. During glycolysis, a six-carbon sugar molecule (glucose) is encouraged to break down by being energized by two ATP molecules. Adding this energy makes some of the bonds unstable. The broken bonds ultimately release enough chemical-bond energy to recharge four ATP molecules. Enzymes speed these oxidation-reduction reactions. Since two ATP

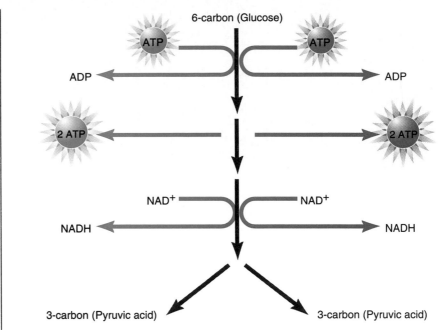

6-carbon (Glucose)

ATP   ATP

ADP   ADP

2 ATP   2 ATP

NAD⁺   NAD⁺

NADH   NADH

3-carbon (Pyruvic acid)   3-carbon (Pyruvic acid)

FIGURE 7.7 Level 2 Glycolysis.

Glycolysis is the biochemical pathway many organisms use to oxidize glucose. During this sequence of chemical reactions, the 6-carbon molecule of glucose is oxidized.

$C_6H_{12}O_6$ (glucose) →

2 $CH_3COCOOH$ (pyruvic acid) + 2 NADH + Energy (2 ATP and heat)

molecules were used to start the reaction and four were produced, there is a net gain of two ATPs from the glycolytic pathway. The sugar is broken down (oxidized) into two three-carbon molecules of **pyruvic acid** (figure 7.7). During glycolysis, the hydrogen ions are not directly added to (reduce) oxygen to form water. Since O_2 is not used as a hydrogen ion and electron acceptor in glycolysis, this pathway is called **anaerobic** (*an-* = without). Instead, the hydrogen ions and electrons are picked up by special carrier molecules known as **NAD⁺** (**nico-tinamide** *adenine* *dinucleotide*). The reduced molecules of NAD⁺ (NADH)* contain a large amount of potential energy that can be used to make ATP in later chemical reactions. The job of NAD⁺ is to safely transport these energy-containing electrons and protons to their final resting place, oxygen. Once they have dropped off their load in the ETS, the NAD⁺ returns to repeat the job.

In summary, the process of glycolysis takes place in the cytoplasm of a cell, where glucose enters a series of reactions that:
1. requires the use of two ATPs,
2. ultimately results in the formation of four ATPs,
3. results in the formation of two NADH, and
4. results in the formation of two molecules of pyruvic acid.

Since two molecules of ATP are used to start the process and a total of four ATPs are generated, each glucose molecule that undergoes glycolysis produces a net yield of two ATPs. Furthermore, the process of glycolysis does not require the presence of oxygen molecules (O_2).

After glucose has been broken down into two pyruvic acid molecules, they are converted into two smaller molecules called acetyl. During the Krebs cycle (figure 7.8), the acetyl is completely oxidized inside the mitochondrion of human cells. In bacteria, this occurs in the cytoplasm. The rest of the hydrogens on the

---

*NADH is actually NADH + H⁺.

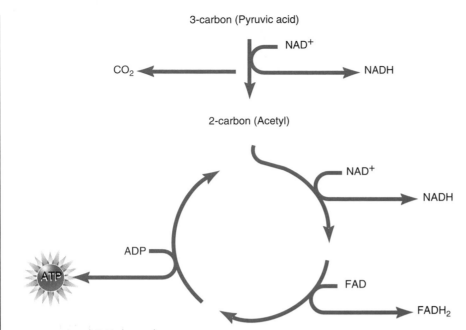

FIGURE 7.8   Level 2 Krebs cycle.

The Krebs cycle is the biochemical pathway performed by some cells to complete the oxidation of glucose. During this sequence of chemical reactions, the pyruvic acid molecules produced from glycolysis are stripped of their hydrogens. The hydrogens are picked up by NAD^+ and FAD for transport to the ETS. The remaining atoms are reorganized into molecules of carbon dioxide. Enough energy is released during the Krebs cycle to charge two ADP molecules to form 2 ATPs.

$$2 \text{ CH}_3\text{COCOOH (pyruvic acid)} \rightarrow$$
$$6 \text{ CO}_2 + 8 \text{ NADH} + 2 \text{ FADH}_2 + \text{Energy (2 ATP + heat)}$$

acetyl molecule are removed and sent to the ETS. The remaining carbon and oxygen atoms are recombined to form CO_2. As in glycolysis, enough energy is released to generate two ATP molecules and the hydrogen ions and electrons are carried to the ETS on NAD^+ and another carrier called **FAD (flavin adenine dinucleotide).** At the end of the Krebs cycle, the acetyl has been completely broken down (oxidized) to CO_2. The energy in the molecule has either been transferred to ATP, NADH, or $FADH_2$. And don't forget, some of the energy has been released as heat.

In summary, the Krebs cycle takes place within the mitochondria. For each pyruvic acid molecule that enters a mitochondrion and is processed through the Krebs cycle:
1. the three carbons of the pyruvic acid are released as carbon dioxide (CO_2),
2. five pairs of hydrogens become attached to hydrogen carriers (four NADH and one $FADH_2$), and
3. one ATP is generated.

Cells generate the greatest amount of ATP from the ETS (figure 7.9). During this step-wise sequence of oxidation-reduction reactions, the energy from the NADH and $FADH_2$ molecules generated in glycolysis and the Krebs cycle is used to recharge the cells' batteries. In a process called *chemiosmosis,* the energy needed to form the high-energy phosphate bonds of ATP comes from electrons that are rich in kinetic energy (figure 7.10). The processes that result in the formation of ATP occur on the membranes of the mitochondrion. Iron-containing *cytochrome* (*cyto* = cell; *chrom* = color) molecules are located on these membranes. The energy-rich electrons are passed (*transported*) from one cytochrome to another, and the energy is used to pump hydrogen ions from one side of the membrane to the other. The result of this is a higher concentration of hydrogen ions on one side of

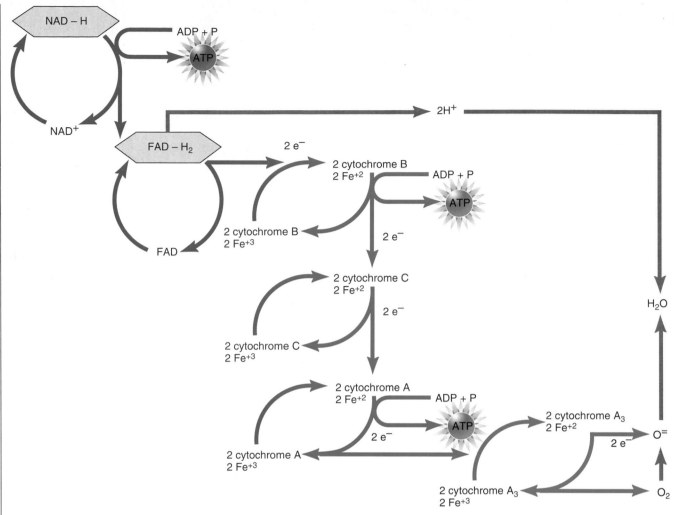

FIGURE 7.9 Level 2 The electron-transport process.

The electron-transport system (ETS) is a series of oxidation-reduction reactions also known as the cytochrome system. The movement of electrons down this biochemical "wire" establishes a kind of electrical current that drives H+ protons to atmospheric oxygen. As the electrons flow through the system, ATPs may be produced.

$$8 \text{ NADH} + 4 \text{ FADH}_2 + 6 \text{ O}_2 \rightarrow 12 \text{ H}_2\text{O} + \text{Energy (32 ATP + heat)} + 8 \text{ NAD}^+ + 4 \text{ FAD}$$

the membrane. As the concentration of hydrogen ions increases on one side, a concentration gradient is established and a "pressure" builds up. This pressure is released when a membrane channel is opened, allowing these hydrogen ions to fly back to the side from which they were pumped. As they streak through the pores an enzyme, ATPase, stimulates the formation of an ATP molecule by bonding a phosphate to an ADP molecule (phosphorylation).

In summary, the electron-transport system takes place within the mitochondrion where:
1. oxygen is used up as oxygen atoms receive the hydrogens from NADH and FADH$_2$ to form water (H$_2$O),
2. NAD$^+$ and FAD are released to be used over again, and
3. 32 ATPs are produced.

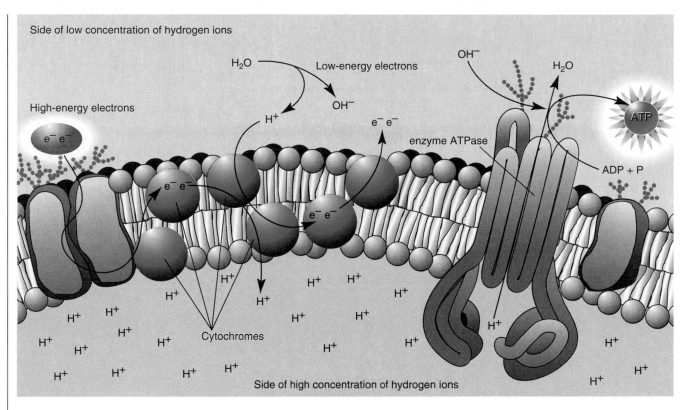

Side of low concentration of hydrogen ions

High-energy electrons

H_2O

Low-energy electrons

OH^-

H^+

OH^-

e^- e^-

OH^-

H_2O

ATP

enzyme ATPase

ADP + P

e^- e^-

e^- e^-

H^+

H^+ H^+

H^+

H^+

H^+ H^+

H^+

H^+

H^+ H^+

H^+

H^+

H^+

Cytochromes

H^+

H^+

H^+

H^+

H^+ H^+

Side of high concentration of hydrogen ions

H^+

H^+

H^+

FIGURE 7.10   Chemiosmosis.

Chemiosmosis is the process of producing ATP by using the energy of hydrogen electrons and protons removed from glucose in glycolysis and the Krebs cycle. These electrons and protons are carried to the electron transport system in the form of NADH and $FADH_2$. The process takes place in the mitochondria of a cell and requires electron transport molecules, the cytochromes. Cytochromes are located on the cristae, the inner folded membrane of the mitochondrion. Each time a pair of electrons is transported from one cytochrome to another, their energy is used to move H^+s into the space between the inner and outer mitochondrial membranes. This establishes a H^+ concentration gradient; i.e., there are more H^+s on one side of the membrane than the other. When these hydrogen ions fly back across the membrane, energy is released and used to synthesize ATP. The enzyme responsible for the phosphorylation (ATP synthetase) is located on the cristae. The electrons used in this process are added to oxygen to form negatively charged $O^=$, which combines with the H^+ to form H_2O.

Level 3

Glycolysis

The first stage of the cellular respiration process takes place in the cytoplasm. This first step, known as **glycolysis,** consists of the enzymatic breakdown of a glucose molecule without the use of molecular oxygen (figure 7.11). Because no oxygen is required, glycolysis is called an **anaerobic** process.

Some energy must be put in to start glycolysis because glucose is a very stable molecule and will not automatically break down to release energy. For each molecule of glucose entering glycolysis, energy is supplied by two ATP molecules. The energy-containing phosphates are released from two ATP molecules and become attached to glucose to form phosphorylated sugar, ($P-C_6-P$). This is a phosphorylation reaction. It is controlled by an enzyme named *phosphorylase.* The phosphorylated glucose is then broken down through several enzymatically controlled reactions into two 3-carbon compounds, each with one attached phosphate, (C_3-P). These 3-carbon compounds are *PGAL, phosphoglyceraldehyde.* Each

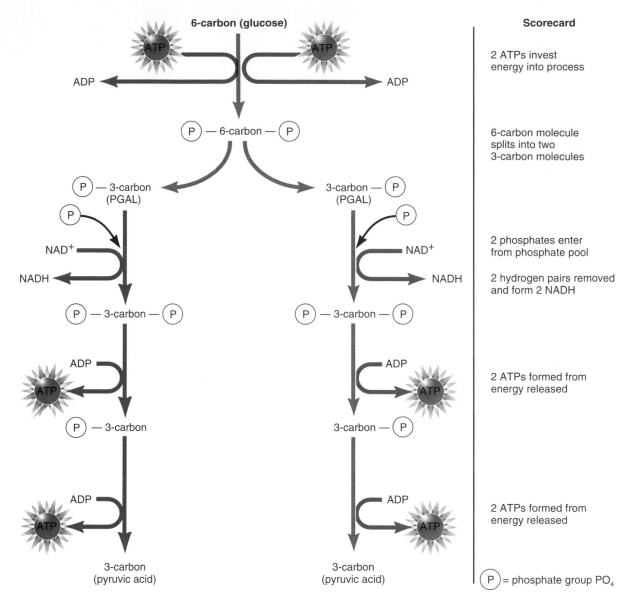

6-carbon (glucose)

2 ATPs invest
energy into process

(P) — 6-carbon — (P)

6-carbon molecule
splits into two
3-carbon molecules

(P) — 3-carbon
(PGAL)

3-carbon — (P)
(PGAL)

2 phosphates enter
from phosphate pool

NAD^+

NAD^+

NADH

NADH

2 hydrogen pairs removed
and form 2 NADH

(P) — 3-carbon — (P)

(P) — 3-carbon — (P)

ADP

ADP

2 ATPs formed from
energy released

ATP

ATP

(P) — 3-carbon

3-carbon — (P)

ADP

ADP

2 ATPs formed from
energy released

ATP

ATP

3-carbon
(pyruvic acid)

3-carbon
(pyruvic acid)

(P) = phosphate group PO_4

Figure 7.11 ▭ Level 3 Glycolysis.
The glycolytic pathway results in the breakdown of 6-carbon sugars under anaerobic conditions. Each molecule of sugar releases enough energy to produce a profit of two ATPs. In addition, two molecules of pyruvic acid and two molecules of hydrogen (carried as NADH) are produced.

Reactants	*Products*
1 glucose	2 pyruvic acid
2 ATP	2 ADP + 2 P
4 ADP + 4 P	4 ATP
$2 NAD^+ + 2 H$	2 NADH

of the two PGAL molecules acquires a second phosphate from a phosphate pool normally found in the cytoplasm. Each molecule now has two phosphates attached ($P–C_3–P$). A series of reactions follows in which energy is released by breaking chemical bonds, causing each of these 3-carbon compounds to lose their phosphates. These high-energy phosphates combine with ADP to form ATP. In addition, four hydrogen atoms detach from the carbon skeleton (oxidation) and become bonded to two hydrogen-carrier molecules (reduction) known as *NAD+*.

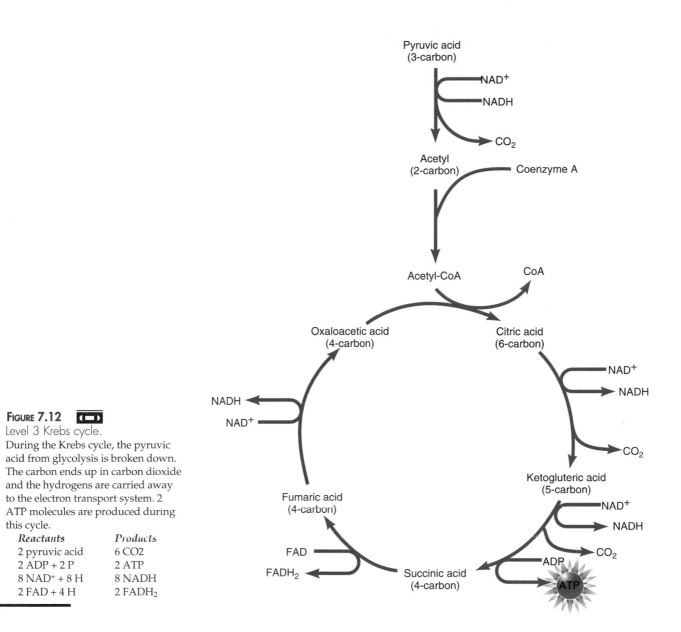

Pyruvic acid
(3-carbon)

NAD$^+$

NADH

CO_2

Acetyl
(2-carbon)

Coenzyme A

Acetyl-CoA

CoA

Oxaloacetic acid
(4-carbon)

Citric acid
(6-carbon)

NAD$^+$

NADH

NADH

NAD$^+$

CO_2

Ketogluteric acid
(5-carbon)

Fumaric acid
(4-carbon)

NAD$^+$

NADH

FAD

CO_2

FADH$_2$

ADP

Succinic acid
(4-carbon)

ATP

FIGURE 7.12

Level 3 Krebs cycle.
During the Krebs cycle, the pyruvic acid from glycolysis is broken down. The carbon ends up in carbon dioxide and the hydrogens are carried away to the electron transport system. 2 ATP molecules are produced during this cycle.

Reactants	Products
2 pyruvic acid	6 CO2
2 ADP + 2 P	2 ATP
8 NAD$^+$ + 8 H	8 NADH
2 FAD + 4 H	2 FADH$_2$

The molecules of NADH contain a large amount of potential energy that may be released in a usable form in later chemical reactions. The 3-carbon molecules that result from glycolysis are called **pyruvic acid.**

In summary, the process of glycolysis takes place in the cytoplasm of a cell. In this process, glucose undergoes reactions requiring the use of two ATPs, leading to the formation of four molecules of ATP, producing two molecules of NADH and two 3-carbon molecules of pyruvic acid.

The Krebs Cycle

The **Krebs cycle** is a series of oxidation-reduction reactions that complete the breakdown of pyruvic acid produced by glycolysis (figure 7.12). In order for pyruvic acid to be used as an energy source, it must enter the mitochondrion. Once inside, an enzyme converts the 3-carbon pyruvic acid molecule to a 2-carbon molecule called **acetyl.** When the acetyl is formed, the carbon removed is released as carbon dioxide. In addition to releasing carbon dioxide, each pyruvic acid molecule is oxidized, since it loses two hydrogens that become attached to NAD^+ molecules (reduction) to form NADH. NAD^+ is serving as a hydrogen carrier.

The carbon dioxide is a waste product that is eventually released by the cell into the atmosphere. The 2-carbon acetyl compound temporarily combines with a large molecule called *coenzyme A (CoA)* to form acetyl-CoA and transfers the acetyl to a 4-carbon compound called *oxaloacetic acid* to become part of a 6-carbon molecule. This new 6-carbon compound is broken down in a series of reactions to regenerate oxaloacetic acid in this cyclic pathway. In the process of breaking down pyruvic acid, three molecules of carbon dioxide are formed. In addition, five pairs of hydrogen are removed and become attached to hydrogen carriers. Four pairs become attached to NAD^+ and one pair becomes attached to a different hydrogen carrier known as **FAD (*f*lavin *a*denine *d*inucleotide).** As the molecules move through the Krebs cycle, enough energy is released to allow the synthesis of one ATP molecule for each acetyl that enters the cycle. The ATP is formed from ADP and a phosphate already present in the mitochondria.

For each pyruvic acid molecule that enters the mitochondrion and is processed through the Krebs cycle, three carbons are released as three carbon dioxide molecules, five pairs of hydrogen atoms are removed and become attached to hydrogen carriers, and one ATP molecule is generated. When both pyruvic acid molecules have been processed through the Krebs cycle,

1. all of the original carbons from the glucose have been released into the atmosphere as six carbon dioxide molecules,
2. all of the hydrogen originally found on the glucose has been transferred to either NAD^+ or FAD to form NADH or $FADH_2$, and
3. two ATPs have been formed from the addition of phosphates to ADPs.

The Electron-Transport System

The series of reactions in which energy is removed from the hydrogens carried by NAD^+ and FAD is known as the **electron-transport system (ETS)** (figure 7.13). This is the final stage of aerobic cellular respiration. The reactions that make up the electron-transport system are a series of oxidation-reduction reactions in which the electrons from the hydrogen atoms are passed from one electron-carrier molecule to another until they ultimately are accepted by oxygen atoms. The negatively charged oxygen combines with the hydrogen ions to form water. It is this step that makes the process aerobic. Water is released into the cytoplasm.

Let's now look at the hydrogen and its carriers in just a bit more detail to account for all of the energy that becomes available to the cell. At three points in the series of oxidation-reductions in the ETS, sufficient energy is released from the NADHs to produce an ATP molecule. Therefore, twenty-four ATPs are released from these eight pairs of hydrogen electrons carried on NADH. In eukaryotic cells, the two pairs of hydrogens released during glycolysis are carried as NADH and converted to $FADH_2$ in order to shuttle them into the mitochondria. Once they are inside the mitochondria, they follow the same pathway as the other $FADH_2$s. The four pairs of hydrogen electrons carried by FAD are lower in energy. When these hydrogen electrons go through the series of oxidation-reduction reactions, they release enough energy to produce ATP at only two points. They produce a total of eight ATPs; therefore, we have a grand total of thirty-two ATPs produced from the hydrogen electrons that enter the ETS.

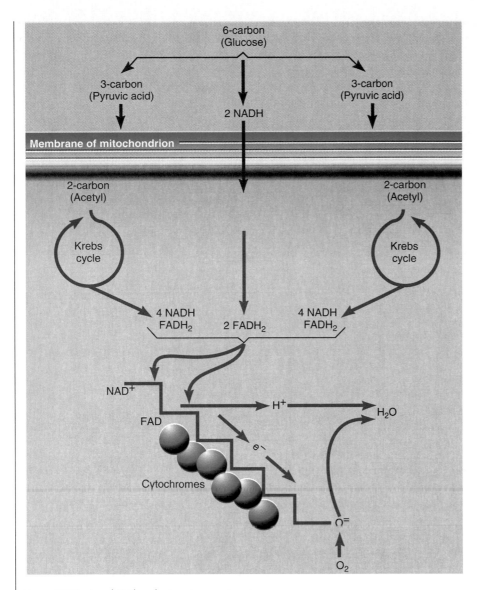

FIGURE 7.13 Level 3 The electron-transport system.
Oxygen is used during this final sequence of oxidation-reduction reactions in aerobic cellular respiration. The electrons that are transported by the ETS arrive in the form of NADH and $FADH_2$ from glycolysis and the Krebs cycle.

Reactants	*Products*
8 NADH + 24 ADP + 24 P	8 NAD^+ + 24 ATP + 8 H
4 $FADH_2$ + 8 ADP + 8 P	4 FAD + 8 ATP + 8 H
6 O_2 + 24 H	12 H_2O

We can now account for all of the ATPs produced during the entire process of aerobic cellular respiration. For each glucose molecule that is completely oxidized:

1. the glycolysis pathway produces two ATPs directly and two NADH molecules,

2. the Krebs cycle produces two ATPs, two $FADH_2$ molecules, and eight NADH molecules, and

3. the ETS produces a total of thirty-two ATPs from the hydrogens obtained from glycolysis and the Krebs cycle.

The grand total of ATPs that results from the complete oxidation of glucose through glycolysis, the Krebs cycle, and the electron-transport system is thirty-six.

Not all organisms use O_2 as their ultimate hydrogen acceptor. Certain cells do not or cannot produce the enzymes needed to run aerobic cellular respiration. Other cells have the enzymes but cannot function aerobically if O_2 is not available. These organisms must use a different biochemical pathway to generate ATP. Some are capable of using other inorganic or organic molecules for this purpose. An organism that uses something other than O_2 as its final hydrogen acceptor is called an **anaerobic** (*an* = without, *aerob* = air) and performs **anaerobic cellular respiration.** The acceptor molecule could be sulfur, nitrogen, or other inorganic atoms or ions. It could also be an organic molecule such as pyruvic acid (CH_3CH_2COOH). Pathways that oxidize glucose to generate ATP energy using something other than O_2 as the ultimate hydrogen acceptor are called **fermentation.** Anaerobic cellular respiration results in the release of less ATP and heat energy than aerobic cellular respiration. Anaerobic respiration is the incomplete oxidation of glucose.

$$C_6H_{12}O_6 + H^+ \text{ \& } e^- \text{ acceptor} \rightarrow \text{Organic molecules} + \text{Energy (ATP + heat)}$$

Many fermentations include glycolysis but are followed by reactions that vary depending on the organism involved and its enzymes. Some organisms are capable of returning the hydrogens removed from sugar to pyruvic acid, forming the products ethyl alcohol and carbon dioxide.

$$C_6H_{12}O_6 + \text{Pyruvic acid (H}^+ \text{ \& } e^- \text{ acceptor)} \rightarrow \text{Ethyl alcohol} + CO_2 \\ + \text{Energy (ATP + heat)}$$

Other organisms produce enzymes that enable the hydrogens to be bonded to pyruvic acid, changing it to lactic acid, acetone, or other organic molecules (figure 7.14).

Although many different products can be formed from pyruvic acid, we will look at only two anaerobic pathways. **Alcoholic fermentation** is the anaerobic respiration pathway that, for example, yeast cells follow when oxygen is lacking in their environment. In this pathway, the pyruvic acid is converted to ethanol (a 2-carbon alcohol) and carbon dioxide. Yeast cells then are only able to generate four ATPs from glycolysis. The cost for glycolysis is still two ATPs; thus, for each glucose a yeast cell oxidizes, it profits by two ATPs.

The products carbon dioxide and ethanol are useful to humans. In making bread, the carbon dioxide is the important end product; it becomes trapped in the bread dough and makes it rise. The alcohol evaporates during the baking process. In the brewing industry, ethanol is the desirable product produced by yeast cells. Champagne, other sparkling wines, and beer are products that contain both carbon dioxide and alcohol. The alcohol accumulates, and the carbon dioxide in the bottle makes them sparkling (bubbly) beverages. In the manufacture of many wines, the carbon dioxide is allowed to escape so they are not sparkling but "still" wines.

Certain bacteria are unable to use oxygen even though it is available, and some bacteria are killed in the presence of O_2. The pyruvic acid that results from glycolysis is converted to lactic acid by the addition of the hydrogens that had been removed from the original glucose.

$$C_6H_{12}O_6 + \text{Pyruvic acid (H}^+ \text{ \& } e^- \text{ acceptor)} \rightarrow \text{Lactic acid} + \text{Energy (ATP + heat)}$$

In this case, the net profit is again only two ATPs per glucose. The lactic acid buildup eventually interferes with normal metabolic functions and the bacteria die. We use the lactic acid waste product from these types of anaerobic bacteria when we make yogurt, cultured sour cream, cheeses, and other fermented dairy products. The lactic acid makes the milk protein coagulate and become pudding-like or solid. It also gives the products their tart flavor, texture, and aroma.

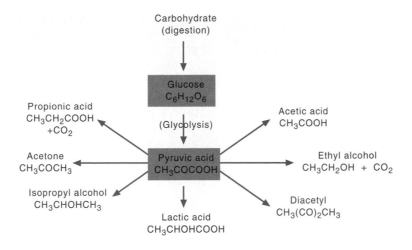

Fermentation product	Possible source	Importance
Acetic acid	Bacteria: *Leuconostoc* sp. *Acetobacter xylenam*	Sours beer Produces vinegar
Ethyl alcohol +CO_2	Yeast: *Saccharomyces* *cerevisiae*	Produces alcohol in beverages
Diacetyl	Bacteria: *Streptococcus* *diacetilactis*	Provides fragrance and flavor to buttermilk
Lactic acid	Bacteria: *Lactobacillus* *bulgaricus*	Aids in changing milk to yogurt
	Human: Muscle cells	Produced when O_2 is limited Results in pain and muscle lethargy
Isopropyl alcohol	Bacteria: *Clostridium* *perfringens*	Causes tissue destruction during gas gangrene
Acetone	Bacteria: *Clostridium* *pasteurinum*	Industrial production for commercial use (fingernail polish remover)
Propionic acid +CO_2	Bacteria: *Propionibacterium* *shermani*	Produces the "eyes" and flavor of Swiss cheese

FIGURE 7.14 A variety of fermentations.

This biochemical pathway illustrates the digestion of a complex carbohydrate to glucose, followed by the glycolytic pathway forming pyruvic acid. Depending on the genetic makeup of the organisms and the enzymes they are able to produce, different end products may be synthesized from the pyruvic acid. The synthesis of these various molecules is the organism's particular way of oxidizing NADH to NAD$^+$ and reducing pyruvic acid to a new end product. Many bacteria use the fermentation process to generate their ATPs and, in the process, produce a variety of end products that are important in our lives.

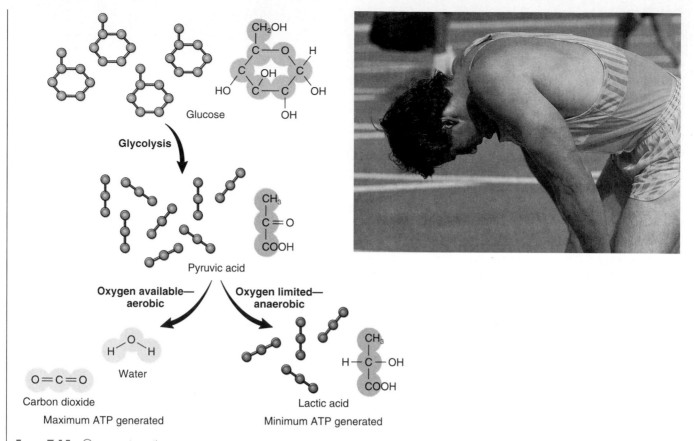

Figure 7.15 Oxygen starvation.
When oxygen is available to all cells, the pyruvic acid from glycolysis is converted into acetyl Co-A, which is sent to the Krebs cycle, and the hydrogens pass through the electron-transport system. When oxygen is not available in sufficient quantities (because of a lack of environmental oxygen or a temporary inability to circulate enough oxygen to cells needing it), some of the pyruvic acid from glycolysis is converted to lactic acid. The lactic acid builds up in cells when this oxygen starvation occurs.

In the human body, different cells have different metabolic capabilities. Red blood cells lack mitochondria and must rely on lactic acid fermentation to provide energy. Nerve cells can only use glucose aerobically. As long as oxygen is available to skeletal muscle cells, they function aerobically. However, when oxygen is unavailable—because of long periods of exercise, or heart or lung problems that prevent oxygen from getting to the skeletal muscle cells—the cells make a valiant effort to meet energy demands by functioning anaerobically.

While skeletal muscle cells are functioning anaerobically, they are building up an oxygen debt. These cells produce lactic acid as their fermentation product. Much of the lactic acid is transported by the bloodstream to the liver, where about 20% is metabolized through the Krebs cycle and 80% is resynthesized into glucose. Even so, there is still a buildup of lactic acid in the muscles. It is the lactic acid buildup that makes the muscles tired when exercising (figure 7.15). When the lactic acid concentration becomes great enough, lactic acid fatigue results. Its symptoms are cramping of the muscles and pain. Due to the pain, we generally stop the activity before the muscle cells die. As a person cools down after a period of exercise, breathing and heart rate stay high until the oxygen debt is repaid and the level of oxygen in muscle cells returns to normal. During this period, the lactic acid that has accumulated is being converted back into pyruvic acid. The pyruvic acid can now continue through the Krebs cycle and the ETS as oxygen becomes available.

Up to this point we have described the methods and pathways that allow organisms to release the energy tied up in carbohydrates. Frequently, cells lack sufficient carbohydrates but have other materials from which energy can be removed. Fats and proteins, in addition to carbohydrates, make up the diet of many organisms. These three foods provide the building blocks for the cells, and all can provide energy. The pathways that organisms use to extract this chemical-bond energy are summarized here.

Fat Respiration

A molecule of true *fat* (*triglyceride*) consists of a molecule of glycerol with three fatty acids attached to it. Before fats can undergo oxidation and release energy, they must be broken down into glycerol and fatty acids. The 3-carbon glycerol molecule can be converted into PGAL, which can then enter the glycolytic pathway (figure 7.16). However, each of the fatty acids must be processed before they can enter the pathway. Each long chain of carbons that makes up the carbon skeleton is hydrolyzed into 2-carbon fragments. Next, each of the 2-carbon fragments is converted into acetyl. The acetyl molecules are carried into the Krebs cycle by coenzyme A molecules. By following the glycerol and each 2-carbon fragment through the cycle, you can see that each molecule of fat has the potential to release several times as much ATP as a molecule of glucose. Each glucose molecule has six pairs of hydrogen, while a typical molecule of fat has up to ten times that number. This is why fat makes such a good long-term energy storage material. It is also why the removal of fat on a weight-reducing diet takes so long! It takes time to use all the energy contained in the hydrogen of fatty acids. On a weight basis, there are twice as many calories in a gram of fat as there are in a gram of carbohydrate. Notice in figure 7.16 that both carbohydrates and fats can enter the Krebs cycle and release energy. Although people require both fat and carbohydrate in their diets, they need not be in precise ratios; the body can make some interconversions. This means that people who eat excessive amounts of carbohydrates will deposit body fat. It also means that people who starve can generate glucose by breaking down fats and using the glycerol to synthesize glucose.

Protein Respiration

Proteins can also be interconverted. The first step in utilizing protein for energy is to digest the protein into individual amino acids. Each amino acid then needs to have the amino group (−NH$_2$) removed. The remaining carbon skeleton, a keto acid, is changed and enters the respiratory cycle as pyruvic acid or as one of the other types of molecules found in the Krebs cycle. These acids have hydrogens as part of their structure. As the acids progress through the Krebs cycle and the ETS, the hydrogens are removed and their energy is converted into the chemical-bond energy of ATP. The amino group that was removed is converted into ammonia. Some organisms excrete ammonia directly, while others convert ammonia into other nitrogen-containing compounds, such as urea or uric acid. All of these molecules are toxic and must be eliminated. They are transported in the blood to the kidneys, where they are eliminated. In the case of a high-protein diet, increasing fluid intake will allow the kidneys to efficiently remove the urea or uric acid.

When proteins are eaten, they are able to be digested into their component amino acids. These amino acids are then available to be used to construct other proteins. If there is no need to construct protein, the amino acids are metabolized to provide energy, or they can be converted to fat for long-term storage. One of the most important concepts you need to recognize from this discussion is that carbohydrates, fats, and proteins can all be used to provide energy. The fate of any type of nutrient in a cell depends on the momentary needs of the cell.

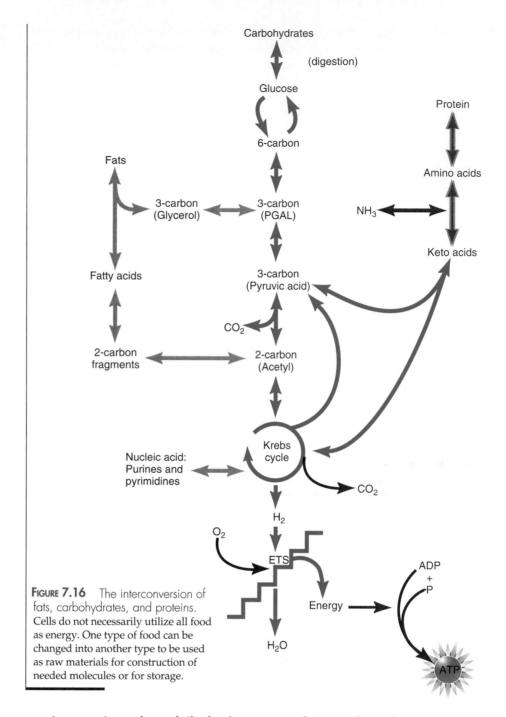

FIGURE 7.16 The interconversion of fats, carbohydrates, and proteins. Cells do not necessarily utilize all food as energy. One type of food can be changed into another type to be used as raw materials for construction of needed molecules or for storage.

An organism whose daily food-energy intake exceeds its daily energy expenditure will convert only the necessary amount of food into energy. The excess food will be interconverted according to the enzymes present and the needs of the organism at that time. In fact, glycolysis and the Krebs cycle allow molecules of the three major food types (carbohydrates, fats, and proteins) to be interconverted.

As long as a person's diet has a certain minimum of each of the three major types of molecules, the cell's metabolic machinery can interconvert molecules to satisfy its needs. If a person is on a starvation diet, the cells will use stored carbohydrates first. Once the carbohydrates are gone (about two days), cells will begin to metabolize stored fat. When the fat is gone (a few days to weeks), the proteins will be used. A person in this condition is likely to die.

If excess carbohydrates are eaten, they are often converted to other carbohydrates for storage or converted into fat. A diet that is excessive in fat results in the storage of fat. Proteins cannot be stored. If they or their component amino acids are not needed immediately, they will be converted into fat, carbohydrates, or energy. This presents a problem for those individuals who do not have ready access to a continuous source of amino acids (i.e., individuals on a low-protein diet). They must convert important cellular components into protein as they are needed. This is the reason why protein and amino acids are considered an important daily food requirement.

Organisms are chemical processors capable of sustaining themselves in a changing environment. All molecules required to support these marvelous reactions are obtained from food and are called **nutrients.** Many of the nutrients that enter living cells undergo chemical change before they are incorporated into the body. These changes are referred to as **assimilation.** Assimilation converts nutrients into specific molecules required by the organism to support its cells and cell activities. These interconversion processes are ultimately under the control of the genetic material, DNA. It is DNA that codes the information necessary to manufacture the enzymes required to extract energy from chemical bonds and to convert raw materials (nutrients) into the structure (anatomy) of the organism.

The amount of food and drink consumed by a person from day to day is a person's **diet.** It must contain the minimal nutrients necessary to manufacture and maintain the body's structure (e.g., bones and muscle) and regulatory molecules (e.g., enzymes), and to supply the energy (ATP) needed to run the body's machinery. If the diet is deficient in nutrients or a person's body cannot process nutrients efficiently, a dietary deficiency and ill health may result. The processes involved in assimilating and utilizing nutrients are collectively known as **nutrition.** A good understanding of nutrition should help one to avoid disease and become healthier. An important concept in nutrition is the amount of energy contained in various foods.

Nutritionists have divided nutrients into six major classes: carbohydrates, lipids, proteins, vitamins, minerals, and water. Chapters 2 and 4 presented the fundamental structures and examples of these types of molecules. A look at each of these classes, from a nutritionist's point of view, should help you to better understand how your body works and how you might best meet your nutritional needs.

Carbohydrates

When the word *carbohydrate* is mentioned, many people think of things like table sugar, pasta, and potatoes. The term *sugar* is usually used to refer to mono- or disaccharides, but the carbohydrate group also includes more complex polysaccharides, such as starch, glycogen, and cellulose. Each of these has a different structural formula, different chemical properties, and plays a different role in the body. Many carbohydrates taste sweet and stimulate the appetite. When complex carbohydrates like starch or glycogen are hydrolyzed to monosaccharides, these may then be utilized in respiration, and the energy of carbohydrates is used to manufacture ATP. Carbohydrates are also converted by the body into molecules that can be used to manufacture necessary components of molecules such as nucleic acids. Carbohydrates can also be a source of fibers that slow the absorption of nutrients and stimulate peristalsis in the intestinal tract (box 7.3).

A diet deficient in carbohydrates results in a condition in which fats are primarily oxidized and converted to ATP. In this situation, fats are metabolized to keto acids, resulting in a potentially dangerous change in the body's pH. A carbohydrate deficiency may also result in the body's use of proteins as a source of energy. In extreme cases this can be fatal, since the oxidation of protein results in an increase in toxic, nitrogen-containing compounds. And don't forget that, as with other nutrients, if there is an excess of carbohydrates in the diet, the body converts them to lipids and stores them in fat cells, and you gain weight.

Box 7.3

Fiber in Your Diet

Fiber has also been called *bulk* and *roughage*. Most fibers are a variety of different kinds of indigestible polysaccharides. The five types of fiber are described in table 7.A.

Most fiber is indigestible by human enzymes, but a small amount is able to be hydrolyzed by beneficial bacteria normally found in the intestinal tract. Since only a negligible amount of kilocalories (kcalories) are obtained through dietary fiber, they are not considered to be a source of energy; however, they do serve other important functions, as shown in table 7.B.

While dietary fiber is of great benefit in many situations, increasing your fiber intake, or increasing it too rapidly, may result in diarrhea, loss of vitamins and minerals, and damage to the lining of the intestinal tract.

BOX TABLE 7.A Five Types of Fiber

Type	Dietary Source	Nature
Cellulose and hemicellulose	Fruits, vegetables, beans, oat and wheat bran, nuts, seeds, whole-grain flour	Wood fiber, plant cell glue, polysaccharide of glucose
Gums, mucilages, and pectins	Vegetables, fruits, seeds, beans, oats, barley	Plant secretions; galactose-containing polysaccharide
Lignin	Seeds, vegetables, whole grains	Stiffens plant cell walls; complex of alcohols and organic acids
Algal polysaccharides	Colloids used in chocolate milk, puddings, pie fillings	Carrageenan; polysaccharide extracted from marine algae and seaweeds
Methyl cellulose	Synthetic products	Polysaccharides

BOX TABLE 7.B Important Functions of Fiber

Benefit	Positive Effect of Dietary Fiber
Relieves constipation/diarrhea	Fiber holds water; softens stool to prevent constipation; forms gels to thicken stool to prevent diarrhea
Controls hemorrhoids	Softer stools ease elimination to prevent weakening of rectal muscles and protrusion of swollen veins
Controls weight	Creates feeling of fullness that promotes weight loss; can be used as replacement for fats and sweets
Reduces colon cancer	Speeds movement through intestinal tract reducing exposure time of cancer-causing agents; does same for bile (associated with cancer risk)
Reduces blood lipids/cardiovascular disease	Binds bile, cholesterol, and other lipids to carry them out of the body
Benefits blood glucose/insulin controls diabetes	Mildly stimulates insulin production and causes a gradual increase in blood glucose
Controls appendicitis	Loosens stool to prevent packing in the appendix and possible infection
Controls diverticulosis	Exercises digestive tract muscles so that they retain their tone; resists bulging of the wall of the intestinal tract into pouches, called diverticula, that could become infected

Lipids

An important class of nutrients is technically known as *lipids*, but many people call them *fats*. This is unfortunate and may lead to some confusion, since fat is only one of three subclasses of lipids. The subclasses, phospholipids, steroids, and true fats, play important roles in human nutrition. Phospholipids are essential components of all cell membranes. Many steroids are hormones that help to regulate a variety of body processes. The lipids sometimes referred to as *true fats* (also called *triglycerides*) are an excellent source of energy. They are able to release 9 kcalories of energy per gram, compared to 4 kcalories per gram of

Table 7.1 Sources of Essential Amino Acids

ESSENTIAL AMINO ACIDS	FOOD SOURCES
Threonine	Dairy products, nuts, soybeans, turkey
Lysine	Dairy products, nuts, soybeans, green peas, beef, turkey
Methionine	Dairy products, fish, oatmeal, wheat
Arginine (essential to infants only)	Dairy products, beef, peanuts, ham, shredded wheat, poultry
Valine	Dairy products, liverwurst, peanuts, oats
Phenylalanine	Dairy products, peanuts, calves' liver
Histidine (essential to infants only)	Human and cow's milk and standard infant formulas
Leucine	Dairy products, beef, poultry, fish, soybeans, peanuts
Tryptophan	Dairy products, sesame seeds, sunflower seeds, lamb, poultry, peanuts
Isoleucine	Dairy products, fish, peanuts, oats, macaroni, lima beans

The essential amino acids are required in the diet for protein building and, along with the nonessential amino acids, allow the body to metabolize all nutrients at an optimum rate. Combinations of different plant foods can provide essential amino acids even if complete protein foods (*e.g., meat, fish, and milk*) are not in the diet.

carbohydrate or protein. A **kilocalorie** is the amount of energy needed to raise the temperature of one kilogram of water one degree Celsius. When hydrolyzed to glycerol and fatty acids, some true fats provide the body with an **essential fatty acid,** linoleic acid. Linoleic acid cannot be synthesized by the human body and, therefore, must be a part of the diet. This essential fatty acid is required by the body for such things as normal growth, blood clotting, and healthy hair and skin. A diet high in linoleic acid has also been shown to help in reducing the amount of the steroid cholesterol in the blood. Some dietary fats also contain dissolved vitamins such as vitamins A, D, E, and K. Therefore, dietary fats can serve as a source of these fat-soluble vitamins.

Fat is an insulator against outside cold and internal heat loss and is an excellent shock absorber. Deposits in back of the eyes serve as cushions when the head suffers a severe blow. During starvation, these deposits are lost, and the eyes become deep-set in the eye sockets, giving the person a ghostly appearance. The pleasant taste and "mouth feel" of many foods is the result of fats. Their ingestion provides that full feeling after a meal, since fats leave the stomach more slowly than other nutrients. You may have heard people say, "When you eat Chinese food, you're hungry a half-hour later." Since Chinese foods contain very little animal fat, it's understandable that after such a meal, the stomach will empty soon, and people don't have that full feeling for very long.

Proteins

Proteins are composed of amino acids linked together by peptide bonds; however, not all proteins contain the same amino acids. Proteins can be divided into two main groups, the **complete proteins** and the **incomplete proteins.** Complete proteins contain all the amino acids necessary for good health, while incomplete proteins lack certain amino acids that the body must have to function efficiently. Table 7.1 lists the **essential amino acids,** those that cannot be synthesized by the human body. Without adequate amounts of these amino acids in the diet, a person may develop protein-deficiency disease. Proteins are essential components of

Table 7.2 Sources and Uses of Vitamins

VITAMIN	FOOD SOURCES	USE IN BODY
Thiamine (B_1)	Peas, beans, eggs, pork, liver	Coenzyme used in Krebs cycle
Riboflavin (B_2)	Milk, whole-grain cereals, green vegetables, liver, eggs	Part of coenzyme used in electron-transport system (FAD)
Niacin (nicotinic acid) (B_3)	Milk, poultry, yeast, cereal	Part of coenzyme used in electron-transport system (NAD^+)
Pyridoxine (B_6)	Most foods	Coenzyme used in synthesis of amino acids
Cyanocobalamin (B_{12})	Meats, dairy products	Used in red blood cell formation
Ascorbic acid (C)	Citrus fruits, vegetables	Part of cell cement used to hold cells together
E	Green vegetables, vegetable oils in most foods	Maintains fertility
D	Dairy products, fish oil	Aids in calcium use in bones
A	Dairy products, vegetables	Used in formation of visual pigment; maintains skin (action not known)

These are only a few of the vitamins used in human metabolism. Notice that a number of them have been referred to earlier in the chapters on enzymes and respiration.

hemoglobin and cell membranes, as well as antibodies, enzymes, some hormones, hair, muscle, and the connective tissue fiber, collagen. Plasma proteins are important because they can serve as buffers. Proteins also provide a last-ditch source of energy when carbohydrate and fat consumption fall below protective levels.

The body's need for a mixture of proteins and carbohydrates is vitally important. Proteins are present in the structures of the human body, but they cannot be stored during times of protein deficiency. If you are on a high-protein diet, the amino acids are not stored; they are either used in protein synthesis or oxidized. A unique relationship called **protein-sparing** exists between carbohydrates and proteins. When adequate amounts of carbohydrates are present in the diet, the body's proteins do not have to be tapped as a source of energy. They are spared from being oxidized. Only when carbohydrate consumption falls below an adequate level will the body use proteins as an energy source. Most people in developed countries have a misconception about the amount of protein necessary in their diets. In actuality, the total amount necessary is quite small and can be easily met.

Vitamins

Vitamins are the fourth class of nutrients. Like essential amino acids and linoleic acid, vitamins cannot be manufactured by the body but are essential in minute amounts to the body's metabolism. Vitamins do not serve as a source of energy, but they help in many enzymatically controlled reactions. They function with specific enzymes to speed the rate of certain chemical reactions. Some enzymes do not function alone but require the attachment of a vitamin to complete their structure. For this reason such vitamins are called *coenzymes*. For example, a B-complex vitamin (niacin) helps enzymes in the respiration of carbohydrates. Most vitamins are acquired from food; however, vitamin D may be formed when ultraviolet light strikes a molecule already in your skin, converting this molecule to vitamin D. This means that vitamin D is not really a vitamin at all. It came to be known as a vitamin because of the mistaken idea that it is only acquired through food rather than being formed in the skin when exposed to sunshine. It would be more correct to call vitamin D a hormone, but most people do not (table 7.2).

Table 7.3 Sources and Uses of Minerals in the Human Body

MINERAL	USE IN BODY	FOOD SOURCE
Calcium	Building of bones and teeth; aids in clotting of blood; regulation of heart, nerve, and muscle activity; enzyme formation; milk production	Asparagus, beans, cauliflower, cheese, cream, egg yolk, milk
Chlorine	Regulation of osmotic pressure; enzyme activities; formation of hydrochloric acid in stomach	Bread, buttermilk, cabbage, cheese, clams, eggs, ham (cured), sauerkraut, table salt
Cobalt	Normal appetite and growth; prevention of a type of anemia; prevention of muscular atrophy	Liver, seafoods, sweetbreads
Copper	Formation of hemoglobin; aids in tissue respiration	Bran, cocoa, liver, mushrooms, oysters, peas, pecans, shrimp
Iodine	Formation of thyroxine; regulation of basal metabolism	Broccoli, fish, iodized table salt, oysters, shrimp
Iron	Formation of hemoglobin; oxygen transport; tissue respiration	Almonds, beans, egg yolk, heart, kidney, liver, meat, soybeans, whole wheat
Magnesium	Muscular activity; enzyme activity; nerve maintenance; bone structure	Beans, bran, brussels sprouts, chocolate, corn, peanuts, peas, prunes, spinach
Phosphorus	Tooth and bone formation; buffer effects in the blood; essential constituent of all cells; muscle contraction	Beans, cheese, cocoa, eggs, liver, milk, oatmeal, peas, whole wheat breads
Potassium	Normal growth; muscle function; maintenance of osmotic pressure; buffer action; regulation of heartbeat	Beans, bran, molasses, olives, oranges, parsnips, potatoes, spinach
Sodium	Regulation of osmotic pressure; buffer action; protection against excessive loss of water	Beef, bread, cheese, oysters, spinach, table salt, wheat germ
Sulfur	Formation of proteins	Beans, bran, cheese, cocoa, eggs, fish, lean meat, nuts, peas
Zinc	Normal growth; tissue respiration	Beans, cress, lentils, liver, peas, spinach

Source: Table, p. 186 from Morrison, et al., *Human Physiology.* Copyright 1977 Holt, Rinehart & Winston, Inc., Orlando, Florida.

Minerals

All members of the **minerals** group are inorganic elements found throughout nature, and they cannot be synthesized by the body. Because they are elements, they cannot be broken down or changed by metabolism or cooking. They commonly occur in many foods and in water. Minerals retain their characteristics whether they are in foods or in the body, and each plays a different role in metabolism. Minerals can function as regulators, activators, transmitters, and controllers of various enzymatic reactions. For example, sodium ions (Na^+) and potassium ions (K^+) are important in the transmission of nerve impulses, while magnesium ions (Mg^{++}) facilitate energy release during reactions involving ATP. Without iron, not enough hemoglobin is formed to transport oxygen, a condition called *anemia.* A lack of calcium may lead to **osteoporosis,** a condition that results from calcium loss, leading to painful, weakened bones. There are twenty-one minerals that are important in your diet. Table 7.3 lists many of these, their functions, and the foods in which they are found.

Water

This last nutrient is crucial to all life and plays many essential roles. You may be able to survive weeks without food, but you would die in a matter of days without water. It is known as the universal solvent because so many types of molecules are soluble in it. The human body is about 65% water. Even dense bone tissue consists of 33% water. All the chemical reactions in living things take place in water. It is the primary component of blood, lymph, and body tissue fluids. Inorganic and organic nutrients and waste molecules are also dissolved in water. Dissolved inorganic ions, such as sodium (Na^+), potassium (K^+), and chloride (Cl^-), are called **electrolytes** because they form a solution capable of conducting electricity. The concentration of these ions in the body's water must be regulated in order to prevent electrolyte imbalances.

Excesses of many types of wastes are eliminated from the body dissolved in water; from the kidneys as urine or in small amounts from the lungs or skin through evaporation. In a similar manner, water acts as a conveyor of heat. Water molecules are also essential reactants in all the various hydrolytic reactions of metabolism. Without it, the breakdown of molecules such as starch, proteins, and lipids would be impossible. With all these important roles played by water, it's no wonder that nutritionists recommend that you drink the equivalent of at least eight glasses each day. This amount of water can be obtained from tap water, soft drinks, juices, and numerous food items, such as lettuce, cucumbers, tomatoes, and applesauce.

SUMMARY

In the process of respiration, organisms convert foods into energy (ATP) and waste materials (carbon dioxide, water, and nitrogen compounds). Organisms that have oxygen (O_2) available can employ the Krebs cycle and electron-transport system (ETS), which yield much more energy per sugar molecule than does fermentation; fermenters must rely entirely on glycolysis. Glycolysis and the Krebs cycle serve as a molecular interconversion system: fats, proteins, and carbohydrates are interconverted depending on the needs of the cell. To be in good health, a person must receive nutrient molecules that can enter the cells and function in metabolic processes. The proper quantity and quality of nutrients are essential to good health. Nutritionists have classified nutrients into six groups: carbohydrates, proteins, lipids, minerals, vitamins, and water. Energy for metabolic processes may be obtained from carbohydrates, lipids, and proteins, and is measured in kilocalories.

QUESTIONS

1. What is a biochemical pathway? Give two examples.
2. What does the term "strict anaerobe" mean?
3. Explain what is meant by fermentation and give an example of a microbe that carries out this process.
4. Why does aerobic respiration yield more energy than anaerobic respiration?
5. Where in a cell do glycolysis, the Krebs cycle, and the electron-transport system take place?
6. Why are some nutrients referred to as essential? Name them.
7. In what way does ATP differ from other organic molecules?
8. Pyruvic acid can be converted into a variety of molecules. Name three.
9. List the six classes of nutrients and give an example of each.
10. Aerobic cellular respiration occurs in three stages. Name these and briefly describe what happens in each stage.

acetyl (ă-sēt′l)   The 2-carbon remainder of the carbon skeleton of pyruvic acid that is able to enter the mitochondrion.

adenosine triphosphate (ATP) (uh-den′o-sēn tri-fos′fāt)   A molecule formed from the building blocks of adenine, ribose, and phosphates. It functions as the primary energy carrier in the cell.

aerobic cellular respiration (a-ro′bik sel′yu-lar res″pĭ-ra′shun)   The biochemical pathway that requires oxygen and converts food, such as carbohydrates, to carbon dioxide and water. During this conversion, it releases the chemical-bond energy as ATP molecules.

alcoholic fermentation (al″ko-hol′ik fer″men-ta′shun)   The anaerobic respiration pathway in yeast cells. During this process, pyruvic acid from glycolysis is converted to ethanol and carbon dioxide.

anaerobic cellular respiration (an′uh-ro″bik sel′yu-lar res″pĭ-ra′shun)   A biochemical pathway that does not require oxygen for the production of ATP and does not use O_2 as its ultimate hydrogen ion acceptor.

assimilation (a-sim′i-la′shun)   The physiological process that takes place in a living cell when converting nutrients in food into specific molecules required by the organism.

biochemical pathway (bi″o-kem′ ĭ-kal path′wa)   A major series of enzyme controlled reactions linked together.

cellular respiration (sel′yu-lar res″pĭ-ra′shun)   A major biochemical pathway along which cells release the chemical-bond energy from food and convert it into a usable form (ATP).

complete protein (kom-plēt pro′te-in)   Protein molecules that provide all the essential amino acids.

diet (di-et)   The amount of food and drink consumed by a person from day to day.

electrolytes (e-lek′tro-līts)   Solutions containing dissolved inorganic ions such as sodium, potassium, and chloride and are capable of conducting electricity.

electron-transport system (ETS) (e-lek′tron trans′port sis′tem)   The series of oxidation-reduction reactions in aerobic cellular respiration in which the energy is removed from hydrogens and transferred to ATP.

essential amino acids (e-sen′shal ah-mēn′o as-ids)   Those amino acids that are unable to be synthesized by the human body and must be part of the diet, such as lysine, tryptophan, and valine.

essential fatty acid (e-sen′shal fat-te as-id)   The fatty acid linoleic acid; it is unable to be synthesized by the human body and must be part of the diet.

FAD (*f***lavin *a*denine *d*inucleotide)** (fla-ven ădd-ă-nen die-new-cle-o-tid)   A hydrogen carrier used in respiration.

fermentation (fir-men-ta-shun)   Pathways that oxidize glucose to generate ATP energy using something other than O_2 as the ultimate hydrogen ion acceptor.

glycolysis (gli-kol′ĭ-sis)   The anaerobic first stage of cellular respiration, consisting of the enzymatic breakdown of a sugar into two molecules of pyruvic acid.

high-energy phosphate bond (hi en′ur-je fos-fāt bond)   The bond between two phosphates in an ADP or ATP molecule that readily releases its energy for cellular processes.

incomplete protein (in-kom-plēt pro′te-in)   Protein molecules that do not provide all the essential amino acids.

kilocalorie (kcalorie) (kil′o-kal″o-re)   The amount of heat energy required to raise the temperature of one kilogram of water one degree Celsius.

Krebs cycle (krebz si′kl)   The series of reactions in aerobic cellular respiration, resulting in the production of two carbon dioxides, the release of four pairs of hydrogens, and the formation of an ATP molecule.

minerals (min′er-als)   Inorganic elements that are not able to be manufactured by the body but are required in low concentrations; essential to metabolism.

NAD+ (*n***icotinamide *a*denine *d*inucleotide)** (nik″o-tin′ah-mīd ădd-ă-nen die-new-klē-o-tid)   An electron acceptor and hydrogen carrier used in respiration.

nutrients (nu′tri-ents)   Molecules required by the body for growth, reproduction, and/or repair.

nutrition (nu′trish-un)   Processes involved in taking in, assimilating, and utilizing nutrients.

osteoporosis (os′te-o-por-o′sis)   A disease condition resulting from the demineralization of the bone resulting in pain, deformities, and fractures. Related to a loss of calcium.

oxidation-reduction (redox) reactions (ok″sĭ-da′shun re-duk′shun re-ak′shuns)   Electron-transfer reactions in which the molecules losing electrons become oxidized and those gaining electrons become reduced.

photosynthesis (fo-to-sin′thuh-sis)   A major biochemical pathway in green plants, resulting in the manufacture of food molecules.

protein-sparing (pro′te-in spar-ing)   The conservation of proteins by first oxidizing carbohydrates and fats as a source of ATP energy.

pyruvic acid (pi-ru′vik as′id)   A 3-carbon carbohydrate that is the end product of the process of glycolysis.

vitamins (vi-tah-mins)   Organic molecules that are not able to be manufactured by the body but are required in very low concentrations.

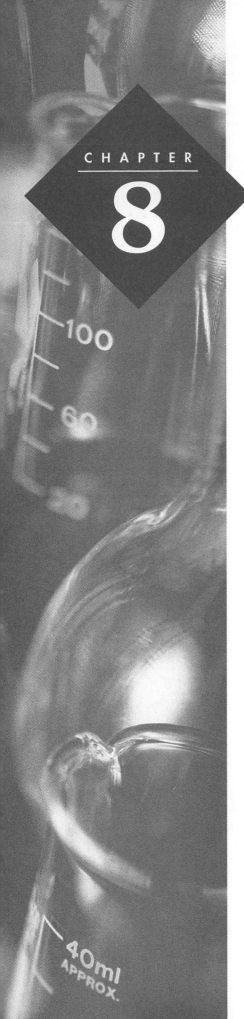

DNA-RNA:
The Molecular Basis of Heredity

CHAPTER OUTLINE

PURPOSE

In previous chapters we have considered a variety of biological structures and their functions. Organic molecules found in living cells are not haphazard arrangements of atoms; they are highly organized and can be classified into major groups. The group known as the *nucleic acids* has a unique structure and is the primary control molecule of the cell. This chapter considers how the structure of these complex molecules is converted into actions by living cells.

CLINICAL VIEWPOINT

Genes within the nucleus of human cells determine the characteristics of each cell and, ultimately, the characteristics of the whole organism. This genetic information is contained in the 46 chromosomes, large organic molecules known as deoxyribonucleic acid (DNA).

 In 1989, scientists began the $3 billion, fifteen-year Human Genome Project aimed at charting the specific arrangement and location of the 100,000 genes estimated to be found on human chromosomes. The methods used to inventory genes have already been used to treat certain genetic diseases. In one case, the gene for tumor necrosis factor (TNF) has been "spliced" into chromosomes of cells lacking a competent TNF gene, thus rendering them "normal." Produced in the proper quantity, TNF is a chemical of the immune system that assists in the killing of cancer cells.

LEARNING OBJECTIVES

- Recognize the structure of DNA and RNA
- Distinguish among DNA, nucleoprotein, chromatin, and chromosome
- Diagram the DNA replication process
- Diagram the DNA transcription process
- Diagram the process of translation
- Give examples of mutagenic agents and how they might affect DNA
- Describe the processes involved in recombinant DNA procedures

In all cells that reproduce, there is a very important library of molecular information. This library contains all the directions for making the structural and regulatory proteins required for life processes. It is like a library of how-to books that does not allow the books to circulate. (If all the DNA in a single human cell were to have its information translated into standard-sized books, the stack would be 15 stories tall.) It is a reference library only. Information can be copied from the books and removed, but the original always stays in the library (the nucleus). It may seem impossible that the directions for growth and development are stored in a place as small as the nucleus of a cell. The secret lies in the language these directions are written in. This language is deoxyribonucleic acid (DNA). DNA has four properties that enable it to function as genetic material. It is able to (1) *replicate* by directing the manufacture of copies of itself; (2) *mutate,* or chemically change, and transmit these changes to future generations; (3) *store* information that determines the characteristics of cells and organisms; and (4) use this information to *direct* the synthesis of structural and regulatory proteins essential to the operation of the cell or organism.

Like the other groups of organic macromolecules, the **nucleic acids** are made up of subunits. The subunits of nucleic acids are called **nucleotides.** Each nucleotide is composed of a *sugar* molecule (S) containing five carbon atoms, a **phosphate group** (P), and a kind of molecule called a **nitrogenous base** (B) (figure 8.1).

Nucleotides differ from one another in the kind of sugar and nitrogenous base they contain. Because of these differences, it is possible to classify nucleic acids into two main groups: ribonucleic acid (RNA) and deoxyribonucleic acid (DNA). The name of each tells about the structure of the molecules. For example, the prefix *ribo-* in RNA tells that the sugar part of this nucleic acid is **ribose.** Similarly, DNA contains a ribose sugar that has been deoxygenated (lost an oxygen atom) **deoxyribose,** (figure 8.2a). The nucleotide units contain nitrogenous bases of two sizes. The larger nitrogenous bases are **adenine** (A) and **guanine** (G), which differ in the kinds of atoms attached to their double-ring structure (figure 8.2b). The smaller nitrogenous bases are **cytosine** (C), **uracil** (U), and **thymine** (T). Each of these differs from the others in the kinds of atoms attached to its single-ring structure (figure 8.2c). These differences in size are important, as you will see later.

DNA is a nucleic acid that functions as the original blueprint for the synthesis of polypeptides. It contains deoxyribose sugar, phosphates, and the nitrogenous bases adenine, thymine, guanine, and cytosine. **RNA** is a type of nucleic acid that is directly involved in the synthesis of polypeptides at ribosomes. It contains ribose sugar, phosphates, and the four nitrogenous bases adenine, guanine,

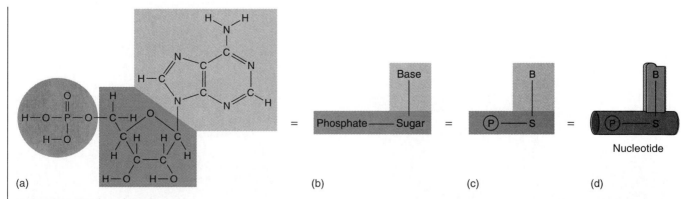

FIGURE 8.1 Nucleotide structure.
(a) All nucleotides are constructed in the basic way shown. The nucleotide is the basic structural unit of all nucleic acid molecules. Notice in (c) that the phosphate group is written in "shorthand" form as a P inside a circle. Part (d) is a stylized version of a nucleotide and will be used throughout the chapter. Remember that this style is only representative of the kind of complex organic molecule shown in (a).

FIGURE 8.2 The building blocks of nucleic acids.

All nucleic acids are composed of two organic components: a 5-carbon sugar molecule and a nitrogenous base. (a) Notice the difference (highlighted in color) between the two sugar molecules. The nitrogenous bases are divided into two groups according to their size. The large *purines*—adenine and guanine molecules—differ from each other in their attached groups (in color), as do the three smaller *pyrimidine* nitrogenous bases—cytosine, uracil, and thymine—in (c). The two types of nucleic acids—DNA and RNA—are composed of these eight building blocks. Note that each building block has a sugar, base, and phosphate component. These nucleotides are color coded throughout the chapter so that you can recognize the difference between DNA and RNA.

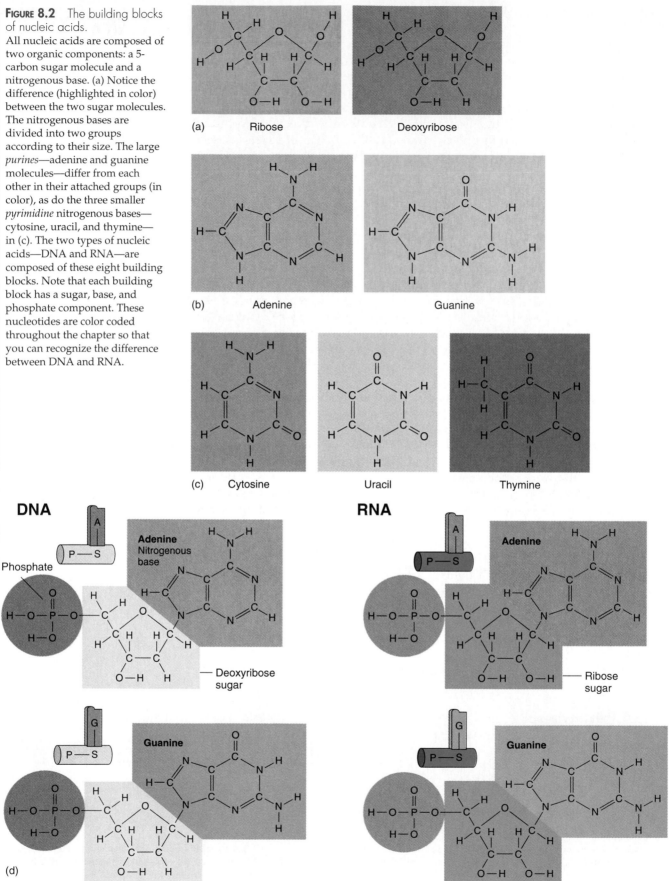

(a) Ribose   Deoxyribose

(b) Adenine   Guanine

(c) Cytosine   Uracil   Thymine

DNA

Phosphate

Adenine
Nitrogenous base

Deoxyribose sugar

Guanine

RNA

Adenine

Ribose sugar

Guanine

(d)

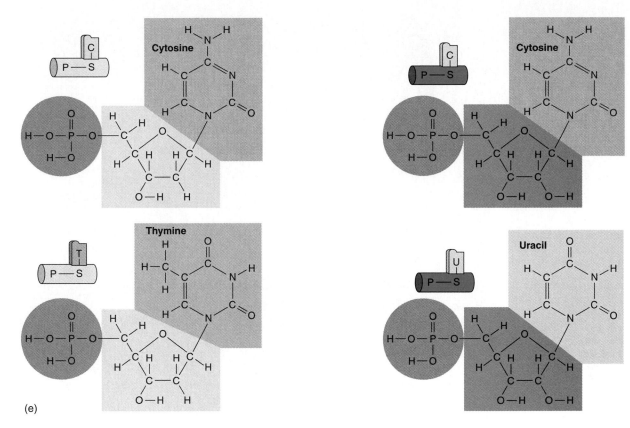

(e)

FIGURE 8.2 CONTINUED

cytosine, and uracil (no thymine in RNA). The construction of a nucleotide involves the bonding of a nitrogenous base to a 5-carbon sugar. For example, when adenine is chemically bonded to ribose sugar, the result is a molecule called *adenosine*. When a phosphate is added to the ribose of the adenosine, a new molecule called *adenosine monophosphate (AMP)* is formed. This is a complete nucleotide. Monophosphate nucleotides are energetically stable, and they are the building blocks of RNA.

Chapter 6 dealt with the function of ATP as a source of chemical-bond energy. Keep in mind that all nucleotides exist in mono-, di-, and triphosphate forms. As in ATP, the other triphosphates contain high-energy phosphate bonds used in the dehydration synthesis reaction that binds nucleotides together as RNA or DNA. The result of this nucleic acid synthesis is a polymer that can be compared to a comb. The protruding "teeth" (different nitrogenous bases) are connected to a common "backbone" (sugar and phosphate molecules). This is the basic structure of both RNA and DNA (figure 8.3).

DNA is actually a double-stranded molecule. It consists of two comblike strands held together between their protruding bases by hydrogen bonds. The two strands are twisted about each other in a double helix known as **duplex DNA** (figure 8.4). This ladderlike molecule has as its "rungs" the hydrogen-bonded base pairs. The four kinds of bases always pair in a definite way: adenine (A) with thymine (T), and guanine (G) with cytosine (C). The bases that pair are said

THE MOLECULAR STRUCTURE OF DNA

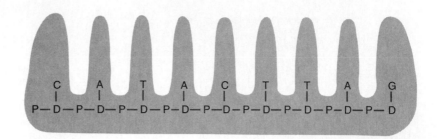

FIGURE 8.3 A single strand of DNA.
A single strand of DNA resembles a comb. The molecule is much longer than pictured here and is composed of a sequence of linked nucleotides.

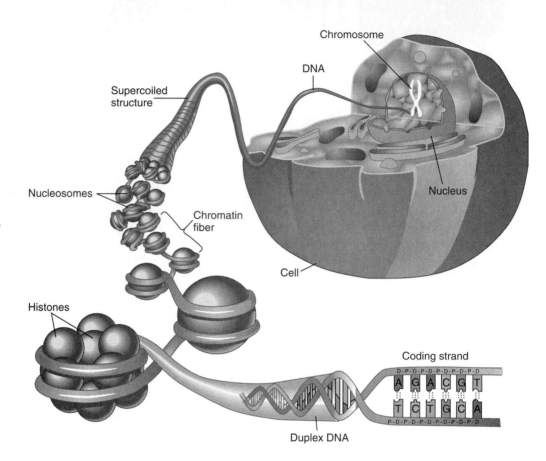

FIGURE 8.4 Duplex DNA. Eukaryotic cells contain duplex DNA in their nuclei, which takes the form of a three-dimensional helix. One strand is a chemical code (the coding strand) that contains the information necessary to control and coordinate the activities of the cell. The two strands are bound together by weak hydrogen bonds formed between the protruding nitrogenous bases according to the base-pairing rule: A pairs with T, and C pairs with G. The length of a DNA molecule is measured in numbers of "base pairs"—the number of rungs on the ladder.

to be **complementary bases.** Notice that the large bases (A and G) pair with the small ones (T and C), thus keeping the backbones of two complementary strands parallel. Three hydrogen bonds are formed between guanine and cytosine:

$$G \vdots C$$

and two between adenine and thymine:

$$A \therefore T$$

It is possible to "write" a message in the form of a stable DNA molecule by combining the four different DNA nucleotides (A, T, G, C) in particular sequences. Notice in figure 8.3 that it is possible to make sense out of the sequence of nitrogenous bases. If the code is "read" from left to right in groups of three, three words can be noted—CAT, ACT, and TAG. In this case, the four DNA nucleotides are being used as an alphabet to construct three-letter words. In order to make sense out of such a code, it is necessary to read in a consistent direction. Reading the sequence in reverse does not always make sense, just as reading this paragraph in reverse would not make sense.

There are two different forms of DNA, eukaryotic and prokaryotic. The genetic material of eukaryotes is duplex DNA, but it has histone proteins attached

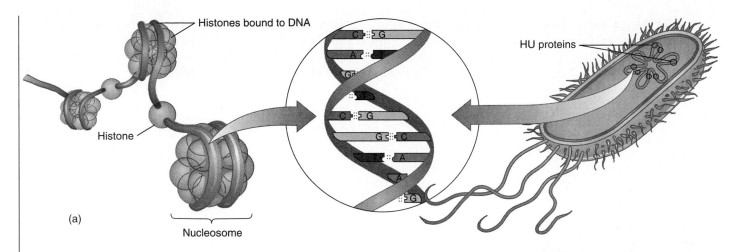

Histones bound to DNA

Histone

(a)

Nucleosome

HU proteins

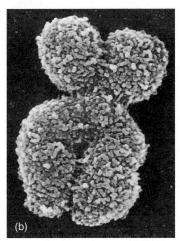

(b)

FIGURE 8.5 The many forms of deoxyribonucleic acid, DNA.
The term *nucleoprotein* is used to describe the combination of DNA and its associated protein in eukaryotic cells. When these giant nucleoprotein molecules are found loose inside of a cell's nucleus, they are called chromatin. (a) Upon close examination of a portion of a eukaryotic nucleoprotein, it is possible to see how the DNA and protein are arranged. The protein component, histone, is found along the DNA in globular masses; they may be individual histones or arranged in groups, the nucleosomes. The nucleic acid of prokaryotic cells (the bacteria) does not have histone protein; rather, it has proteins called HU proteins. In addition, the ends of the giant nucleoprotein molecule overlap and bind with one another to form a loop. (b) During certain stages in the reproduction of a eukaryotic cell, the nucleoprotein coils and "supercoils," forming tightly bound masses. When stained, these are easily seen through the microscope. In their supercoiled form, they are called chromosomes, meaning colored bodies.

along its length. The duplex DNA strands, with attached proteins, are called **nucleoproteins,** or **chromatin fibers.** Histone and DNA are not arranged haphazardly, but come together in a highly organized pattern. The duplex DNA spirals around repeating clusters of eight histone spheres. Histone clusters with their encircling DNA are called **nucleosomes** (figure 8.5a). When eukaryotic chromatin coils into condensed, highly knotted bodies, they are easily seen through a microscope after staining with dye. Condensed like this, a chromatin fiber is referred to as a **chromosome** (figure 8.5b). The genetic material in prokaryotic cells is also duplex DNA, with the ends of the polymer connected to form a loop (figure 8.5c). While prokaryotic cells do not have histone protein, they do have an attached protein called *HU protein.*

Each chromatin strand is different because each strand has a different chemical code. Coded DNA serves as a central cell library. Tens of thousands of messages are in this storehouse of information. This information tells the cell such things as (1) how to produce enzymes required for the digestion of nutrients, (2) how to manufacture enzymes that will metabolize the nutrients and eliminate harmful wastes, (3) how to repair and assemble cell parts, (4) how to reproduce healthy offspring, (5) when and how to react to favorable and unfavorable changes in the environment, and (6) how to coordinate and regulate all of life's essential functions. If any of these functions are not performed, the cell will die. The importance of maintaining essential DNA in a cell becomes clear when we consider cells that have lost it. For example, human red blood cells lose their nuclei as they become specialized for carrying oxygen and carbon dioxide throughout the body. Without DNA they are unable to manufacture the essential cell components needed to sustain themselves. They continue to exist for about 120 days, functioning only on enzymes manufactured earlier in their lives. When these enzymes are gone, the cells die. Since these specialized cells begin to die the moment they lose their DNA, they are more accurately called *red blood corpuscles* (*RBCs*): "little dying red bodies."

Once scientists began to understand the chemical makeup of the nucleic acids, an attempt was made to understand how DNA and RNA relate to cell structure and activities. The concept that resulted is known as the *central dogma,* main belief, or "source of all information." It is most easily written in this form:

$$\text{DNA} \Leftarrow (\text{replication}) \Leftarrow \textbf{\textit{DNA}} \Rightarrow (\text{transcription}) \Rightarrow \text{RNA} \Rightarrow (\text{translation}) \Rightarrow \text{Proteins} \begin{smallmatrix} \nearrow \text{structural} \\ \searrow \text{regulatory} \end{smallmatrix}$$

What this says is that DNA is the genetic material of the cell and (going to the left) it is capable of reproducing itself, a process called *DNA replication.* Going to the right, DNA is capable of supervising the manufacture of RNA (a process known as *transcription*), which in turn is involved in the production of protein molecules, a process known as *translation.*

DNA replication occurs in cells in preparation for mitosis and meiosis. Without this process, daughter cells would not receive the library of information required to sustain life. The transcription process results in the formation of a strand of RNA that is a copy of a piece of the DNA on which it is formed. Some of the RNA molecules become involved in various biochemical processes, while others are used in the translation of the RNA information into proteins. Structural proteins are used by the cell as building materials (feathers, hair), while regulatory proteins are used to direct and control chemical reactions (enzymes, some hormones).

DNA REPLICATION

Since all cells must maintain a complete set of genetic material, there must be a doubling of DNA in order to have enough to pass on to the offspring. **DNA replication** is the process of duplicating the genetic material prior to its distribution to daughter cells. When a cell divides into two daughter cells, each new cell must receive a complete copy of the parent cell's genetic information, or it will not be able to manufacture all proteins vital to its existence. Accuracy of duplication is essential in order to guarantee the continued existence of that type of cell. Should the daughters not receive exact copies, they may be unable to manufacture the structural and regulatory proteins essential for their survival.

The DNA replication process requires many enzymes. It begins when an enzyme breaks the hydrogen bonds between the bases of the two strands of DNA. In eukaryotic cells, this occurs in hundreds of different "forks" or places along the length of the DNA. Moving along the DNA, the enzyme "unzips" the halves of the duplex DNA. Proceeding in opposite directions on each side, enzymes known as **DNA polymerase** proceed down the length of the DNA, bonding new DNA nucleotides into position. In addition, DNA polymerase, which speeds the addition of new nucleotides to the growing chain, works along with another enzyme called *exonuclease* to make sure that no mistakes are made. Mismatched nucleotides are either prevented from being bonded into the wrong position or misplaced nucleotides are cut out and replaced with the proper unit. When cells age, this repair process may not be as efficient and can contribute to cell death. Generally, replication proceeds in both directions from every fork, appearing as replication "bubbles" (figure 8.6). The complementary bases

$$(A ::: T, G :::: C)$$

pair with the exposed nitrogenous bases of both DNA strands by forming new hydrogen bonds. Once properly aligned, a covalent bond is formed between the sugars and phosphates of the newly positioned nucleotides using DNA polymerase. A strong sugar and phosphate backbone is formed in the process. This process continues until all the replication "bubbles" join. In prokaryotic cells, replication of the circular DNA molecule begins at one point and proceeds in opposite directions until the circle is completely replicated.

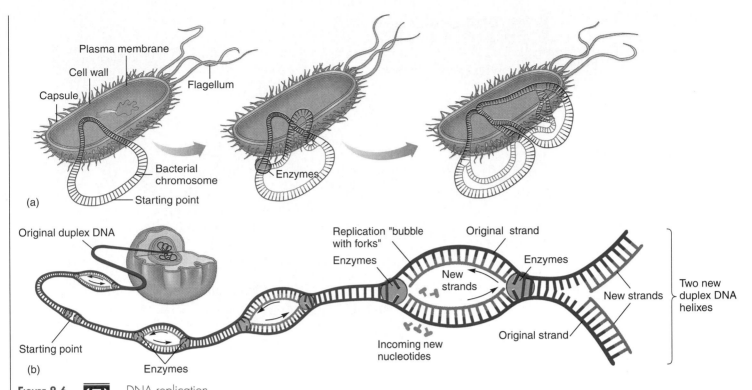

FIGURE 8.6 〔▭〕 DNA replication.

These illustrations summarize the basic events that occur during the replication of duplex DNA. (a) In prokaryotic cells "unzipping" enzymes attach to the DNA as it replicates in many places, forming a "fuzzy" mass of partially replicated strands. As these enzymes move in both directions down the duplex DNA, new complementary DNA nucleotides are base-paired on the exposed strands and linked together by other enzymes (DNA polymerase and exonuclease), forming new strands that are identical to the originals and appear as ever-enlarging double loops. (b) In eukaryotic cells the "unzipping" enzymes attach to the DNA at numerous points, breaking the hydrogen bonds that bind the complementary strands. As the DNA replicates, numerous replication "bubbles" or "forks" appear along the length of the duplex DNA. Eventually all the forks come together, completing the replication process.

A new complementary strand of DNA forms on each of the old DNA strands, resulting in the formation of two double-stranded duplex DNA molecules. In this way, the exposed nitrogenous bases of the original DNA serve as a **template,** or pattern, for the formation of the new DNA. As the new DNA is completed, it twists into its double-helix shape.

The completion of the process yields two double helices that are identical in their nucleotide sequences. The DNA replication process is highly accurate. It has been estimated that there is only one error made for every 2×10^9 nucleotides. A human cell contains 46 chromosomes consisting of about 5,000,000,000 (5 billion) base pairs. This averages to about five errors per cell! Don't forget that this figure is an estimate. While some cells may have five errors per replication, others may have more, and some may have no errors at all. It is also important to note that some errors may be major and deadly, while others are insignificant. Since this error rate is so small, DNA replication is considered by most to be essentially error-free. Following DNA replication, the cell now contains twice the amount of genetic information and is ready to begin the process of distributing one set of genetic information to each of its two daughter cells.

The distribution of DNA involves splitting the cell and distributing a set of genetic information to the two new daughter cells. In this way, each new cell has the necessary information to control its activities. The mother cell ceases to exist when it divides its contents between the two smaller daughter cells (figure 8.7).

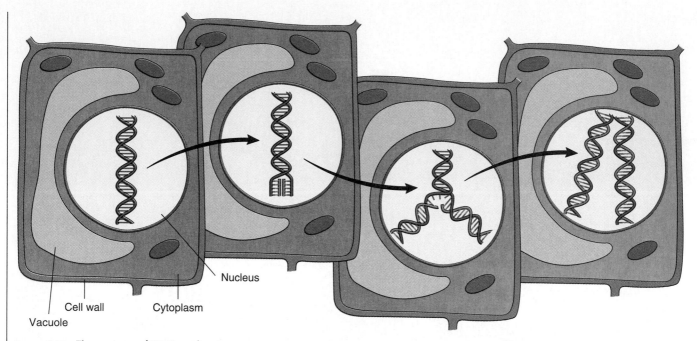

FIGURE 8.7 The process of DNA replication.

These are the generalized events in the nucleus of a eukaryotic cell during the process of DNA replication. Notice that the final cell has two double helices; they are identical to each other and identical to the original duplex strands.

A cell does not really die when it reproduces itself; it merely starts over again. This is called the *life cycle* of a cell. A cell may divide and redistribute its genetic information to the next generation in a number of ways. These processes will be dealt with in detail in chapters 9 and 10.

DNA TRANSCRIPTION

As noted earlier, DNA functions in the manner of a reference library that does not allow its books to circulate. Information from the originals must be copied. The second major function of DNA is to make a single-stranded, complementary RNA copy of DNA. This operation is called **transcription** (*scribe* = to write), which means to transfer data from one form to another. In this case, the data is copied from DNA language to RNA language. The same base-pairing rules that control the accuracy of DNA replication apply to the process of transcription. Using this process, the genetic information stored as a DNA chemical code is carried in the form of an RNA copy to other parts of the cell. It is RNA that is used to guide the assembly of amino acids into structural and regulatory proteins. Without the process of transcription, genetic information would be useless in directing cell functions. Although many types of RNA are synthesized from the genes, the three most important are messenger RNA (mRNA), transfer RNA (tRNA), and ribosomal RNA (rRNA).

$$\text{DNA} \longrightarrow \begin{cases} \text{mRNA} \\ \text{tRNA} \\ \text{rRNA} \end{cases} \longrightarrow \text{Protein} \begin{cases} \longrightarrow \text{Structural protein} \\ \longrightarrow \text{Regulatory proteins} \end{cases}$$
$$\text{Other types of RNA} \longrightarrow \text{Various biochemical reactions}$$

Transcription begins in a way that is similar to DNA replication. The duplex DNA is separated by an enzyme, exposing the nitrogenous-base sequences of the two strands. However, unlike DNA replication, transcription only occurs on one of the two DNA strands, which serves as a template, or pattern, for the synthesis of RNA (box 8.1). But which strand is copied? Where does it start and when does it stop? Where along the sequence of thousands of nitrogenous bases does the chemical

Box 8.1

HIV Infection (AIDS) and Reverse Transcriptase

AIDS is an acronym for *acquired immuno deficiency syndrome* and is caused by human immunodeficiency viruses. They are members of the *retrovirus* family (see box figure 8.1). HIV is a spherical virus with an outer membrane, inside protein coat, and RNA core. Its genetic material is RNA, not DNA. Genes are carried from one generation to the next as RNA molecules. This is not the case in humans and many other organisms where DNA is the genetic material.

human sequence:

$$\text{DNA} \xrightarrow{\text{transcriptase}} \text{RNA} \longrightarrow \text{protein.}$$

However, once having entered a suitable, susceptible host cell, HIV must convert its RNA to a DNA genome in order to integrate into the host cell's chromosome. Only then can it become an active, disease-causing parasite. This conversion of RNA to DNA is contrary, reverse, or *retro* to the RNA-forming process controlled by the enzyme transcriptase. Humans do not have the genetic capability to manufacture the enzyme necessary to convert RNA to DNA, *reverse transcriptase*.

retrovirus sequence:

$$\text{RNA} \xrightarrow{\text{reverse transcriptase}} \text{DNA.}$$

When HIV carries out gene replication and protein synthesis, the process is diagrammed:

$$\text{RNA} \xrightarrow{\text{reverse transcriptase}} \text{DNA} \xrightarrow{\text{transcriptase}} \text{RNA} \longrightarrow \text{protein.}$$

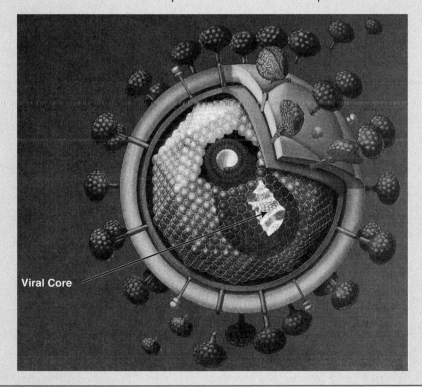

Viral Core

This has two important implications. First, the presence of reverse transcriptase in a human can be looked upon as an indication of retroviral infection because it is not manufactured by human cells. However, since HIV is only one type of several retroviruses, the presence of the enzyme in an individual does not necessarily indicate an HIV infection. It does indicate "some type" of retroviral infection. Second, interference with reverse transcriptase will frustrate the virus's attempt to integrate into the host chromosome. This may prevent disease caused by viral replication within the host cell. This is the principal means by which the drug AZT operates. AZT, azidothymidine (or Zodovudine) and DDC, dideoxycytosine, disrupt the operation of reverse transcriptase.

Box Figure 8.1

code for the manufacture of a particular enzyme begin and where does it end? If transcription begins randomly, the resulting RNA may not be an accurate copy of the code, and the enzyme product may be useless or deadly to the cell. To answer these questions, it is necessary to explore the nature of the genetic code itself.

We know that genetic information is in chemical-code form in the DNA molecule. When the coded information is used or *expressed*, it guides the assembly of particular amino acids into structural and regulatory polypeptides and proteins. If DNA is molecular language, then each nucleotide in this language can be thought of as a letter within a four-letter alphabet. Each word, or code, is always three letters (nucleotides) long, and only three-letter words can be written. A **DNA code** is a triplet nucleotide sequence that codes for one of the twenty common amino acids. The number of codes in this language is limited because there are only four different nucleotides, which are used only in groups of three. The order of these three letters is just as important in DNA language as it is in our language. We recognize that CAT is not the same as TAC. If all the possible three-letter codes were written using only the four DNA nucleotides for letters, there would be a total of sixty-four combinations. When codes are found at a particular place along a coding strand of DNA, and the sequence has meaning, the sequence is called a **gene.** "Meaning" in this case refers to the fact that the gene can be transcribed into an RNA molecule, which in turn may control the assembly of individual amino acids into a polypeptide.

Prokaryotic Transcription

Each bacterial gene is made of attached nucleotides that are transcribed in order into a single strand of RNA. This RNA molecule is used to direct the assembly of a specific sequence of amino acids to form a polypeptide. This system follows the pattern of:

one DNA gene → one RNA → one polypeptide

The beginning of each gene on a DNA strand is identified by the presence of a region known as the **promoter,** just ahead of an **initiation code** that has the base sequence TAC. The gene ends with a terminator region, just in back of one of three possible **termination codes**—ATT, ATC, or ACT. These are the "start reading here" and "stop reading here" signals. The actual genetic information is located between initiation and termination codes:

promoter::initiator code:::::gene:::::terminator code::terminator region

When a bacterial gene is transcribed into RNA, the duplex DNA is "unzipped," and an enzyme known as **RNA polymerase** attaches to the DNA at the promoter region (figure 8.8). It is from this region that the enzymes will begin to assemble RNA nucleotides into a complete, single-stranded copy of the gene, including initiation and termination codes. Triplet RNA nucleotide sequences complementary to DNA codes are called **codons.** Remember that there is no thymine in RNA molecules; it is replaced with uracil. Therefore, the initiation code in DNA (TAC) would be base-paired by RNA polymerase to form the RNA codon AUG. When transcription is complete, the newly assembled RNA is separated from its DNA template and made available for use in the cell; the DNA recoils into its original double-helix form.

As previously mentioned, three general types of RNA are produced by transcription: messenger RNA, transfer RNA, and ribosomal RNA. Each kind of RNA is made from a specific gene and performs a specific function in the synthesis of polypeptides from individual amino acids at ribosomes. **Messenger RNA (mRNA)** is a mature, straight-chain copy of a gene that describes the exact sequence in which amino acids should be bonded together to form a polypeptide.

Transfer RNA (tRNA) molecules are responsible for picking up particular amino acids and transferring them to the ribosome for assembly into the polypeptide. All tRNA molecules are shaped like a cloverleaf. This shape is formed when they fold and some of the bases form hydrogen bonds that hold the molecule together. One end of the tRNA is able to attach to a specific amino acid. Toward the midsection of the molecule, a triplet nucleotide sequence can base-pair with a codon on mRNA. This triplet nucleotide sequence on tRNA that is complementary to a codon of mRNA is called an **anticodon. Ribosomal RNA (rRNA)** is a highly coiled molecule and is used, along with protein molecules, in the manufacture of all ribosomes, the cytoplasmic organelles where tRNA, mRNA, and rRNA come together to help in the synthesis of proteins.

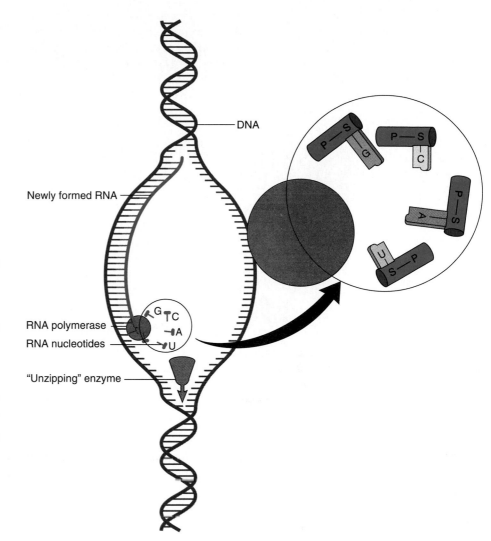

FIGURE 8.8

Transcription of mRNA in prokaryotic cells.

This is a summary that illustrates the basic events that occur during the transcription of one side (the coding strand) of duplex DNA. The "unzipping" enzyme attaches to the DNA at a point that allows it to break the hydrogen bonds that bind the complementary strands. As this enzyme moves down the duplex DNA, new complementary RNA nucleotides are base-paired on one of the exposed strands and linked together by another enzyme (RNA polymerase), forming a new strand that is complementary to the nucleotide sequence of the DNA. The newly formed RNA is then separated from its DNA complement. Depending on the DNA segment that has been transcribed, this RNA molecule may be a messenger RNA (mRNA), a transfer RNA (tRNA), a ribosomal RNA (rRNA), or an RNA molecule used for other purposes within the cell.

Labels in figure:
- DNA
- Newly formed RNA
- RNA polymerase
- RNA nucleotides
- "Unzipping" enzyme

Eukaryotic Transcription

The transcription system is different in eukaryotic cells. A eukaryotic gene begins with a promoter region and an initiation code and ends with a termination code and region. However, the intervening gene sequence contains patches of nucleotides that have no meaning but do serve important roles in maintaining the cell. If they were used in protein synthesis, the resulting proteins would be worthless. To remedy this problem, eukaryotic cells prune these segments from the mRNA after transcription. When such *split genes* are transcribed, RNA polymerase synthesizes a strand of pre-mRNA that initially includes copies of both *exons* (meaningful mRNA coding sequences) and *introns* (meaningless mRNA coding sequences). Soon after its manufacture, this pre-mRNA molecule has the meaningless introns clipped out and the exons spliced together into the final version, or *mature = mRNA*, which is used by the cell (figure 8.9). The molecules that are responsible for cutting the pre-mRNA are RNA-protein complexes called *"snurps."*

The mRNA molecule is a coded message written in the biological world's universal nucleic acid language. The code is read in one direction starting at the initiator. The information is used to assemble amino acids into protein by a process

TRANSLATION, OR PROTEIN SYNTHESIS

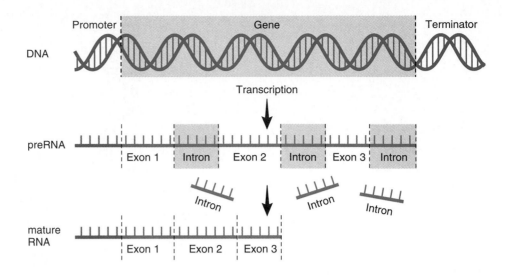

Figure 8.9 Transcription of mRNA in eukaryotic cells. This is a summary of the events that occur in the nucleus during the manufacturing of mRNA in a eukaryotic cell. Notice that the original nucleotide sequence is first transcribed into an RNA molecule that is later "clipped" with "snurp" molecules and then rebonded to form a shorter version of the original. It is during this time that the introns are removed.

Table 8.1 Amino Acids

AMINO ACID	ABBREVIATION
Alanine	Ala
Arginine	Arg
Asparagine	AspN
Aspartic acid	Asp
Cysteine	Cys
Glutamic acid	Glu
Glutamine	GluN
Glycine	Gly
Histidine	His
Isoleucine	Ileu
Leucine	Leu
Lysine	Lys
Methionine	Met
Phenylalanine	Phe
Proline	Pro
Serine	Ser
Threonine	Thr
Tryptophan	Trp
Tyrosine	Tyr
Valine	Val

called **translation.** The word *translation* refers to the fact that nucleic acid language is being changed to protein language. To translate mRNA language into protein language, a dictionary is necessary. Remember, the four letters in the nucleic acid alphabet yield sixty-four possible three-letter words. The protein language has twenty words in the form of twenty common amino acids (table 8.1). Thus, there are more than enough nucleotide words for the twenty amino acid molecules because each nucleotide triplet codes for an amino acid.

Table 8.2 is an amino acid–nucleic acid dictionary. Notice that more than one codon may code for the same amino acid. Some would contend that this is needless repetition, but such "synonyms" can have survival value. If, for example,

Table 8.2 Amino Acid–Nucleic Acid Dictionary

Second letter

First Letter	U	C	A	G	Third Letter
U	UUU ⎤ Phe UUC ⎦ UUA ⎤ Leu UUG ⎦	UCU ⎤ UCC ⎥ Ser UCA ⎥ UCG ⎦	UAU ⎤ Tyr UAC ⎦ UAA Stop UAG Stop	UGU ⎤ Cys UGC ⎦ UGA Stop UGG Trp	U C A G
C	CUU ⎤ CUC ⎥ Leu CUA ⎥ CUG ⎦	CCU ⎤ CCC ⎥ Pro CCA ⎥ CCG ⎦	CAU ⎤ His CAC ⎦ CAA ⎤ Gln CAG ⎦	CGU ⎤ CGC ⎥ Arg CGA ⎥ CGG ⎦	U C A G
A	AUU ⎤ AUC ⎥ Ile AUA ⎦ AUG Met	ACU ⎤ ACC ⎥ Thr ACA ⎥ ACG ⎦	AAU ⎤ Asn AAC ⎦ AAA ⎤ Lys AAG ⎦	AGU ⎤ Ser AGC ⎦ AGA ⎤ Arg AGG ⎦	U C A G
G	GUU ⎤ GUC ⎥ Val GUA ⎥ GUG ⎦	GCU ⎤ GCC ⎥ Ala GCA ⎥ GCG ⎦	GAU ⎤ Asp GAC ⎦ GAA ⎤ Glu GAG ⎦	GGU ⎤ GGC ⎥ Gly GGA ⎥ GGG ⎦	U C A G

A dictionary can come in handy for learning any new language. This one is used to translate nucleic acid language into protein language.

the gene or the mRNA becomes damaged in a way that causes a particular nucleotide base to change to another type, the chances are still good that the proper amino acid will be read into its proper position. But not all such changes can be compensated for by the codon system, and an altered protein may be produced (figure 8.10). Changes can occur that cause great harm. Some damage is so extensive that the entire strand of DNA is broken, resulting in improper **protein synthesis,** or a total lack of synthesis. Any change in DNA is called a **mutation.**

The construction site of the protein molecules (i.e., the translation site) is on the ribosome, a cellular organelle that serves as the meeting place for mRNA and the tRNA that is carrying amino acid building blocks. Ribosomes can be found free in the cytoplasm or attached to the ER. Proteins destined to be part of the cell membrane or packaged for export from the cell are synthesized on ribosomes attached to the endoplasmic reticulum. Proteins that are to perform their function in the cytoplasm are synthesized on unattached or free ribosomes. The mRNA molecule is placed on the ribosome two codons (six nucleotides) at a time (figure 8.11). The tRNA, which is carrying an amino acid, forms hydrogen bonds with the mRNA (between the codon and anticodon) long enough only for certain reactions to occur. The ribosome tRNA-mRNA complex is formed. Both RNA molecules combine first with the smaller of the two ribosomal units, and then the larger ribosomal unit is added. The molecules of tRNA carrying amino acids move in to combine with the mRNA on the ribosome.

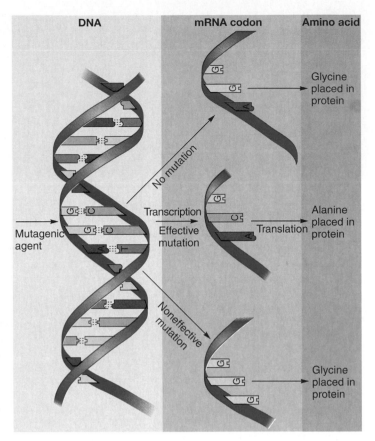

FIGURE 8.10
Noneffective and effective mutation. A nucleotide substitution changes the genetic information only if the changed codon results in a different amino acid being substituted into a protein chain. This feature of DNA serves to better ensure that the synthesized protein will be functional.

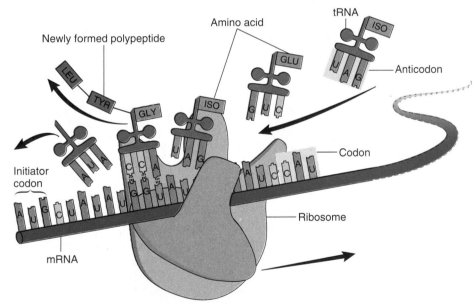

FIGURE 8.11 Translation.
Translation results in the formation of a specific sequence of amino acids, each covalently bonded to another by a peptide bond. This amino acid aligning-and-bonding process takes place on the ribosomes. Each amino acid is brought into its proper position by a particular tRNA molecule. Each tRNA molecule has its own particular coded message that enables it to bind to a specific amino acid. As a result, a particular tRNA will only pick up one type of amino acid for transport to the ribosomes.

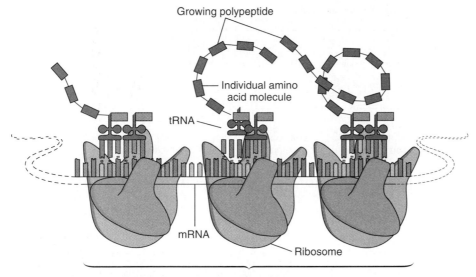

Growing polypeptide

Individual amino
acid molecule

tRNA

mRNA

Ribosome

Polysome complex

FIGURE 8.12 A polysome.

Any single mRNA molecule can be translated on a series of ribosomes. The mRNA and its several attached translating ribosomes are called a polysome. The mRNA moves along and through the ribosomes in a way similar to an audiocassette tape moving between the heads of a cassette player. As the tape passes through, the music signals on the tape are translated into audible sounds. The translation process used to assemble amino acids into protein would be comparable to feeding a single cassette tape through a series of cassette players. The first player would broadcast the music first and finish first, while the last one would start playing the music last and would finish last. Within the polysome complex, the first ribosome to bind to the mRNA will complete the translation of a polypeptide first, and the last ribosome to bind to the mRNA will synthesize the polypeptide last. Both the tape and the mRNA can be "played" again.

Amino acids are transferred to the ribosome by tRNA molecules that are so specific that they are only capable of transferring one particular amino acid. There are at least twenty different coding types of tRNA, and each tRNA transfers a specific amino acid to a ribosome for synthesis into a polypeptide. The tRNA properly aligns each amino acid so that it may be chemically bonded to another amino acid to form a long chain.

Each amino acid is bonded in sequence to form the new protein. As each is bonded in order, the ribosomal unit is moved along the mRNA to allow the next molecule of tRNA and its amino acid to fit into position. Once the final amino acid is bonded into position, all the molecules (mRNA, tRNA, and the newly formed polypeptide) are released from the ribosome. The termination codons signal this action. The intact ribosome is again free to become engaged in another protein-synthesis operation. In most cells the mRNA travels through more than one ribosome at a time. When viewed with the electron microscope, this appears as a long thread (mRNA) with several dark knots (ribosomes) along its length. This sequence of several translating ribosomes attached to the same mRNA is known as a **polysome** (figure 8.12). The newly synthesized chains of amino acids leave the ribosomes and fold into their typical three-dimensional structure for use in the cell.

Thus, the mRNA moves through the ribosomes, its specific codon sequence allowing for the chemical bonding of a specific sequence of amino acids. Remember that the sequence was originally determined by the DNA. Figure 8.13 shows a possible result of protein synthesis. After transcribing the DNA code, the mRNA delivers its message to a ribosome, where a protein is made. In the case of figure 8.13, the amino acid sequence contains phenylalanine, serine, lysine, and arginine.

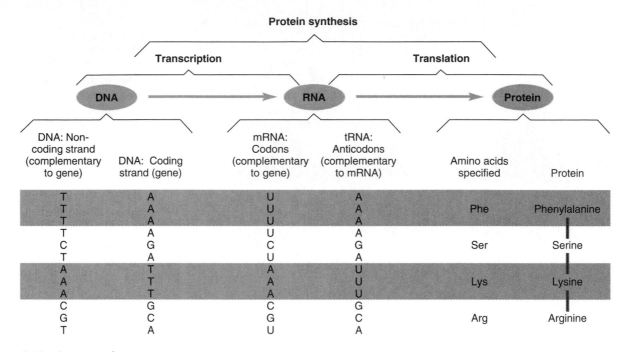

Protein synthesis

Transcription		Translation	
DNA	RNA	Protein

DNA: Non-coding strand (complementary to gene)	DNA: Coding strand (gene)	mRNA: Codons (complementary to gene)	tRNA: Anticodons (complementary to mRNA)	Amino acids specified	Protein
T T T	A A A	U U U	A A A	Phe	Phenylalanine
T C T	A G A	U C U	A G A	Ser	Serine
A A A	T T T	A A A	U U U	Lys	Lysine
C G T	G C A	C G U	G C A	Arg	Arginine

FIGURE 8.13 Protein synthesis.
There are several steps involved in protein synthesis. (1) mRNA is manufactured from a DNA molecule in the transcription operation; (2) the mRNA enters the cytoplasm and attaches to ribosomes; (3) the tRNA carries amino acids to the ribosome and positions them in the order specified by the mRNA in the translation operation; (4) the amino acids are combined chemically to form a protein.

Each protein has a specific sequence of amino acids that determines its three-dimensional shape. This shape determines the activity of the protein molecule. The protein may be a structural component of a cell or a regulatory protein, such as an enzyme. Any changes in amino acids or their order changes the action of the protein molecule. The protein insulin, for example, has a different amino acid sequence than the digestive enzyme trypsin. Both proteins are essential to human life and must be produced constantly and accurately. The amino acid sequence of each is determined by a different gene. Each gene is a particular sequence of DNA nucleotides. Any alteration of that sequence can directly alter the protein structure and, therefore the survival, of the organism.

ALTERATIONS OF DNA

Several kinds of changes to DNA may result in mutations. Phenomena that are either known or suspected causes of DNA damage are called **mutagenic agents.** Two such agents known to cause damage to DNA are x-radiation (X rays) and the chemical nicotine, found in tobacco. Both have been studied extensively, and there is little doubt that they cause mutations. *Jumping genes,* yet another cause of mutation, are segments of DNA capable of moving from one position in a strand of DNA to another. When the jumping gene is spliced into its new location, it alters the normal nucleotide sequence, causing normally stable genes to be misread during transcription. The result may be a mutant gene (figure 8.14).

Changes in the structure of DNA may have harmful effects on the next generation if they occur in the sex cells. Some damage to DNA is so extensive that the entire strand of DNA is broken, resulting in improper protein synthesis or a total lack of synthesis. This changes more than just a nucleotide base and is called a **chromosomal mutation.** In some cases the damage is so extensive that cells die. If enough cells are destroyed, the whole organism will die. A number of experiments indicate that many street drugs such as LSD (lysergic acid diethylamide) are mutagenic agents and cause DNA to break into smaller pieces.

Another example of the effects of altered DNA may be seen in human red blood cells. Red blood cells contain the oxygen-transport molecule, hemoglobin. Normal hemoglobin molecules are composed of 150 amino acids in four

Duplex DNA

FIGURE 8.14 Jumping genes. Alteration in the sequence of DNA nucleotides occurs when one segment of DNA "jumps" out of its original position in the duplex DNA and inserts itself into a different position in the strand. This changes the original nucleotide sequence and, therefore, the encoded message.

FIGURE 8.15 Normal and sickled red blood cells. (a) Normal red blood cells are shown in comparison with (b) cells having the sickle shape. This sickling is the result of a single amino acid change in the hemoglobin molecule.

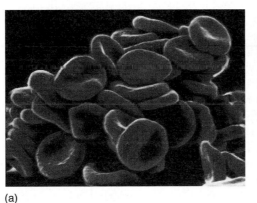
(a)

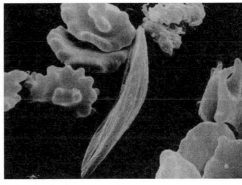
(b)

chains—two alpha and two beta chains. The nucleotide sequence of the gene for the beta chain is known, as is the amino acid sequence for this chain. In normal individuals, the sequence begins like this:

Val-His-Leu-Thr-Pro-*Glu*-Glu-Lys . . . .

In some individuals, a single nucleotide of the gene that controls synthesis of the beta chain changes. This type of mutation is called a **point mutation.** The result is a new amino acid sequence in all the red blood cells:

Val-His-Leu-Thr-Pro-***Val***-Glu-Lys . . . .

This single nucleotide change, which causes a single amino acid to change, may seem minor. However, it is the cause of **sickle-cell anemia,** a disease that affects the red blood cells by changing them from a circular to a sickle shape when oxygen levels are low (figure 8.15). When this sickling occurs, the red blood cells do not flow smoothly through capillaries. Their irregular shapes cause them to clump, clogging the blood vessels. This prevents them from delivering their oxygen load to the oxygen-demanding tissues. A number of physical disabilities may result, including physical weakness, brain damage, pain and stiffness of the joints, kidney damage, rheumatism, and in severe cases, death.

There is no cure for this disease because all of the individual's cells contain the same wrong genetic information. However, a powerful new science of gene manipulation, **biotechnology,** suggests that in the future, genetic diseases may be controlled or cured. Since 1953, when the structure of the DNA molecule was first described, there has been a rapid succession of advances in the field of genetics. It is now possible to transfer the DNA from one organism to another. This has made possible the manufacture of human genes and gene products by bacteria.

MANIPULATING DNA TO OUR ADVANTAGE

Biotechnology includes the use of a method of splicing genes from one organism into another, resulting in a new form of DNA called **recombinant DNA.** This process is accomplished using enzymes that are naturally involved in the DNA-replication process and others naturally produced by bacteria. When genes are spliced from different organisms into host cells, the host cell replicates these new, "foreign" genes and synthesizes proteins encoded by them. Gene splicing begins with the laboratory isolation of DNA from an organism that contains the desired gene; for example, from human cells that contain the gene for the manufacture of insulin. If the gene is short enough and its base sequence is known, it may be synthesized in the laboratory from separate nucleotides. If the gene is too long and complex, it is cut from the chromosome with enzymes called *restriction endonucleases.* They are given this name because these enzymes (*-ases*) only cut DNA (*nucle-*) at certain base sequences (restricted in their action) and work inside (*endo-*) the DNA. These particular enzymes do not cut the DNA straight across, but in a zig-zag pattern that leaves one strand slightly longer than its complement. The short nucleotide sequence that sticks out and remains unpaired is called a *sticky end* because it can be reattached to another complementary strand. DNA segments have been successfully cut from rats, frogs, bacteria, and humans.

This isolated gene with its "sticky end" is spliced into microbial DNA. The host DNA is opened up with the proper restriction endonuclease, and ligase (i.e., tie together) enzymes are used to attach the sticky ends into the host DNA. This gene-splicing procedure may be performed with small loops of bacterial DNA that are not part of the main chromosome. These small DNA loops are called *plasmids.* Once the splicing is completed, the plasmids can be inserted into the bacterial host by treating the cell with special chemicals that encourage it to take in these large chunks of DNA. A more efficient alternative is to splice the desired gene into the DNA of a bacterial virus so that it can carry the new gene into the bacterium as it infects the host cell. Once inside the host cell, the genes may be replicated, along with the rest of the DNA to clone the "foreign" gene, or they may begin to synthesize the encoded protein.

As this highly sophisticated procedure has been refined, it has become possible to quickly and accurately splice genes from a variety of species into host bacteria, making possible the synthesis of large quantities of medically important products. For example, recombinant DNA procedures are responsible for the production of human insulin, used in the control of diabetes; interferon, used as an antiviral agent; human growth hormone, used to stimulate growth in children lacking this hormone; and somatostatin, a brain hormone also implicated in growth. Over 200 such products have been manufactured using these methods.

The possibilities that open up with the manipulation of DNA are revolutionary (box 8.2). These methods enable cells to produce molecules that they would not normally make. Some research laboratories have even spliced genes into laboratory-cultured human cells. Should such a venture prove to be practical, genetic diseases

Box 8.2

The PCR and Genetic Fingerprinting

In 1989, the American Association for the Advancement of Science named DNA polymerase "Molecule of the Year." The value of this enzyme in the polymerase chain reaction (PCR) is so great that it could not be ignored. Just what is the PCR, how does it work, and what can you do with it?

The PCR is a laboratory procedure for copying selected segments of DNA. A single cell can provide enough DNA for analysis and identification! Having a large number of copies of a "target sequence" of nucleotides enables biochemists to more easily work with DNA. This is like increasing the one "needle in the haystack" to such large numbers (*100 billion in only a matter of hours*) that they're not hard to find, recognize, and work with. The types of specimens that can be used include semen, hair, blood, bacteria, protozoa, viruses, mummified tissue, and frozen cells. The process requires the DNA specimen, free DNA nucleotides, synthetic "primer" DNA, DNA polymerase, and simple lab equipment, such as a test tube and a source of heat.

Having decided which target sequence of nucleotides (which "needle") is to be replicated, scientists heat the specimen of DNA to separate the coding and noncoding strands. Molecules of synthetic "primer" DNA are added to the specimen. These primer molecules are specifically designed to attach to the ends of the target sequence. Next, a mixture of triphosphorylated nucleotides is added so that they can become the newly replicated DNA. The presence of the primer, attached to the DNA and added nucleotides, serves as the substrate for the DNA polymerase. Once added, the polymerase begins making its way down the length of the DNA from one attached primer end to the other. The enzyme bonds the new DNA nucleotides to the strand, replicating the molecule as it goes. It stops when it reaches the other end, having produced a new copy of the target sequence. Since the enzyme will continue to operate as long as enzymes and substrates are available, the process continues, and in a short time there are billions of small pieces of DNA, all replicas of the target sequence.

So what, you say? Well, consider the following. Using the PCR, scientists have been able to:

1. more accurately diagnose such diseases as sickle-cell anemia, cancer, Lyme disease, AIDS, and Legionnaires disease;

2. perform highly accurate tissue typing for matching organ-transplant donors and recipients;

3. help resolve criminal cases of rape, murder, assault, and robbery by matching suspect DNA to that found at the crime scene;

4. detect specific bacteria in environmental samples;

5. monitor the spread of genetically engineered microorganisms in the environment;

6. check water quality by detecting bacterial contamination from feces;

7. identify viruses in water samples;

8. identify disease-causing protozoa in water;

9. determine specific metabolic pathways and activities occurring in microorganisms;

10. determine races, distribution patterns, kinships, migration patterns, evolutionary relationships, and rates of evolution of long-extinct species;

11. accurately settle paternity suits;

12. confirm identity in amnesia cases;

13. identify a person as a relative for immigration purposes;

14. provide the basis for making human antibodies in specific bacteria;

15. possibly provide the basis for replicating genes that could be transplanted into individuals suffering from genetic diseases; and

16. identify nucleotide sequences peculiar to the human genome (an application currently underway as part of the Human Genome Project).

such as sickle-cell anemia could be controlled. The process of recombinant DNA gene splicing also enables cells to be more efficient at producing molecules that they normally synthesize. Some of the likely rewards are (1) production of additional, medically useful proteins; (2) mapping of the locations of genes on human chromosomes; (3) more complete understanding of how genes are regulated; (4) production of crop plants with increased yields; and (5) development of new species of garden plants.

The discovery of the structure of DNA over forty years ago seemed very far removed from the practical world. The importance of this "pure" or "basic" research is just now being realized. Many companies are involved in recombinant DNA research with the aim of alleviating or curing disease.

SUMMARY

The successful operation of a living cell depends on its ability to accurately reproduce genes and control chemical reactions. DNA replication results in an exact doubling of the genetic material. The process virtually guarantees that identical strands of DNA will be passed on to the next generation of cells.

The enzymes are responsible for the efficient control of a cell's metabolism. However, the production of protein molecules is under the control of the nucleic acids, the primary control molecules of the cell. The structure of the nucleic acids DNA and RNA determine the structure of the proteins, while the structure of the proteins determines their function in the cell's life cycle. Protein synthesis involves the decoding of the DNA into specific protein molecules and the use of the intermediate molecules, mRNA and tRNA, at the ribosome. Errors in any of the codons of these molecules may produce observable changes in the cell's functioning and lead to cell death.

Methods of manipulating DNA have led to the controlled transfer of genes from one kind of organism to another. This has made it possible for bacteria to produce a number of human gene products.

QUESTIONS

1. What is the difference between a nucleotide, a nitrogenous base, and a codon?
2. What are the differences between DNA and RNA?
3. List the sequence of events that takes place when a DNA message is translated into protein.
4. Chromosomal and point mutations both occur in DNA. In what ways do they differ? How is this related to recombinant DNA?
5. Why is DNA replication necessary?
6. What is polymerase and how does it function?
7. How does DNA replication differ from the manufacture of an RNA molecule?
8. If a DNA nucleotide sequence is CATAAAGCA, what is the mRNA nucleotide sequence that would base-pair with it?
9. What amino acids would occur in the protein chemically coded by the sequence of nucleotides in question 8?
10. How do tRNA, rRNA, and mRNA differ in function?

CHAPTER GLOSSARY

adenine (ad'ĕ-nēn) A double-ring nitrogenous-base molecule in DNA and RNA. It is the complementary base of thymine or uracil.

anticodon (an"te-ko'don) A sequence of three nitrogenous bases on a tRNA molecule capable of forming hydrogen bonds with three complementary bases on an mRNA codon during translation.

biotechnology (bi-o-tek-nol'uh-je) The science of gene manipulation.

chromatin fibers (kro'mah-tin fi'bers) *See* **nucleoproteins.**

chromosomal mutation (kro-mo-sōm'al miu-ta´shun) A change in the gene arrangement in a cell as a result of breaks in the DNA molecule.

chromosome (kro'mo-sōm) A duplex DNA molecule with attached protein (nucleoprotein) coiled into a short, compact unit.

codon (ko'don) A sequence of three nucleotides of an mRNA molecule that directs the placement of a particular amino acid during translation.

complementary base (kom"plĕ-men'tah-re bās) A base that can form hydrogen bonds with another base of a specific nucleotide.

cytosine (si'to-sēn) A single-ring nitrogenous-base molecule in DNA and RNA. It is complementary to guanine.

deoxyribonucleic acid (DNA) (de-ok"se-ri-bo-nu-kle'ik ă'sid) A polymer of nucleotides that serves as genetic information. In prokaryotic cells, it is a duplex DNA (double-stranded) loop and contains attached HU proteins. In eukaryotic cells, it is found in strands with attached histone proteins. When tightly coiled, it is known as a chromosome.

deoxyribose (de-ok"se-ri'b⁻os) A 5-carbon sugar molecule; a component of DNA.

DNA code (D-N-A cōd) A sequence of three nucleotides of a DNA molecule.

DNA polymerase (po-lim'er-ās) An enzyme that bonds DNA nucleotides together when they base pair with an existing DNA strand.

DNA replication (rep"lĭ-ka'shun) The process by which the genetic material (DNA) of the cell reproduces itself prior to its distribution to the next generation of cells.

duplex DNA (du'pleks) DNA in a double-helix shape.

gene (jēn) Any molecule, usually a segment of DNA, that is able to (1) replicate by directing the manufacture of copies of itself; (2) mutate, or chemically change, and transmit these changes to future generations; (3) store information that determines the characteristics of cells and organisms; and (4) use this information to direct the synthesis of structural and regulatory proteins.

guanine (gwah'nēn) A double-ring nitrogenous-base molecule in DNA and RNA. It is the complementary base of cytosine.

initiation code (ĭ-nĭ'she-a"shun cōd) The code on DNA with the base sequence TAC that begins the process of transcription.

messenger RNA (mRNA) (mes'en-jer) A molecule composed of ribonucleotides that functions as a copy of the gene and is used in the cytoplasm of the cell during protein synthesis.

mutagenic agent (miu-tah-jen´ik a-jent) Anything that causes permanent change in DNA.

mutation (miu-ta'shun) Any change in the genetic information of a cell.

nitrogenous base (ni-trah'jen-us bās) A category of organic molecules found as components of the nucleic acids. There are five common types: thymine, guanine, cytosine, adenine, and uracil.

nucleic acids (nu'kle-ik ă'sids) Complex molecules that store and transfer information within a cell. They are constructed of fundamental monomers known as nucleotides.

nucleoproteins (nu-kle-o-pro'te-inz) The duplex DNA strands with attached proteins; also called chromatin fibers.

nucleosomes (nu'kle-o-sōmz) Histone clusters with their encircling DNA.

nucleotide (nu'kle-o-tīd) The building block of the nucleic acids. Each is composed of a 5-carbon sugar, a phosphate, and a nitrogenous base.

phosphate (fos-fāt) Part of a nucleotide; composed of phosphorus and oxygen atoms.

point mutation (point miu-ta'shun) A change in the DNA of a cell as a result of a loss or change in a nitrogenous-base sequence.

polysome (pah'le-sōm) A sequence of several translating ribosomes attached to the same mRNA.

promoter (pro-mo'ter) A region of DNA at the beginning of each gene, just ahead of an initiator code.

protein synthesis (pro'te-in sin'thĕ-sis) The process whereby the tRNA utilizes the mRNA as a guide to arrange the amino acids in their proper sequence according to the genetic information in the chemical code of DNA.

recombinant DNA (re-kom'bĭ-nant) DNA that has been constructed by inserting new pieces of DNA into the DNA of another organism, such as a bacterium.

ribonucleic acid (RNA) (ri-bo-nu-kle'ik ă'sid) A polymer of nucleotides formed on the template surface of DNA by transcription. Three forms that have been identified are mRNA, rRNA, and tRNA.

ribose (ri'bōs) A 5-carbon sugar molecule that is a component of RNA.

ribosomal RNA (rRNA) (ri-bo-sōm'al) A globular form of RNA; a part of ribosomes.

RNA polymerase (po-lim'er-ās) An enzyme that attaches to the DNA at the promoter region of a gene when the genetic information is transcribed into RNA.

sickle-cell anemia (sĭ-kul sel ah-ne'me-ah) A disease caused by a point mutation. This malfunction produces sickle-shaped red blood cells.

template (tem'plet) A model from which a new structure can be made. This term has special reference to DNA as a model for both DNA replication and transcription.

termination code (ter-mĭ-na'shun cōd) The DNA nucleotide sequence just in back of a gene with the code ATT, ATC, or ACT that signals "stop here."

thymine (thi'mēn) A single-ring nitrogenous-base molecule in DNA but not in RNA. It is complementary to adenine.

transcription (tran-skrip'shun) The process of manufacturing RNA from the template surface of DNA. Three forms of RNA that may be produced are mRNA, rRNA, and tRNA.

transfer RNA (tRNA) (trans'fur) A molecule composed of ribonucleic acid. It is responsible for transporting a specific amino acid into a ribosome for assembly into a protein.

translation (trans-la'shun) The assembly of individual amino acids into a polypeptide.

uracil (yu'rah-sil) A single-ring nitrogenous-base molecule in RNA but not in DNA. It is complementary to adenine.

 THE DYNAMIC HUMAN   Correlations to Chapter Eight:

Immune and Lymphatic Systems → Clinical Concepts → HIV/AIDS

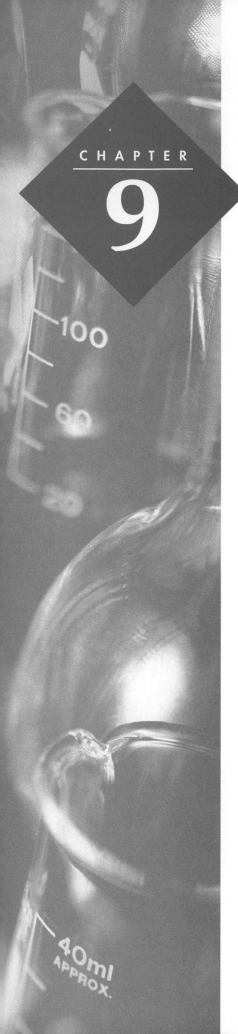

CHAPTER
9

Mitosis— The Cell-Cloning Process

CHAPTER OUTLINE

PURPOSE

In the previous chapter we saw how the molecule DNA replicates. Once this process is complete, doubled DNA is distributed to two newly produced daughter cells. The way in which this cell-splitting process occurs ensures that the daughter cells will have the same genetic message as the original DNA molecule. However, cells with identical genetic messages may differ in how they are built and how they function. The relationships among DNA, genes, and chromosomes are concepts for later consideration of genetics and sex-cell formation.

CLINICAL VIEWPOINT

As you grow up, cell division results in an increase in the number of cells that make up your body. Many tissues, such as nerve and muscle tissue, stop dividing early in childhood. Other tissues, such as skin and blood, continue to divide throughout your life. As we pass middle age, we become smaller. This is the result of a decrease in the rate of cell division. Cells are dying faster than they can be replaced. This is made more obvious by the fact that muscle tone is lost as the cells die and are replaced by connective tissue. Cell division is, therefore, one of the areas currently being researched in the area of gerontology.

LEARNING OBJECTIVES

- List the purposes of cell division
- Explain the cell cycle
- State the processes that occur during interphase
- Name the stages of mitosis and explain what is happening during each stage
- Define differentiation
- Explain how cancer is caused and treated

Even though individual cells may die, the process of cell division replaces dead cells with new ones, repairs damaged tissues, and allows living organisms to grow. For example, you began as a single cell that resulted from the union of a sperm and an egg. One of the *first* activities of this single cell was to divide. As this process continued, the number of cells in your body increased, so that, as an adult, your body consists of several trillion cells. The *second* function of cell division is to provide for the maintenance of the body. Certain cells in your body, such as red blood cells, gut lining, and skin, wear out. As they do, they must be replaced with new cells. All together, you lose about fifty million cells per second; this means that millions of cells are dividing in your body at any given time. A *third* purpose of cell division is repair. When a bone is broken, the break heals because cells divide, increasing the number of cells available to knit the broken pieces together. If some skin cells are destroyed by a cut or abrasion, cell division produces new cells to repair the damage.

During cell division, two events occur. The replicated genetic information of a cell is equally distributed to two daughter nuclei in a process called **mitosis.** As the nucleus goes through its division, there is also a division of the cytoplasm into two new cells. This division of the cell's cytoplasm is called **cytokinesis**—cell splitting. Each new cell gets one of the two daughter nuclei so that both have a complete set of genetic information.

All cells go through a basic life cycle, but they vary in the amount of time they spend in the different stages. A generalized picture of a cell's life cycle may help you to understand it better (figure 9.1). Once begun, cell division is a continuous process without a beginning or an end. It is a cycle in which cells continue to grow and divide. There are four stages to the life cycle of a eukaryotic cell: (1) G_1, gap (growth)-phase one; (2) S, synthesis; (3) G_2, gap (growth)-phase two; and (4) cell division (mitosis and cytokinesis).

The first three phases of the cell cycle—G_1, S, and G_2—occur during a period of time known as interphase. **Interphase** is the stage between cell divisions. During the G_1 stage, the cell grows in volume as it produces tRNA, mRNA, ribosomes, enzymes, and other cell components. During the S stage, DNA replication occurs in preparation for the distribution of genes to daughter cells. During the G_2 stage that follows, final preparations are made for mitosis with the synthesis of spindle-fiber proteins.

During interphase, the cell is not dividing but is engaged in metabolic activities, such as muscle-cell contractions, photosynthesis, or glandular-cell secretion. During interphase, the nuclear membrane is intact and the individual chromosomes are not visible (figure 9.2). The individual chromatin strands are too thin and tangled to be seen. Remember that **chromosomes** include various kinds of histone proteins as well as DNA, the cell's genetic information. The double helix of DNA and the nucleosomes are arranged as a chromatid, and there are two attached chromatids for each replicated chromosome. It is these chromatids (chromosomes) that will be distributed during mitosis.

All stages in the life cycle of a cell are continuous; there is no precise point when the G_1 stage ends and the S stage begins, or when the interphase period ends and mitosis begins. Likewise, in the individual stages of mitosis, there is a gradual transition from one stage to the next. However, to enable communication, scientists have subdivided the process into four stages based on recognizable events. These four phases are prophase, metaphase, anaphase, and telophase.

Prophase

As the G_2 stage of interphase ends, mitosis begins. **Prophase** is the first stage of mitosis. One of the first noticeable changes is that the individual chromosomes

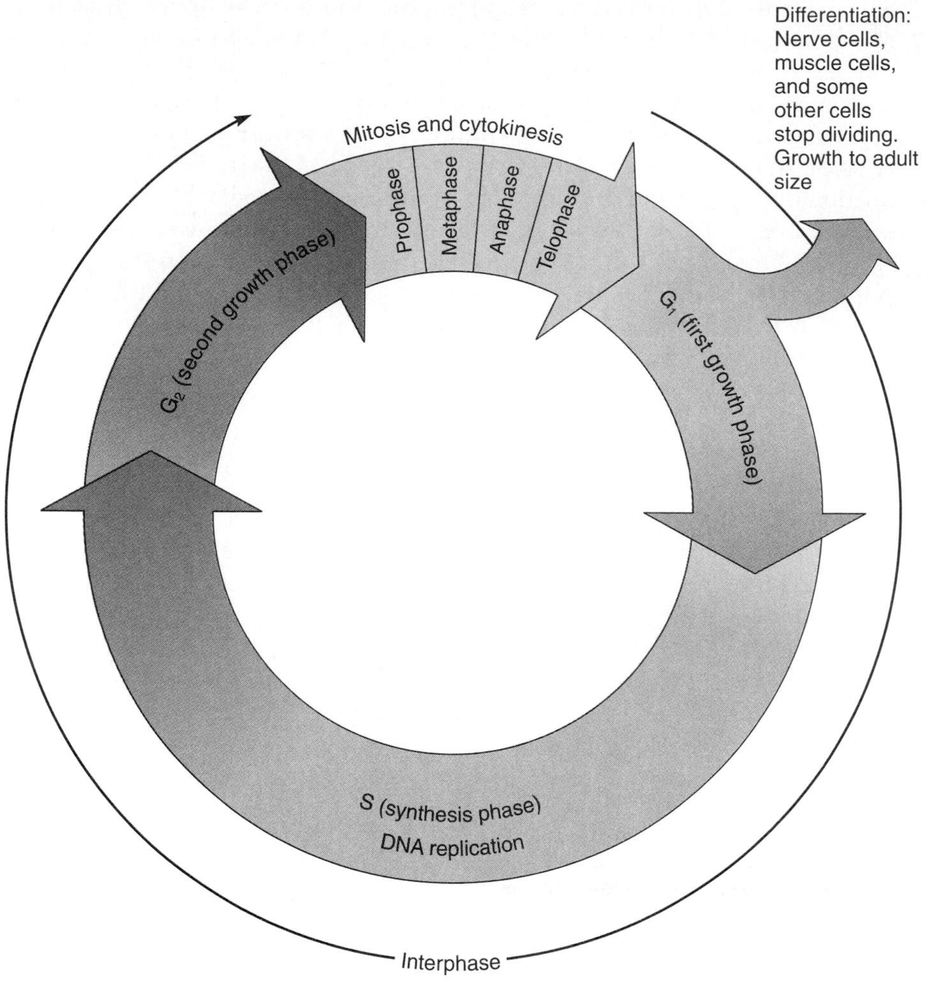

FIGURE 9.1

The cell cycle.

During the cell cycle, tRNA, mRNA, ribosomes, and enzymes are produced in the G_1 stage. DNA replication occurs in the S stage. Proteins required for the spindles are synthesized in the G_2 stage. The nucleus is replicated in mitosis, and two cells are formed by cytokinesis. Once some organs, such as the brain, have completely developed, certain types of cells, such as nerve cells, remain in the G_2 stage. The time periods indicated are relative and vary depending on the type of cell and the age of the organism.

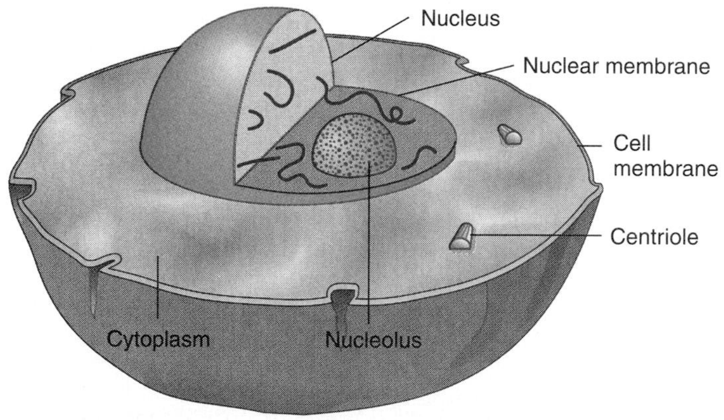

FIGURE 9.2 Interphase.

Growth and the production of necessary organic compounds occur during this phase. If the cell is going to divide, DNA replication also occurs during interphase. The individual chromosomes are not visible, but a distinct nuclear membrane and nucleolus are present.

become visible (figure 9.3). The thin, tangled chromatin present during interphase gradually coils and thickens, becoming visible as separate chromosomes. The DNA portion of the chromosome has genes that are arranged in a specific order. Each chromosome carries its own set of genes that is different from the sets of genes on other chromosomes.

As prophase proceeds, and as the chromosomes become more visible, we recognize that each chromosome is made of two parallel, threadlike parts lying side by side. Each parallel thread is called a **chromatid** (figure 9.4). These chro-

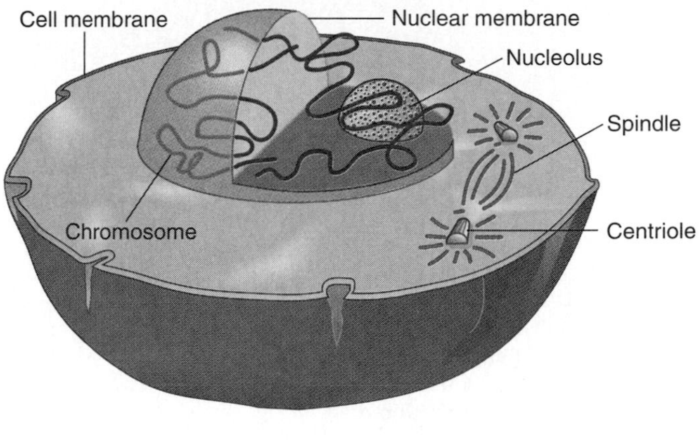

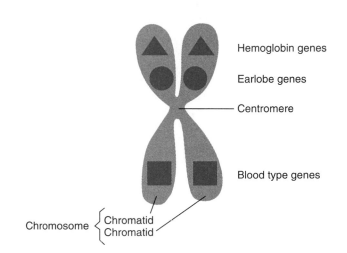

FIGURE 9.3 Early prophase.
Chromosomes begin to appear as thin, tangled threads, and the nucleolus and nuclear membrane are present. The two sets of microtubules known as the centrioles begin to separate and move to opposite poles of the cell. A series of fibers known as the spindle will soon begin to form.

Cell membrane
Nuclear membrane
Nucleolus
Spindle
Chromosome
Centriole

FIGURE 9.4 Chromosomes.
During interphase, when chromosome replication occurs, the original duplex DNA unzips to form two identical double strands that are attached at the centromere. Each of these double strands is a chromatid. The two identical chromatids of the chromosome are sometimes termed a dyad, to reflect that there are two duplex DNA molecules, each located in a chromatid. The DNA contains the genetic data. (The examples presented here are for illustrative purposes only. Do not assume that the traits listed are actually located in the positions shown on these hypothetical chromosomes.)

Hemoglobin genes
Earlobe genes
Centromere
Blood type genes
Chromosome { Chromatid / Chromatid

matids were formed during the S stage of interphase, when DNA synthesis occurred. The two identical chromatids are attached at a region called the **centromere.** This portion of the DNA is not replicated during prophase, but remains base-paired as in the original duplex DNA.

In the diagrams in this text, a few genes are shown as they might occur on human chromosomes. The diagrams show fewer chromosomes and fewer genes on each chromosome than are actually present. Normal human cells have ten billion nucleotides arranged into forty-six chromosomes, each chromosome with thousands of genes. In this book, smaller numbers of genes and chromosomes are used to make it easier to follow the events that happen in mitosis.

Several other events occur as the cell proceeds to the late prophase stage (figure 9.5). One of these events is the duplication of the **centrioles.** Remember that human and many other eukaryotic cells contain centrioles, microtubule-containing organelles located just outside the nucleus. As they duplicate, they move to the poles of the cells. As the centrioles move to the poles, the microtubules are assembled into the *spindle.* The **spindle** is an array of microtubules extending from pole to pole that is used in the movement of chromosomes.

In most eukaryotic cells as prophase is occurring, the nuclear membrane is gradually disassembled. Although it is present at the beginning of prophase, it disappears by the time this stage is completed. In addition to the nuclear membrane, the nucleoli within the nucleus disappear. Because of the disassembly of the nuclear membrane, the chromosomes are free to move anywhere within the cytoplasm of the cell. As this movement occurs, the cell enters into the next stage of mitosis.

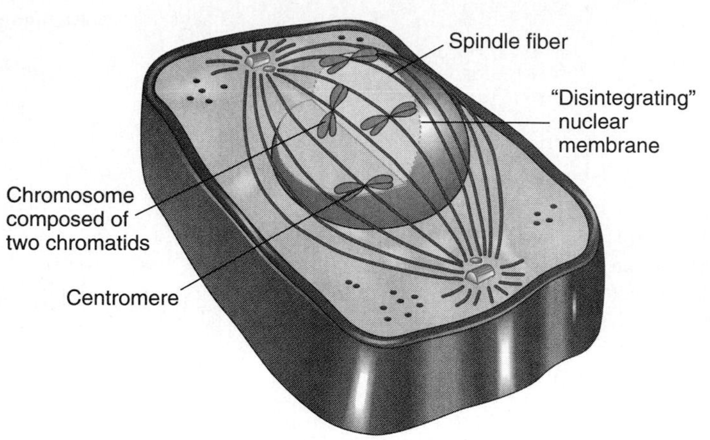

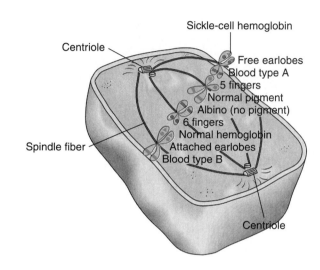

FIGURE 9.5 Late prophase.
In late prophase, the chromosomes appear as two chromatids (a dyad) connected at a centromere. The nucleolus and the nuclear membrane have disassembled. The centrioles have moved farther apart, and the spindle is produced.

Spindle fiber

"Disintegrating" nuclear membrane

Chromosome composed of two chromatids

Centromere

Sickle-cell hemoglobin

Centriole

Free earlobes
Blood type A
5 fingers
Normal pigment
Albino (no pigment)
6 fingers
Normal hemoglobin
Attached earlobes
Blood type B

Spindle fiber

Centriole

FIGURE 9.6 Metaphase.
During metaphase the chromosomes travel along the spindle and align at the equatorial plane. Notice that each chromosome still consists of two chromatids.

Metaphase

During **metaphase,** the second stage in mitosis, the chromosomes align at the equatorial plane. There is no nucleus present during metaphase, and the spindle, which started to form during prophase, is completed. The centrioles are at the poles, and the microtubules extend between them to form the spindle. At the beginning of metaphase, the chromosomes become attached to the spindle fibers at their centromeres. Initially they are distributed randomly throughout the cytoplasm. Then the chromosomes move until all their centromeres align themselves along the equatorial plane at the equator of the cell (figure 9.6). At this stage in mitosis, each chromosome still consists of two chromatids attached at a centromere. In a human cell, there are forty-six chromosomes or ninety-two chromatids aligned at the cell's equatorial plane during metaphase.

If we view a cell in the metaphase stage from the side (*see* figure 9.6), it is an equatorial view. In this view, the chromosomes appear as if they were in a line. If we view the cell from the pole, it is a polar view. The chromosomes are seen on the equatorial plane (figure 9.7). Chromosomes viewed from this direction look like hot dogs scattered on a plate.

Anaphase

Anaphase is the third stage of mitosis. The nuclear membrane is still absent and the spindle extends from pole to pole. In anaphase, each chromosome splits as

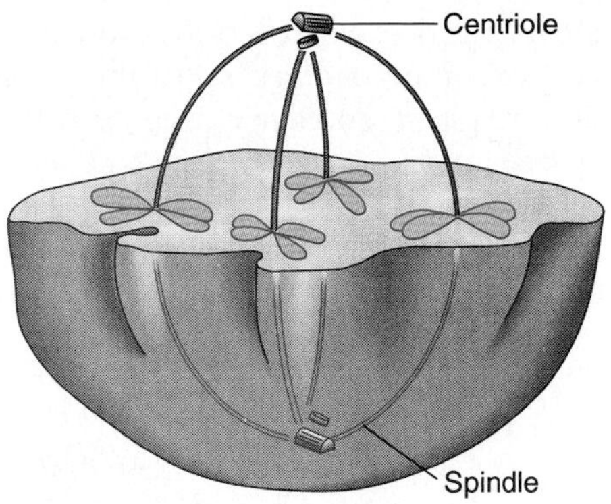

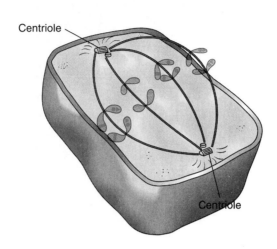

FIGURE 9.7 A polar view of metaphase.
The polar view shows the chromosomes spread out on the equatorial plane.

FIGURE 9.8 Anaphase.
The pairs of chromatids separate as the centromeres replicate. The chromatids, now called daughter chromosomes, are separating and moving toward the poles.

the centromere is replicated, and the two chromatids within the chromosome separate as they move along the spindle fibers toward the opposite ends of the poles (figure 9.8). Although this movement of chromosomes has been observed repeatedly, no one knows the exact mechanism of its action. After this separation of chromatids occurs, the chromatids are called **daughter chromosomes.** Daughter chromosomes contain identical genetic information.

Examine figure 9.8 closely and notice that the four chromosomes moving to one pole have exactly the same genetic information as the four moving to the opposite pole. It is the alignment of the chromosomes in metaphase, and their separation in anaphase, that causes this type of distribution. At the end of anaphase, there are two identical groups of chromosomes, one group at each pole. The next stage completes the mitosis process.

Telophase

Telophase is the last stage in mitosis. It is during telophase that daughter nuclei are formed. Each set of chromosomes becomes enclosed by a nuclear membrane and the nucleoli reappear. Now the cell has two identical **daughter nuclei** (figure 9.9). In addition, the microtubules are disassembled, so the spindle disappears. With the formation of the daughter nuclei, mitosis, the first process in cell division, is completed and the second process, cytokinesis, can occur. Cytokinesis divides the cytoplasm of the original cell and forms two smaller daughter cells. **Daughter cells** are two cells formed by cell division that have identical genetic information. Each of the newly formed daughter cells then enters the G_1 stage of interphase. These cells can grow, replicate their DNA, and enter another round of mitosis and cytokinesis to continue the cell cycle.

Mitosis—The Cell-Cloning Process   **165**

DIFFERENTIATION

Because of the two processes in cell division, mitosis and cytokinesis, the daughter cells have the same genetic composition. You received a set of genes from your father in his sperm, and a set of genes from your mother in her egg. By cell division, this cell formed two daughter cells. This process was repeated, and there were four cells, all of which had the same genes. All the trillions of cells in your body were formed by the process of cell division. This means that, except for mutations, all the cells in your body have the same genes (figure 9.10).

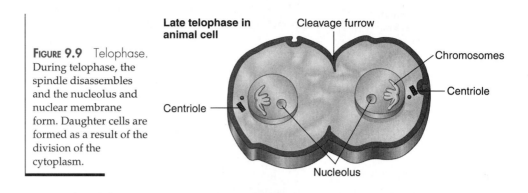

FIGURE 9.9 Telophase. During telophase, the spindle disassembles and the nucleolus and nuclear membrane form. Daughter cells are formed as a result of the division of the cytoplasm.

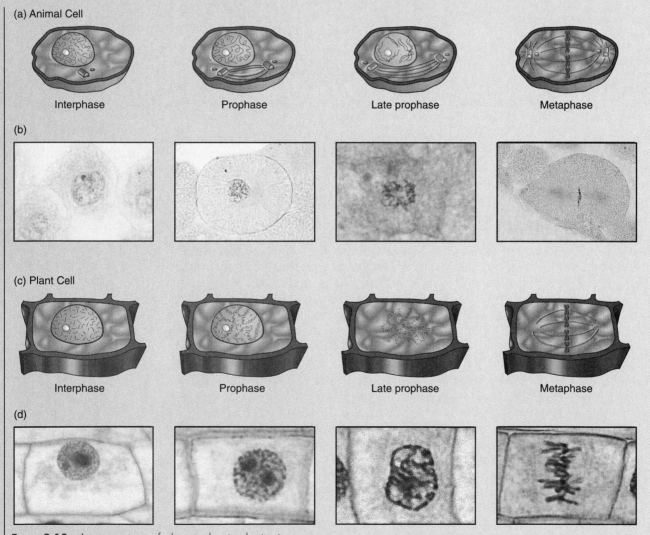

FIGURE 9.10 A comparison of plant and animal mitosis.
(a) Illustration of mitosis in an animal cell. (b) Photographs of mitosis in a whitefish blastula. (c) Drawing of mitosis in a plant cell.
(d) Photographs of mitosis in an onion root tip.

However, all the cells in your body are not the same. There are nerve cells, muscle cells, bone cells, skin cells, and many other types. How is it possible that cells with the same genes can produce different types of cells? Think of the genes in a cell as individual recipes in a cookbook. You could give a copy of the same cookbook to one hundred people and, although they all have the same book, each person could prepare a different dish. If you use the recipe to make a chocolate cake, you ignore the directions for making salads, fried chicken, and soups, although these recipes also are in the book.

It is the same with cells. Although some genes are used by all cells, some cells only activate certain genes. Muscle cells produce proteins capable of contraction. Most other cells do not use these genes. Pancreas cells use genes that result in the formation of digestive enzymes, but they never produce contractile proteins. **Differentiation** is the process of forming specialized cells within a multicellular organism. Some cells, such as muscle and nerve cells, lose their ability to divide; they remain permanently in the interphase condition. Other cells retain their ability to divide as their form of specialization. Cells that line the digestive tract or form the surface of your skin are examples of dividing cells. In growing organisms such as infants, seedlings, or embryos, most cells are capable of division and divide at a rapid rate. In older organisms, many cells lose their ability to divide as a result of

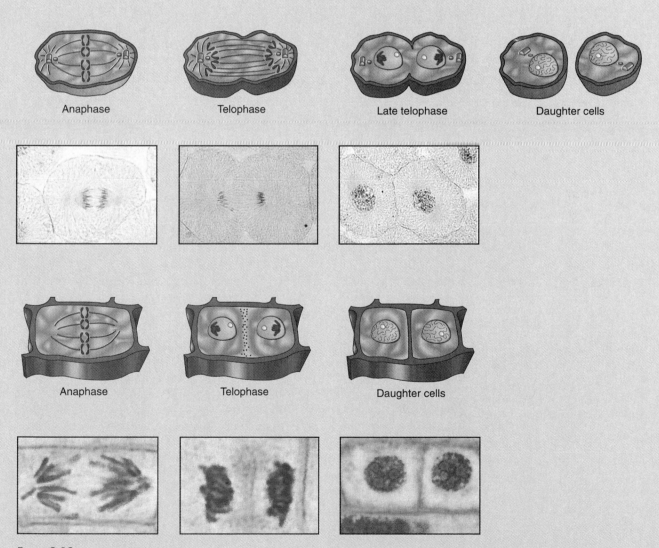

FIGURE 9.10   CONTINUED

FIGURE 9.11 Cytokinesis.
In animal cells there is a pinching
in of the cytoplasm that
eventually forms two daughter
cells. Daughter cells in plants are
formed when a cell plate
separates the cell into two cells.

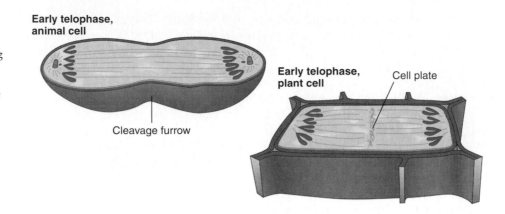

Early telophase,
animal cell

Cleavage furrow

Early telophase,
plant cell

Cell plate

FIGURE 9.12
Multinucleated cells.
Many types of fungi
including bread molds,
water molds, *Penicillium,* and
Aspergillus, are comprised of
multinucleated cells. As the
organism grows, nuclei
undergo mitosis but not
cytokinesis. As a result, each
cell contains tens of nuclei.
This multinucleate condition
provides each cell with a
large amount of DNA, which
fungi are capable of
regulating.

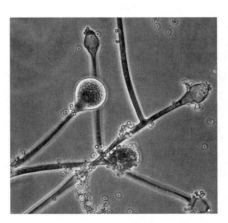

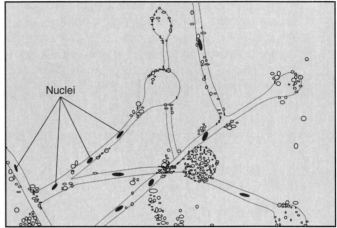

Nuclei

differentiation, and the frequency of cell division decreases. As the organism ages, the lower frequency of cell division may affect many bodily processes, including healing. In some older people, there may be so few cells capable of dividing that a broken bone may never heal. It is also possible for a cell to undergo mitosis but not cytokinesis (figure 9.11). In many types of fungi the cells undergo mitosis but not cytokinesis, which results in multinucleated cells (figure 9.12).

ABNORMAL CELL DIVISION

Understanding mitosis can help you understand certain biological problems and how to solve them. All cells do not divide at the same rate, but each kind of cell has a regulated division rhythm. Regulation of the cycle can come from inside or outside the cell. When human white blood cells are grown outside the body under special conditions, they develop a regular cell-division cycle. The cycle is determined by the DNA of the cells. However, white blood cells in the human body may increase their rate of mitosis as a result of outside influences. Disease organisms entering the body, tissue damage, and changes in cell DNA all may alter the rate at which white blood cells divide. An increase in white blood cells in response to the invasion of disease organisms is valuable because these white blood cells are capable of destroying the disease-causing organisms.

On the other hand, an uncontrolled increase in the rate of mitosis in white blood cells causes a kind of cancer known as *leukemia.* In some forms, this condition causes a general weakening of the body, because the excess number of white blood cells diverts necessary nutrients from other cells of the body and interferes with their normal activities.

Normally, cells become specialized for a particular function. Each cell type has its cell-division process regulated so that it does not interfere with the activities of

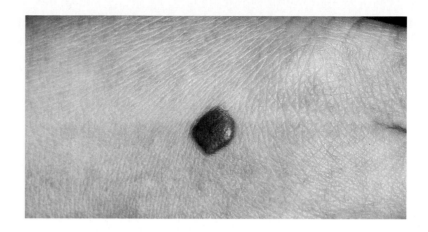

Figure 9.13 Cancer.
Malignant melanoma is a type of skin cancer. It forms as a result of a mutation in a pigmented skin cell. Only the dark area in the photograph is the cancer; the surrounding cells have the genetic information to develop into normal, healthy skin.

other cells or the whole organism. However, some cells may revert to an embryonic state and begin to divide. Sometimes this division occurs in an uncontrolled fashion. When this happens, a group of cells forms what is known as a *tumor* (figure 9.13). A *benign* tumor is a cell mass that does not fragment and spread beyond its original area of growth. A benign tumor can become harmful by growing to a point at which it interferes with normal body functions. Some tumors are *malignant*. Cells of these tumors move from the original site (metastasize) and establish new colonies in other regions of the body. **Cancer** is an abnormal growth of cells that has a malignant potential. Cancer cells break off from the original tumor and enter the bloodstream. When they get stuck to the inside of a capillary, the cancer cells move through the wall of the blood vessel and invade the tissue, where it begins to reproduce by mitosis. This tumor causes new blood vessels to grow into this new cancerous site, which will carry nutrients to this growing mass. These vessels can also bring other spreading cancer cells to the new tumor site.

Once cancer has been detected, treatment requires the elimination of the tumor. There are three kinds of treatment. If the cancer is confined to one or a few specific locations, it may be possible to surgically remove it. However, there are cases where surgery is impractical. If the tumor is located where it can't be removed without destroying healthy vital tissue, surgery may not be used. For example, the removal of certain brain cancers could severely damage the brain. In these cases, two other methods may be used to treat cancer.

Chemotherapy uses various types of chemicals to destroy cancer cells. This treatment may be used without knowing exactly where the cancer is located. However, it has negative effects on normal cells. Chemotherapy affects all actively dividing cells including hair follicles, intestinal mucosa, and bone marrow, where blood cells are produced. It lowers the body's immune reaction because it decreases its ability to produce white blood cells. Other side effects include intestinal disorders and the loss of hair, which are caused by damage to healthy dividing cells in the scalp and the intestinal tract.

Radiation therapy uses large amounts of X rays or gamma rays. Since this treatment damages surrounding healthy cells, it is used very cautiously when surgery is impractical. Radiation therapy can be effective because cells undergoing division are usually not in the G_1 stage. Nondividing cells pause in the G_1 stage and are less likely to be damaged by treatment. Cancer cells are usually in the S or G_2 stage. In these stages, DNA replication or protein synthesis is occurring and the cell is more subject to damage. Therefore, while radiation therapy may destroy healthy cells, it usually destroys more cancer cells.

Chemotherapy and radiation treatment are often used to control leukemia by taking advantage of the fact that these cells are undergoing an unusual mitosis. Dividing cells are likely to be damaged by x-radiation because the radiation can

Mitosis—The Cell-Cloning Process **169**

more easily destroy essential molecules (DNA) of the cell. Since cancer cells spend more time dividing than normal cells, they have a greater chance of being killed by radiation. Physicians, therefore, often prescribe cobalt therapy for certain patients with widely dispersed cancers such as leukemia. Cobalt is radioactive and releases radiation.

As a treatment for cancer, radiation is dangerous for the same reasons that it is beneficial. In cases of extreme exposure to radiation, people develop what is called *radiation sickness.* The symptoms of this disease include loss of hair, bloody vomiting and diarrhea, and a reduced white blood cell count. These symptoms occur in parts of the body where mitosis is common. The lining of the intestine is constantly being lost as food travels through and it must be replaced by the process of mitosis. Hair growth is the result of the continuous division of cells at the roots. White blood cells are also continuously reproduced in the bone marrow and lymph nodes. When radiation strikes these rapidly dividing cells and kills them, the lining of the intestine wears away and bleeds, hair falls out, and few new white blood cells are produced to defend the body against infection.

SUMMARY

Cell division is necessary for growth, repair, and reproduction. Cells go through a cell cycle that includes cell division (mitosis and cytokinesis) and interphase. Interphase is the period of growth and preparation for division. Mitosis is divided into four stages: prophase, metaphase, anaphase, and telophase. During mitosis, two daughter nuclei are formed from one parent nucleus. These nuclei have identical sets of chromosomes and genes that are exact copies of those of the parent. Although the process of mitosis has been presented as a series of phases, you should realize that it is a continuous, flowing process from prophase through telophase. Following mitosis, cytokinesis divides the cytoplasm, and the cell returns to interphase.

The regulation of mitosis is important if organisms are to remain healthy. Regular divisions are necessary to replace lost cells and allow for growth. However, uncontrolled cell division may result in cancer and disruption of the total organism's well-being.

QUESTIONS

1. Name the four stages of mitosis and describe what occurs in each stage.
2. What is meant by cell cycle?
3. During which stage of a cell's cycle does DNA replication occur?
4. At what phase of mitosis does the DNA become most visible?
5. What is cytokinesis?
6. Why can X-ray treatment be used to control cancer?
7. What is the purpose of mitosis?
8. What is the difference between a cell plate and a cell wall?
9. What types of activities occur during interphase?
10. List five differences between an interphase cell and a cell in mitosis.

anaphase (an'ă-fāz)   The third stage of mitosis, characterized by dividing the centromeres and movement of the chromosomes to the poles.

cancer (kan'sur)   A tumor that is malignant.

centrioles (sen'tre-ōls)   Organelles containing microtubules located just outside the nucleus.

centromere (sen'tro-mēr)   The unreplicated region where two chromatids are joined.

chromatid (kro'mah-tid)   One of two component parts of a chromosome formed by replication and attached at the centromere.

chromosomes (kro'mo-sōmz)   Complex structures within the nucleus composed of various kinds of histone proteins and DNA that contains the cell's genetic information.

cytokinesis (si-to-kǐ-ne'sis)   Division of the cytoplasm of one cell into two new cells.

daughter cells (daw'tur sels)   Two cells formed by cell division.

daughter chromosomes (daw'tur kro'mo-sōmz)   Chromosomes produced by DNA replication that contain identical genetic information; formed after chromosome division in anaphase.

daughter nuclei (daw'tur nu'kle-i)   Two nuclei formed by mitosis.

differentiation (dif"fur-ent-she-a'shun)   The process of forming specialized cells within a multicellular organism.

interphase (in'tur-fāz)   The stage between cell divisions in which the cell is engaged in metabolic activities.

metaphase (me'tah-fāz)   The second stage in mitosis, characterized by alignment of the chromosomes at the equatorial plane.

mitosis (mi-to'sis)   A process that results in equal and identical distribution of replicated chromosomes into two newly formed nuclei.

prophase (pro'fāz)   The first phase of mitosis during which individual chromosomes become visible.

spindle (spin'dul)   An array of microtubules extending from pole to pole; used in the movement of chromosomes.

telophase (tel'uh-fāz)   The last phase in mitosis characterized by the formation of daughter nuclei.

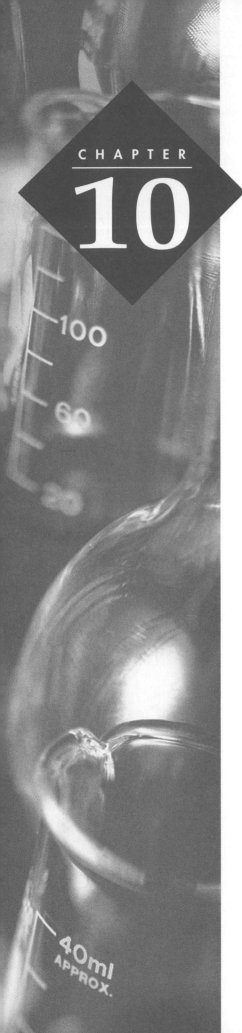

Meiosis—Sex-Cell Formation

CHAPTER OUTLINE

PURPOSE

How can the chromosome number in humans remain at forty-six generation after generation if both parents contribute equally to the genetic information of the child? In this chapter, we will discuss the mechanics of the process of meiosis. Meiosis is a specialized cell division that results in the formation of sex cells. Knowing the mechanics of this process is essential to understanding how genetic variety can occur in sex cells. This variety ultimately shows up as differences in offspring.

CLINICAL VIEWPOINT

Professional biologists, medical professionals, and others use symbols to represent the males and females of a species. The symbol for the male (♂) represents the shield and spear of the Greek god Zeus and the female symbol (♀) represents the vanity mirror of the goddess, Aphrodite. While their origins were certainly sexist, the symbols have persisted in Western culture and are universally recognized. Biologists also use a variety of other terms to refer to males and females (i.e., boys and girls; + and − strains), all of which can become pretty confusing after a while. To help keep things clear in your mind, just remember that the male donates or contributes genetic material into the female gamete, who accepts or receives the genetic material.

LEARNING OBJECTIVES

- Explain why sexually reproducing organisms must form cells with the haploid number of chromosomes
- Describe the stages in meiosis I
- Describe the stages in meiosis II

- Diagram how trisomy results from errors in the meiotic process
- Understand how genetic variety in offspring is generated by mutation, crossing-over, segregation, independent assortment, and fertilization
- Explain the similarities and differences between mitosis and meiosis

The most successful kinds of plants and animals are those that have developed a method of shuffling and exchanging genetic information. This usually involves organisms that have two sets of genetic data, one inherited from each parent. **Sexual reproduction** is the formation of a new individual by the union of two sex cells. Before sexual reproduction can occur, the two sets of genetic information must be reduced to one set. This is somewhat similar to shuffling a deck of cards and dealing out hands: the shuffling and dealing assure that each hand will be different. An organism with two sets of chromosomes can produce many combinations of chromosomes when it produces sex cells, just as many different hands can be dealt from one pack of cards. When one of these sex cells unites with another, a new organism containing two sets of genetic information is formed. This new organism's information might very well be superior to the information found in either parent; this is the value of sexual reproduction.

In chapter 9, we discussed the cell cycle and pointed out that it is a continuous process, without a beginning or an end. The process of mitosis, followed by growth, is important in the life cycle of any organism. Thus, the *cell cycle* is part of an organism's *life cycle* (figure 10.1).

The sex cells produced by male organisms are called **sperm,** and those produced by females are called **eggs.** A general term sometimes used to refer to either eggs or sperm is the term **gamete.** The cellular process that is responsible for generating gametes is called **gametogenesis.** The uniting of an egg and sperm (gametes) is known as **fertilization.**

In many organisms the **zygote,** which results from the union of an egg and a sperm, divides repeatedly by mitosis to form the complete organism. Notice in figure 10.1 that the zygote and its descendants have two sets of chromosomes. However, the male gamete and the female gamete each contain only one set of chromosomes. These sex cells are said to be **haploid.** The haploid number of chromosomes is noted as *n.* A zygote contains two sets and is said to be **diploid.** The diploid number of chromosomes is noted as $2n$ ($n + n = 2n$). Diploid cells have two sets of chromosomes, one set from each parent. Remember, a chromosome is composed of two chromatids, each containing duplex DNA. These two chromatids are attached to each other at a point called the *centromere.* In a diploid nucleus, the chromosomes occur as **homologous chromosomes**—a pair of chromosomes in a diploid cell that contain similar genes throughout their length. One of the chromosomes of a homologous pair was donated by the father, the other by the mother (figure 10.2). Different species of organisms vary in the number of chromosomes they contain. Table 10.1 lists several different organisms and their haploid and diploid chromosome numbers.

It is necessary for organisms that reproduce sexually to form gametes having only one set of chromosomes. If gametes contained two sets of chromosomes, the zygote resulting from their union would have four sets of chromosomes. The number of chromosomes would continue to double with each new generation, which could result in death. However, this does not happen; the number of

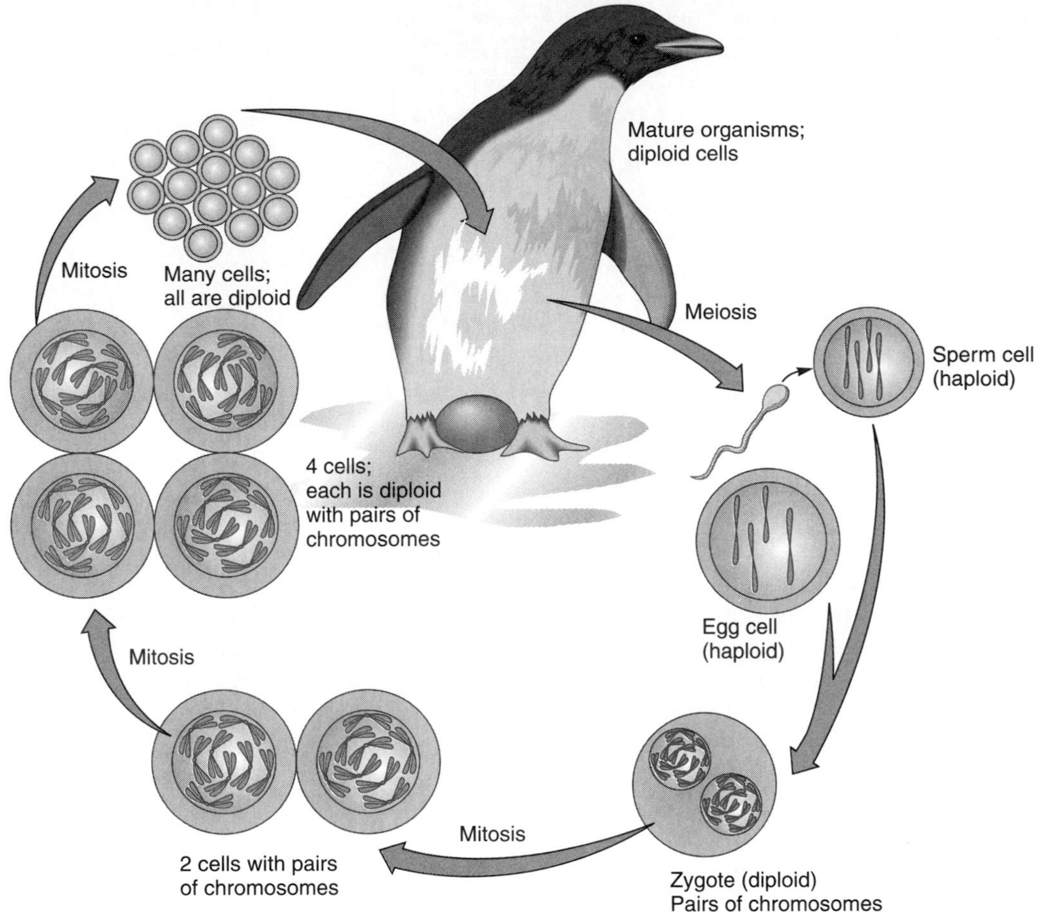

Figure 10.1
Life cycle.
The cells of this adult penguin have, for our purpose, eight chromosomes in their nuclei. In preparation for sexual reproduction, the number of chromosomes must be reduced by half so that fertilization will result in the original number of eight chromosomes in the new individual. The offspring will grow and produce new cells by mitosis. (The actual number of chromosomes has not been shown.)

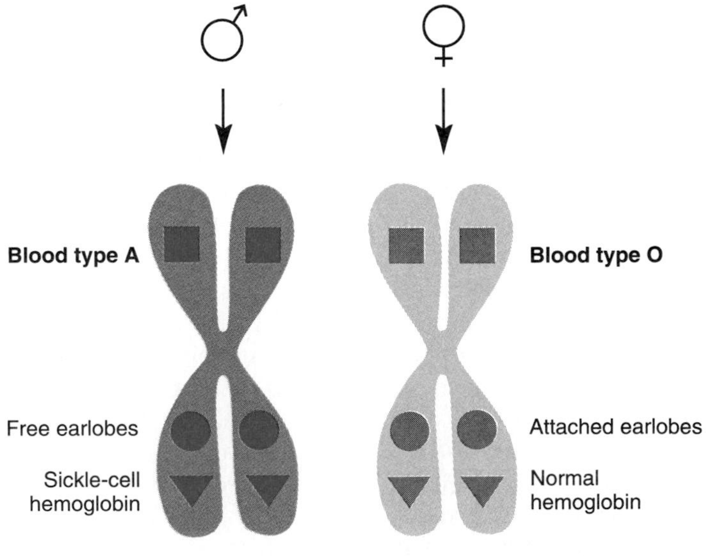

Mature organisms; diploid cells

Meiosis

Sperm cell (haploid)

Egg cell (haploid)

Zygote (diploid) Pairs of chromosomes

Mitosis

2 cells with pairs of chromosomes

Mitosis

4 cells; each is diploid with pairs of chromosomes

Mitosis

Many cells; all are diploid

Mitosis

Figure 10.2 A pair of homologous chromosomes.
A pair of chromosomes of similar size and shape that have genes for the same traits are said to be homologous. Notice that the genes may not be identical but code for the same type of information. Homologous chromosomes are of the same length, have the same types of gene in the same sequence, their centromeres in the same location, and one has come from the male parent while the other has been contributed from the female parent.

Blood type A

Blood type O

Free earlobes

Attached earlobes

Sickle-cell hemoglobin

Normal hemoglobin

chromosomes remains constant generation after generation. Since cell division by mitosis and cytokinesis results in cells that have the same number of chromosomes as the parent cell, two questions arise: how are sperm and egg cells formed, and how do they get only one-half the chromosomes of the diploid cell? The answers lie in the process of **meiosis,** the specialized pair of cell divisions that reduce the

Table 10.1 Chromosome Numbers

ORGANISM	HAPLOID NUMBER	DIPLOID NUMBER
Mosquito	3	6
Fruit fly	4	8
Housefly	6	12
Toad	18	36
Cat	19	38
Human	23	46
Hedgehog	23	46
Chimpanzee	24	48
Horse	32	64
Dog	39	78
Onion	8	16
Kidney bean	11	22
Rice	12	24
Tomato	12	24
Potato	24	48
Tobacco	24	48
Cotton	26	52

chromosome number from diploid ($2n$) to haploid (n). The major function of meiosis is to produce cells that have one set of genetic information. Therefore, when fertilization occurs, the zygote will have two sets of chromosomes, as did each parent.

Not every cell goes through the process of meiosis. Only specialized organs are capable of producing haploid cells (figure 10.3). In animals, the organs in which meiosis occurs are called **gonads.** The female gonads that produce eggs are called **ovaries.** The male gonads that produce sperm are called **testes.**

To illustrate meiosis in this chapter, for clarity we have chosen to show only 8 chromosomes (figure 10.4). In reality, humans have 46 chromosomes (23 pairs). The haploid number of chromosomes in this cell is four, and these haploid cells contain only one complete set of four chromosomes. As you can see, there are eight chromosomes in this cell—four from the mother and four from the father. A closer look at figure 10.4 shows you there are only four types of chromosomes, but two of each type:

1. Long chromosomes consisting of chromatids attached at the centromeres near the center;
2. Long chromosomes consisting of chromatids attached near one end;
3. Short chromosomes consisting of chromatids attached near one end; and
4. Short chromosomes consisting of chromatids attached near the center.

We can therefore talk about the number of chromosomes in two ways. We can say that our hypothetical diploid cell has eight chromosomes, or we can say that it has four pairs of homologous chromosomes.

Haploid cells, on the other hand, do not have homologous chromosomes. They have one of each type of chromosome. The whole point of meiosis is to distribute the chromosomes and the genes they carry so that each daughter cell gets one member of each homologous pair. In this way, each daughter cell gets one complete set of genetic information.

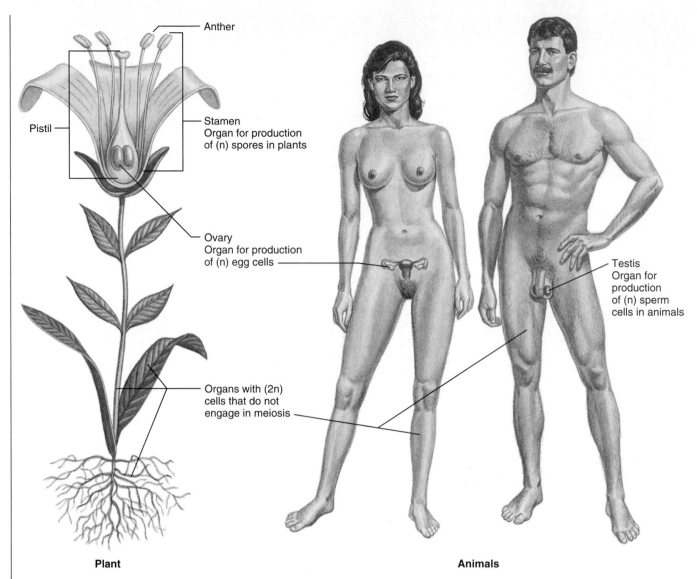

Anther

Pistil

Stamen
Organ for production
of (n) spores in plants

Ovary
Organ for production
of (n) egg cells

Organs with (2n)
cells that do not
engage in meiosis

Testis
Organ for
production
of (n) sperm
cells in animals

Plant

Animals

FIGURE 10.3 Haploid and diploid cells.
Both plants and animals produce cells with a haploid number of chromosomes. The male anther in plants and the testes in animals produce haploid male cells, sperm. In both plants and animals, the ovaries produce haploid female cells, eggs.

THE MECHANICS OF MEIOSIS: MEIOSIS I

Meiosis is preceded by an interphase stage when DNA replication occurs. In a sequence of events called *meiosis I*, members of homologous pairs of chromosomes divide into two complete sets. This is sometimes called a **reduction division,** a type of cell division in which daughter cells get only half the chromosomes from the parent cell. The division begins with chromosomes composed of two chromatids. The sequence of events in meiosis I is artificially divided into four phases: prophase I, metaphase I, anaphase I, and telophase I.

Prophase I

During prophase I, the cell is preparing itself for division (figure 10.5). The chromatin material coils and thickens into chromosomes, the nucleoli disappear, the nuclear membrane is disassembled, and the spindle begins to form. The spindle is formed in human cells when the centrioles move to the poles. However, there is an important difference between the prophase stage of mitosis and prophase I

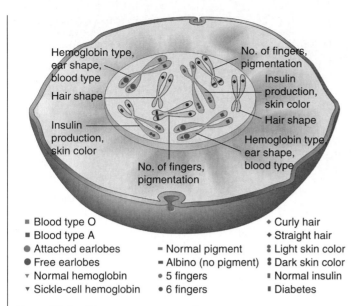

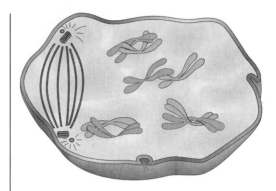

- ■ Blood type O
- ■ Blood type A
- ● Attached earlobes
- ● Free earlobes
- ▾ Normal hemoglobin
- ▾ Sickle-cell hemoglobin

- = Normal pigment
- ▬ Albino (no pigment)
- ● 5 fingers
- ● 6 fingers

- ◆ Curly hair
- ◆ Straight hair
- ⁑ Light skin color
- ⁑ Dark skin color
- ▌ Normal insulin
- ▌ Diabetes

FIGURE 10.4 Chromosomes in a cell.
In this diagram of a cell, the eight chromosomes are scattered in the nucleus. Even though they are not arranged in pairs, note that there are four pairs (each pair consisting of one colored and one gray chromosome) of homologous chromosomes. Check to be sure you can pair them up using the list of characteristics.

FIGURE 10.5 Prophase I.
During prophase I, the cell is preparing for division. A unique event that occurs in prophase I is the synapsis of the chromosomes. Notice that the nuclear membrane is no longer apparent and that the paired homologues are free to move about the cell.

of meiosis. During prophase I, homologous chromosomes come to lie next to each other in a process called **synapsis.** While the chromosomes are synapsed, a unique event called *crossing-over* may occur. **Crossing-over** is the exchange of equivalent sections of DNA on homologous chromosomes. We will fit crossing-over into the whole picture of meiosis later.

Metaphase I

The synapsed pair of homologous chromosomes now move into position on the equatorial plane of the cell. In this stage, the centromere of each chromosome attaches to the spindle. The synapsed homologous chromosomes move to the equator of the cell as single units. How they are arranged on the equator (which one is on the left and which one is on the right) is determined by chance (figure 10.6). In the cell in figure 10.6, three colored chromosomes from the father and one gray chromosome from the mother are lined up on the left. Similarly, one colored chromosome from the father and three gray chromosomes from the mother are on the right. They could have aligned themselves in several other ways. For instance, they could have lined up as shown on the right in figure 10.6.

Anaphase I

Anaphase I is the stage during which homologous chromosomes separate (figure 10.7). During this stage, the chromosome number is reduced from diploid to haploid. The two members of each pair of homologous chromosomes move away from each other toward opposite poles. The centromeres do not replicate during this phase. The direction each takes is determined by how each pair was originally arranged on the spindle. Each chromosome is independently attached to a spindle fiber at its centromere. Unlike the anaphase stage of mitosis, *the centromeres that hold the chromatids together do not divide during anaphase I of meiosis.*

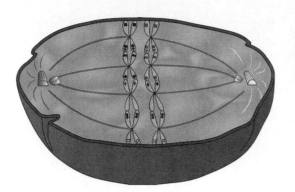

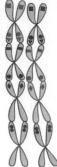

FIGURE 10.6 Metaphase I.
Notice that the homologous chromosome pairs are arranged on the equatorial plane in the synapsed condition. The cell at the left shows one way the chromosomes could be lined up. The chromosomes on the right shows a second arrangement. How many other ways can you diagram?

- ■ Blood type A
- ■ Blood type O
- ● Free earlobes
- ● Attached earlobes
- ▼ Sickle-cell hemoglobir
- ▼ Normal hemoglobin
- ▬ Albino (no pigment)
- ▬ Normal pigment
- ● 6 fingers
- ● 5 fingers
- ◆ Straight hair
- ◆ Curly hair
- 🕴 Dark skin color
- 🕴 Light skin color
- □ Diabetes
- □ Normal insulin

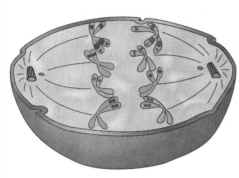

- ■ Blood type O
- ■ Blood type A
- ● Attached earlobes
- ● Free earlobes
- ▼ Normal hemoglobin
- ▼ Sickle-cell hemoglobin
- ▬ Normal pigment
- ▬ Albino (no pigment)
- ● 5 fingers
- ● 6 fingers
- ◆ Curly hair
- ◆ Straight hair
- 🕴 Light skin color
- 🕴 Dark skin color

FIGURE 10.7 Anaphase I.
During this phase, one member of each homologous pair is segregated from the other member of the pair. Notice that the centromeres of the chromosomes do not replicate.

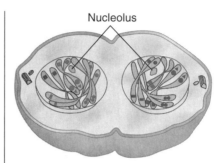

Nucleolus

FIGURE 10.8 Telophase I.
What activities would you expect during the telophase stage of cell division? What term is used to describe the fact that the cytoplasm is beginning to split the parent cell into two daughter cells?

Each chromosome still consists of two chromatids. Because the homologous chromosomes and the genes they carry are being separated from one another, this process is called **segregation.** The way in which a single pair of homologous chromosomes segregates does not influence how other pairs of homologous chromosomes segregate. That is, each pair segregates independently of other pairs. This is known as **independent assortment** of chromosomes.

Telophase I

Telophase I consists of changes that return the cell to an interphase-like condition (figure 10.8). The chromosomes uncoil and become long, thin threads, the nuclear membrane re-forms around them, and nucleoli reappear. During this activity, cytokinesis divides the cytoplasm into two separate cells.

Because of meiosis I, the total number of chromosomes is divided equally, and each daughter cell has one member of each homologous chromosome pair. This means that the genetic data each cell receives is one-half of the total, but each cell still has a complete set of the genetic information. Each individual chromosome is still composed of two chromatids joined at the centromere, and the chromosome number is reduced from diploid ($2n$) to haploid (n). In the cell we have been using as our example, the number of chromosomes is reduced from eight to four. The four pairs of chromosomes have been distributed to the two daughter cells.

FIGURE 10.9 Meiosis I.
The stages in meiosis I result in
reduction division. This reduces the
number of chromosomes in the
parental cell from the diploid
number to the haploid number in
each of the two daughter cells.

Prophase I

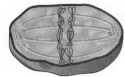

Metaphase I

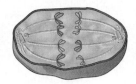

Anaphase I

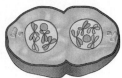

Telophase I

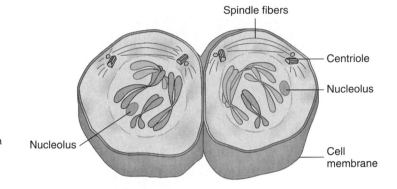

Spindle fibers

Centriole

Nucleolus

Nucleolus

Cell
membrane

FIGURE 10.10 Prophase II.
The two daughter cells are preparing for the second division
of meiosis. Study this diagram carefully. Solely from your
observations, can you list the events of this stage?

Depending on the type of cell, there may be a time following telophase I
when a cell engages in normal metabolic activity that corresponds to an interphase stage. However, the chromosomes do not replicate before the cell enters
meiosis II. Figure 10.9 shows the events in meiosis I.

Meiosis II includes four phases: prophase II, metaphase II, anaphase II, and
telophase II. The two daughter cells formed during meiosis I continue through
meiosis II, so that usually four cells result from the two divisions.

THE MECHANICS OF MEIOSIS: MEIOSIS II

Prophase II

Prophase II is similar to prophase in mitosis; the nuclear membrane is disassembled, nucleoli disappear, and the spindle apparatus begins to form. However, it
differs from prophase I because these cells are haploid, not diploid (figure 10.10).
Also, synapsis, crossing-over, segregation, and independent assortment do not
occur during prophase II.

Metaphase II

The metaphase II stage is typical of any metaphase stage because the chromosomes attach by their centromeres to the spindle at the equatorial plane of the
cell. Since pairs of chromosomes are no longer together in the same cell, each
chromosome moves as a separate unit (figure 10.11).

Anaphase II

Anaphase II differs from anaphase I because the centromere of each chromosome
replicates in two, and the chromatids, now called *daughter chromosomes,* move to
the poles (figure 10.12). Remember, there are no paired homologs in this stage;
therefore, segregation and independent assortment cannot occur.

Telophase II

During telophase II, the cell returns to a nondividing condition. As cytokinesis
occurs, new nuclear membranes form, chromosomes uncoil, nucleoli re-form,

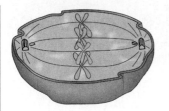 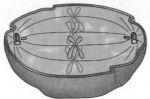

FIGURE 10.11 Metaphase II.
During this metaphase, each chromosome lines up on the equatorial plane. Each chromosome is composed of two chromatids joined at a centromere. How does metaphase II of meiosis compare to metaphase of mitosis?

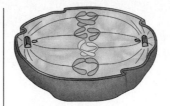 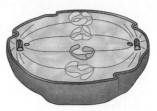

FIGURE 10.12 Anaphase II.
This anaphase stage is very similar to the anaphase of mitosis. The centromere of each chromosome divides and one chromatid separates from the other. As soon as this happens, we no longer refer to them as chromatids; we now call each strand of nucleoprotein a chromosome.

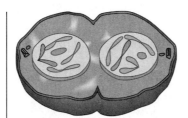 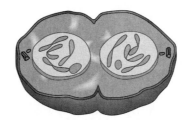

FIGURE 10.13 Telophase II.
During the telophase stage, what events would you expect?

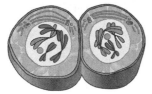 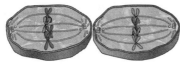 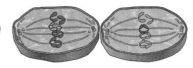 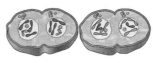

| Prophase II | Metaphase II | Anaphase II | Telophase II |

FIGURE 10.14 Meiosis II.
During meiosis II, the centromere replicates and each chromosome divides into separate chromatids. Four haploid cells are produced from one diploid parent cell.

and the spindles disappear (figure 10.13). This stage is followed by differentiation; the four cells mature into gametes—either sperm or eggs. The events of meiosis II are summarized in figure 10.14.

In many organisms, egg cells are produced in such a manner that three of the four cells resulting from meiosis in a female disintegrate. However, since the one that survives is randomly chosen, the likelihood of any one particular combination of genes being formed is not affected. *The whole point of learning the mechanism of meiosis is to see how variation happens.* Now we can look at variation and how it comes about.

SOURCES OF VARIATION

The formation of a haploid cell by meiosis, and the combination of two haploid cells to form a diploid cell by sexual reproduction, result in variety in the offspring. There are five factors that influence genetic variation in offspring: mutations, crossing-over, segregation, independent assortment, and fertilization.

Two types of mutations were discussed in chapter 8: point mutations and chromosomal mutations. In point mutations, there is a change in a DNA nucleotide that results in the production of a different protein. In chromosomal mutations, genes are rearranged. By causing the production of different proteins, both types of mutations increase variation. The second source of variation is crossing-over.

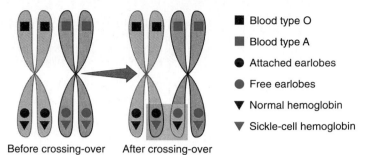

FIGURE 10.15 [icon] Synapsis and crossing-over.
While pairs of homologous chromosomes are in synapsis, one part of one chromatid can break off and be exchanged for an equivalent part of its homologous chromatid. List the new combination of genes on each chromatid that have resulted from the crossing-over.

Before crossing-over   After crossing-over

- ■ Blood type O
- ■ Blood type A
- ● Attached earlobes
- ● Free earlobes
- ▼ Normal hemoglobin
- ▼ Sickle-cell hemoglobin

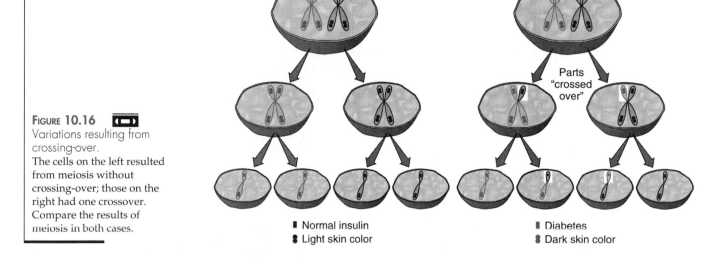

FIGURE 10.16 [icon]
Variations resulting from crossing-over.
The cells on the left resulted from meiosis without crossing-over; those on the right had one crossover. Compare the results of meiosis in both cases.

Parts "crossed over"

- ▮ Normal insulin
- ▰ Light skin color

- ▮ Diabetes
- ▰ Dark skin color

Crossing-Over

Crossing-over is the exchange of a part of a chromatid from one homologous chromosome with an equivalent part of a chromatid from the other homologous chromosome. This exchange results in a new gene combination. Crossing-over occurs during meiosis I while homologous chromosomes are synapsed. Remember that a chromosome is a double strand of DNA. To break a chromosome, bonds between sugars and phosphates are broken. This is done at the same spot on both chromatids, and the two pieces switch places. After switching places, the two pieces of DNA are bonded together by re-forming the bonds between the sugar and the phosphate molecules. Examine figure 10.15 carefully to note precisely what occurs during crossing-over.

This figure shows a pair of homologous chromosomes close to each other. Notice that each gene occupies a specific place on the chromosome. This is the *locus*, a place on a chromosome where a gene is located. Homologous chromosomes contain an identical order of genes. For the sake of simplicity, only a few loci are labeled on the chromosomes used as examples. Actually, the chromosomes contain hundreds or possibly thousands of genes.

What does crossing-over have to do with the possible kinds of cells that result from meiosis? Consider figure 10.16. Notice that without crossing-over, only two kinds of genetically different gametes result. Two of the four gametes have one type of chromosome, while the other two have the other type of chromosome. With crossing-over, four genetically different gametes are formed. With just one crossover, we double the number of kinds of gametes possible from meiosis. Since crossing-over can occur at almost any point along the length of the

Meiosis—Sex-Cell Formation **181**

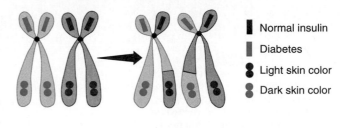

Figure 10.17 Multiple crossovers.
Crossing-over can occur several times between one pair of homologous chromosomes. List the new combination of genes on each chromatid that have resulted from the crossing-over.

Normal insulin
Diabetes
Light skin color
Dark skin color

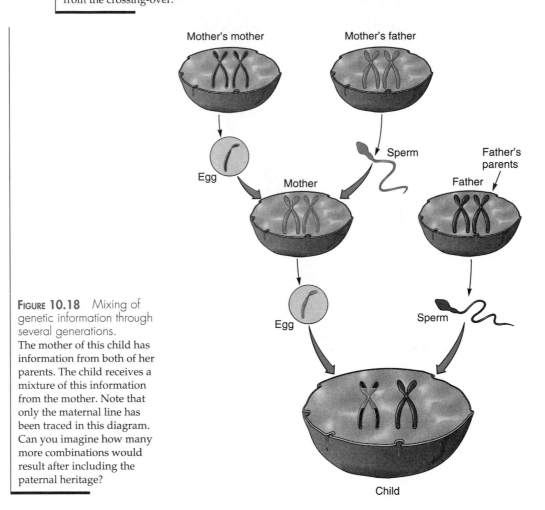

Mother's mother

Mother's father

Egg

Sperm

Mother

Father's parents

Father

Egg

Sperm

Child

Figure 10.18 Mixing of genetic information through several generations.
The mother of this child has information from both of her parents. The child receives a mixture of this information from the mother. Note that only the maternal line has been traced in this diagram. Can you imagine how many more combinations would result after including the paternal heritage?

chromosome, great variation is possible. In fact, crossing-over can occur at a number of different points on the same chromosome; that is, there can be more than one crossover per chromosome pair (figure 10.17).

Crossing-over helps to explain why a child can show a mixture of family characteristics (figure 10.18). If the colored chromosome was the chromosome that a mother received from her mother, the child could receive some genetic information not only from the mother's mother, but also from the mother's father. When crossing-over occurs during the meiotic process, pieces of genetic material are exchanged between the chromosomes. This means that genes that were originally on the same chromosome become separated. They are moved to their synapsed homolog, and therefore into different gametes. The closer two genes are to each other on a chromosome (i.e., the more closely they are *linked*), the more likely they will stay together and not be separated during crossing-over. Thus, there is a high probability that they will be inherited together. The further apart two genes are, the more likely it is that they will be separated during crossing-over. This fact enables biologists to construct chromosome maps (*see* box 10.1).

Box 10.1

The Human Genome Project

The human genome project was first proposed in 1986 and is one of the most ambitious projects ever undertaken in the biological sciences. The goal is nothing less than the complete characterization of the genetic makeup of humans. If the effort is successful, scientists will have produced a map of each of the twenty-three pairs of human chromosomes that will show the names and places of all of our genes. This international project involving about one hundred laboratories is expected to take fifteen years. Work began in many of these labs in 1990. Powerful computers are used to store and share the enormous amount of information derived from the analyses of human DNA. To get an idea of the size of this project, a human Y chromosome (one of the smallest of the human chromosomes) is estimated to be composed of 28 million chemical subunits called *nitrogenous bases*. The larger X chromosome may be composed of 160 million bases (box figure 10.1). It is the sequence of these bases that determine the genes.

Two kinds of work are progressing simultaneously. Physical maps are being constructed by determining the location of specific "markers" (known sequences of bases) and their closeness to genes. A kind of chromosome map already exists that pictures patterns of colored bands on chromosomes, a result of chromosome-staining procedures. Using these banded chromosomes, the markers can then be related to these colored bands on a specific region of a chromosome. Work is continuing on the human genome project to identify the location of genes. Each year a more complete picture is revealed.

The second goal—to determine the exact order of nitrogenous bases of the DNA for each chromosome—will take longer. Techniques exist for determining base sequences, but it is a time-consuming job to sort out the several million bases that may be found in any one chromosome. It is estimated, for example, that there are over 100,000 genes yet to have their base sequences determined and their exact positions identified. At the end of 1992, certain chromosomes had some of their base sequences identified, and over 2,000 genes (about 2% of the entire human genome) had been located at specific places.

When the maps are completed for all of the human chromosomes, it will be possible to examine a person's DNA and identify genetic abnormalities. This could be extremely useful in diagnosing diseases and providing genetic counseling to carriers of genetic defects who are considering having children. This kind of information would also create possibilities for new gene therapies. Once it is known where an abnormal gene is located and how it differs in base-sequence from the normal DNA sequence, steps could be taken to correct the abnormality. However, there is also a concern that, as knowledge of our genetic makeup becomes easier to determine, some people may attempt to use this information for profit or political power. This is a real concern since some insurance companies refuse to insure people at "genetic risk." Refusing to provide coverage would save these companies the expense of future medical bills incurred by "less-than-perfect" people. Another fear is that attempts may be made to "breed out" certain genes and people from the human population in order to create a "perfect race."

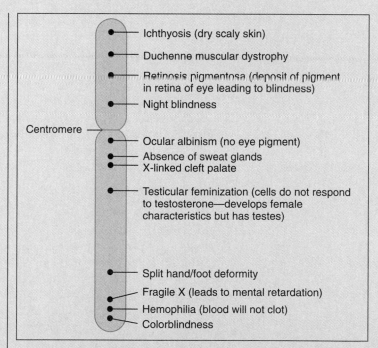

BOX FIGURE 10.1 **Genes known to be on the X chromosome.** This gene map shows the approximate position of several genes known to be on the human X chromosome.

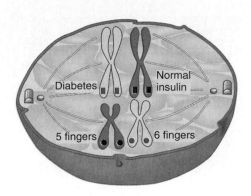

FIGURE 10.19 The independent orientation of homologous chromosome pairs. The orientation of one pair of chromosomes on the equatorial plane does not affect the orientation of a second pair of chromosomes. This results in increased variety in the haploid cells.

Segregation

After crossing-over has taken place, segregation occurs. This involves the separation and movement of homologous chromosomes to the poles. Let's say a person has one form of a gene for normal insulin production on one chromosome and an abnormal form of this gene on the other. Such a person would produce enough insulin to be healthy and would not be diabetic. When this pair of chromosomes segregates during anaphase I, one daughter cell receives a chromosome with a normal gene for insulin production and the second daughter cell receives a chromosome with an abnormal gene for diabetes. The process of segregation causes genes to be separated from one another so that they have an equal chance of being transmitted to the next generation. If the mate also has one normal gene for insulin production and one abnormal for diabetes, that person also produces two kinds of gametes.

Both of the parents have normal insulin production. If one or both of them contributed a gene for normal insulin production during fertilization, the offspring would produce enough insulin to be healthy. However, if, by chance, both parents contributed the gamete with the abnormal gene for diabetes, the child would be a diabetic. Thus, parents may produce offspring with traits different from their own. In this variation, no new genes are created; they are simply redistributed in a fashion that allows for the new combination of genes in the offspring to be different from the parents' gene combinations. This will be explored in greater detail in chapter 11.

Independent Assortment

So far in discussing variety, we have only dealt with one pair of chromosomes, which allows two varieties of gametes. Now let's consider how variation increases when we add a second pair of chromosomes (figure 10.19).

In figure 10.19, chromosomes carrying insulin-production information always separate from each other. The second pair of chromosomes with the information for the number of fingers also separates. Since the pole to which a chromosome moves is a chance event, half of the time the chromosomes divide so that insulin production and six-fingeredness move in one direction, while diabetes and five-fingeredness move in the opposite direction. The other half of the time, insulin production and five-fingeredness go together, while diabetes and six-fingeredness go to the other pole. With four chromosomes (two pair), four kinds of gametes are possible (figure 10.20). With three pairs of homologous chromosomes, there are eight possible kinds of cells with respect to chromosome combinations resulting from meiosis. See if you can list them. The number of possible chromosomal combinations of gametes is found by the expression 2^n, where n equals the number of pairs of chromosomes. With three pairs of chromosomes, n equals 3, and so $2^n = 2^3 = 2 \times 2 \times 2 = 8$. With 23 pairs of chromosomes, as in the human cell, $2^n = 2^{23} = 8,388,608$. More than eight million kinds of sperm cells or egg cells are possible

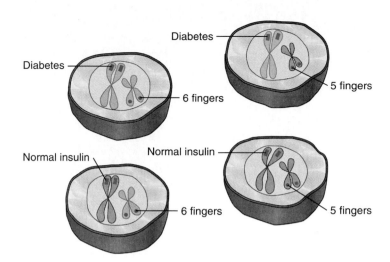

FIGURE 10.20 *Variation resulting from independent assortment.*
When a cell has two pairs of homologous chromosomes, four kinds of haploid cells can result from independent assortment. How many kinds of haploid cells could result if the parental cell had three pairs? Four pairs?

from a single human parent organism. This number is actually smaller than the maximum variety that could be produced, since it only takes into consideration the variety generated as a result of independent assortment. This huge variation is possible because each pair of homologous chromosomes assorts independently of the other pairs of homologous chromosomes (independent assortment). In addition to this variation, crossing-over creates new gene combinations, and mutation can cause the formation of new genes, thereby increasing this number greatly.

Fertilization

Because of the large number of possible gametes resulting from independent assortment, segregation, mutation, and crossing-over, an incredibly large number of types of offspring can result. Since human males can produce millions of genetically different sperm and females can produce millions of genetically different eggs, the number of kinds of offspring possible is infinite for all practical purposes. With the possible exception of identical twins, every human that has ever been born is genetically unique.

In the normal process of meiosis, diploid cells have their number of chromosomes reduced to haploid. This involves segregating homologous chromosomes into separate cells during the first meiotic division. Occasionally, a pair of homologous chromosomes does not segregate properly during gametogenesis and both chromosomes of a pair end up in the same gamete. This kind of division is known as **nondisjunction** (figure 10.21). As you can see in this figure, two cells are missing a chromosome and the genes that were carried on it. This usually results in the death of the cells. The other cells have a double dose of one chromosome. Apparently the genes of an organism are balanced against one another. A double dose of some genes and a single dose of others results in abnormalities that may lead to the death of the cell. Some of these abnormal cells, however, do live and develop into sperm or eggs. If one of these abnormal sperm or eggs unites with a normal gamete, the offspring will have an abnormal number of chromosomes. There will be three of one of the kinds of chromosomes instead of the normal two, a condition referred to as **trisomy.** All the cells that develop by mitosis from that zygote will also be trisomic.

It is possible to examine cells and count chromosomes. Among the easiest cells to view are white blood cells. They are dropped onto a microscope slide so that the cells are broken open and the chromosomes separated. Computerized images are made of chromosomes from cells in the metaphase stage of mitosis.

NONDISJUNCTION

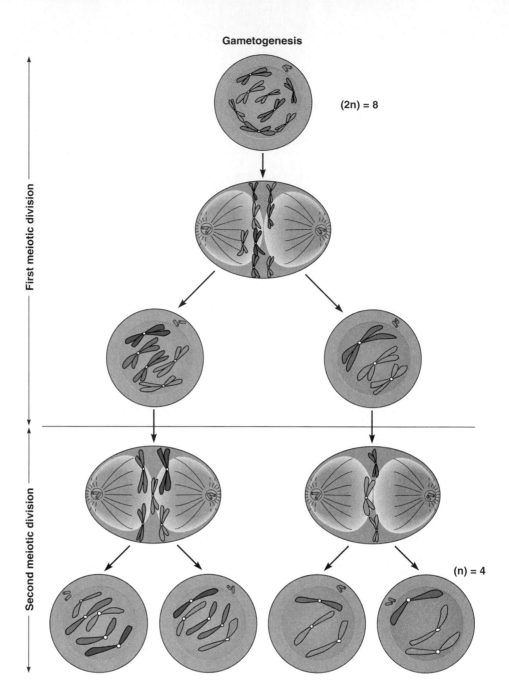

Gametogenesis

(2n) = 8

First meiotic division

Second meiotic division

(n) = 4

FIGURE 10.21 Nondisjunction during gametogenesis. When a pair of homologous chromosomes fails to separate properly during meiosis I, gametogenesis results in gametes that have an abnormal number of chromosomes. Notice that two of the highlighted cells have an additional chromosome, while the other two are deficient by that same chromosome.

The chromosomes in the pictures are arranged for comparison to known samples (figure 10.22). This picture of an individual's chromosomal makeup is referred to as their *karyotype*.

One example of the effects of nondisjunction is the condition known as **Down syndrome** (mongolism). If a gamete with two number 21 chromosomes has been fertilized by another containing the typical one copy of chromosome number 21, the resulting zygote would have forty-seven chromosomes (for example, twenty-four from the female plus twenty-three from the male parent) (figure 10.23). The child who developed from this fertilization would have forty-seven chromosomes in every cell of his or her body as a result of mitosis, and the symptoms characteristic of Down syndrome. These could include thickened eyelids, some mental impairment, and faulty speech (figure 10.24). Premature aging is probably the most significant impact of this genetic disease.

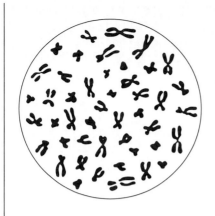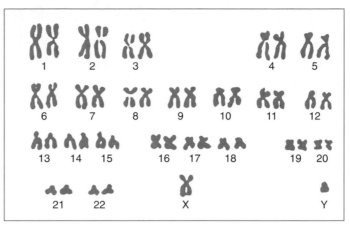

FIGURE 10.22 Human male chromosomes.
The randomly arranged human male chromosomes shown on the left were photographed from metaphase cells spattered onto a microscope slide. Those on the right are the result of arranging them into pairs of homologous chromosomes.

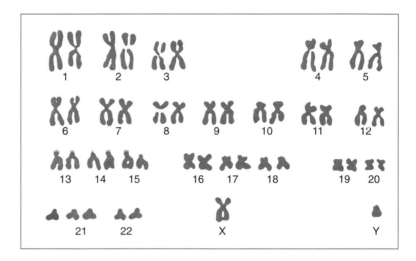

FIGURE 10.23 Chromosomes from an individual displaying Down syndrome.
Notice that each pair of chromosomes has been numbered and that the person from whom these chromosomes were taken has an extra chromosome number 21. The person with this trisomic condition could display a variety of physical characteristics, including slightly slanted eyes, flattened facial features, a large tongue, and a tendency toward short stature and fingers. Most individuals also display mental retardation.

It was thought that the woman's age played an important part in the occurrence of trisomies such as Down syndrome. In women, gametogenesis begins early in life, but cells destined to become eggs are put on hold during meiosis I. One of these cells completes the meiotic process monthly, beginning at puberty and ending at menopause. This means that eggs released for fertilization later in life are older than those released earlier in life. Therefore, it was believed that the chances of abnormalities such as nondisjunction increase as the age of the mother increases. However, the evidence no longer supports this age-egg-related link. Currently, the increase in frequency of trisomies with age has been correlated with a decrease in the activity of a woman's immune system. As she ages, her immune system is less likely to recognize the difference between an abnormal and normal embryo. This means that she is more likely to carry an abnormal fetus to full term. Figure 10.25 illustrates the frequency of occurrence of nondisjunction at different ages in women. Notice that the frequency of nondisjunction increases very rapidly after age thirty-seven. For this reason, many physicians encourage couples to have their

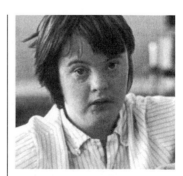

FIGURE 10.24 Down syndrome. Every downic child's body has one extra chromosome. With special care, planning, and training, people with this syndrome can lead useful, productive lives.

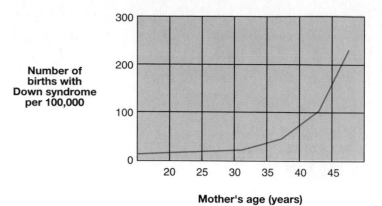

Figure 10.25 Nondisjunction as a function of a mother's age.

Notice that as the age of the female increases, the rate of nondisjunction increases only slightly until the age of approximately thirty-seven. From that point on, the rate increases drastically. This increase is most likely due to women experiencing fewer miscarriages of abnormal embryos.

children in their early to mid-twenties and not in their late thirties or early forties. Physicians normally encourage older women who are pregnant to have the cells of their fetus checked to see if they have the normal chromosome number. It is important to know that the male parent can also contribute the extra chromosome 21. However, it appears that this occurs less than 30% of the time.

Sometimes two separate chromosomes may be joined to one another. (Chromosome 21 may be joined to chromosome 14.) Therefore, whenever an individual is born with a trisomic condition, it is recommended that both parents have a karyotype in an attempt to identify the possible source of the extra chromosome. This is not to fix blame but to provide information on the likelihood that a next pregnancy would also result in a trisomic child.

CHROMOSOMES AND SEX DETERMINATION

You already know that there are several different kinds of chromosomes, that each chromosome carries genes unique to it, and that these genes are found at specific places. Furthermore, diploid organisms have homologous pairs of chromosomes. Sexual characteristics are determined by genes in the same manner as other types of characteristics. In many organisms, sex-determining genes are located on specific chromosomes known as **sex chromosomes.** All other chromosomes not involved in determining the sex of an individual are known as **autosomes** (box 10.2). The biological mechanism that determines female or male gender in humans has been well documented. When a human egg or sperm cell is produced, it contains twenty-three chromosomes, one of which is a sex-determining chromosome.

There are two kinds of sex-determining chromosomes: the X chromosome and the Y chromosome. The two sex-determining chromosomes, X and Y, do not carry equivalent amounts of information, nor do they have equal functions. In addition to their function in determining sex, the X chromosome carries typical information about the production of specific proteins. The Y chromosome carries information for determining maleness as well as a few other genes.

When a human sperm cell is produced, it carries twenty-three chromosomes, one of which is a sex-determining chromosome. Unlike eggs, which always carry an X chromosome, half of the sperm cells carry an X chromosome and the other half carry a Y chromosome. If an X-carrying sperm cell fertilizes the X-containing

Box 10.2

The Birds, Bees, . . . and Alligators and What???

The determination of the sex of an individual depends on the kind of organism you are! For example, in humans, the physical features that result in maleness are triggered by a gene on the Y chromosome. Lack of a Y chromosome results in an individual that is female. In other organisms, sex may be determined by other combinations of chromosomes or environmental factors.

Organism	Sex Determination
Birds	Chromosomally determined: XY individuals are female.
Bees	Males (the drones) are haploid and females (workers or queens) are diploid females.
Certain species of alligators, turtles, and lizards	Egg incubation temperatures cause hormonal changes in the developing embryo; higher incubation temperatures cause the developing brain to shift sex in favor of the individual becoming a female. (Placing a drop of the hormone estrogen on the developing egg also causes the embryo to become female!)
Boat shell snails	Males can become females; however, they will remain male if they mate and remain in one spot
Shrimp, orchids, and some tropical fish	Males convert to females; on occasion females convert to males. Reason? Probably to maximize breeding!
African reed frog	Females convert to males. Reason? Probably to maximize breeding!

egg cell, the resulting embryo will develop into a female. It is the absence of the Y chromosome that determines femaleness. Femaleness appears to be the "preset" condition. A typical human female has an X chromosome from each parent. If a Y-carrying sperm cell fertilizes the egg, a male embryo develops.

The embryo becomes male or female based on the sex-determining chromosomes that control the differentiation of the sex organs, the testes and ovaries. If the Y chromosome is present, the embryonic gonads begin to differentiate into testes about seven weeks after conception. If the embryo does not have a Y chromosome, the gonads differentiate into female sex organs later.

Researchers are interested in how females, with two X chromosomes, handle the double dose of genetic material in comparison to males, who have only one X chromosome. M. L. Barr discovered that a dark-staining body was generally present in female cells but was not present in male cells. It was postulated, and has since been confirmed, that this structure is an X chromosome that is largely nonfunctional. Therefore, although female cells have two X chromosomes, only one is functional; the other X chromosome coils up tightly and does not direct the manufacture of proteins. The one X chromosome of the male functions as expected, and the Y chromosome directs the expression of traits that occur only in males. The tightly coiled structure in the cells of female mammals is called a *Barr body*.

A COMPARISON OF MITOSIS AND MEIOSIS

Some of the similarities and differences between mitosis and meiosis were pointed out earlier in this chapter. Study table 10.2 to familiarize yourself with the differences between these two processes.

Table 10.2 A Comparison of Mitosis and Meiosis

MITOSIS	MEIOSIS
1. One division completes the process.	1. Two divisions are required to complete the process.
2. Chromosomes do not synapse.	2. Homologous chromosomes synapse in prophase I.
3. Homologous chromosomes do not cross over.	3. Homologous chromosomes do cross over.
4. Centromeres divide in anaphase.	4. Centromeres divide in anaphase II, but not in anaphase I.
5. Daughter cells have the same number of chromosomes as the parent cell ($2n \rightarrow 2n$ or $n \rightarrow n$).	5. Daughter cells have half the number of chromosomes as the parent cell ($2n \rightarrow n$).
6. Daughter cells have the same genetic information as the parent cell.	6. Daughter cells are genetically different from the parent cell.
7. Results in growth, replacement of worn-out cells, and repair of damage.	7. Results in sex cells.

SUMMARY

Meiosis is a specialized process of cell division resulting in the production of four cells, each of which has the haploid number of chromosomes. The total process involves two sequential divisions during which one diploid cell reduces to four haploid cells. Since the chromosomes act as carriers for genetic information, genes separate into different sets during meiosis. Crossing-over and segregation allow hidden characteristics to be displayed, while independent assortment allows characteristics donated by the mother and the father to be mixed in new combinations.

Together, crossing-over, segregation, and independent assortment ensure that all sex cells are unique. Therefore, when any two cells unite to form a zygote, the zygote will also be one of a kind. The sex of many kinds of organisms is determined by the specific genetic composition of chromosomes. In humans, females have two X chromosomes, while males have an X and a Y chromosome.

QUESTIONS

1. List three differences between mitosis and meiosis.
2. How do haploid cells differ from diploid cells?
3. What are the major sources of variation in the process of meiosis?
4. Can a haploid cell undergo meiosis?
5. What is unique about prophase I?
6. Why is meiosis necessary in organisms that reproduce sexually?
7. Define the terms *zygote, fertilization,* and *homologous chromosomes.*
8. How much variation as a result of independent assortment can occur in cells with the following diploid numbers: 2, 4, 6, 8, and 22?
9. Diagram the metaphase I stage of a cell with the diploid number of 8.
10. Diagram fertilization as it would occur between a sperm and an egg with the haploid number of 3.

autosomes (aw'to-sōmz) Chromosomes not involved in determining the sex of individuals.

crossing-over (kros'sing o-ver) The exchange of a part of a chromatid from one chromosome with an equivalent part of a chromatid from a homologous chromosome.

diploid (dip'loid) Having two sets of chromosomes: one set from the maternal parent and one set from the paternal parent.

Down syndrome (down sin'drōm) A genetic disorder resulting from the presence of an extra chromosome number 21. Symptoms include slightly slanted eyes, flattened facial features, a large tongue, and a tendency toward short stature and fingers. Some individuals also display mental retardation.

egg cells (eg sels) The haploid sex cells produced by sexually mature females.

fertilization (fer"tĭ-lĭ-za'shun) The joining of haploid nuclei, usually from an egg and a sperm cell, resulting in a diploid cell called the zygote.

gamete (gam'ēt) A haploid sex cell.

gametogenesis (ga-me"to-jen'e-sis) The generating of gametes; the meiotic cell-division process that produces sex cells; oogenesis and spermatogenesis.

gonad (go-nad) A generalized term for the organs in which meiosis occurs; ovaries or testes.

haploid (hap'loid) Having a single set of chromosomes resulting from the reduction division of meiosis.

homologous chromosomes (ho-mol'o-gus kro'mo-sōmz) A pair of chromosomes in a diploid cell that contain similar genes at corresponding loci throughout their length.

independent assortment (in"de-pen'dent ă-sort'ment) The segregation, or assortment, of one pair of homologous chromosomes, independently of the segregation, or assortment, of any other pair of chromosomes.

meiosis (mi-o'sis) The specialized pair of cell divisions that reduce the chromosome number from diploid ($2n$) to haploid (n).

nondisjunction (non"dis-junk'shun) An abnormal meiotic division that results in sex cells with too many or too few chromosomes.

ovaries (o'var-ēz) The female sex organs that produce haploid sex cells—the eggs or ova.

reduction division (re-duk'shun dĭ-vĭ'zhun) A type of cell division in which daughter cells get only half the chromosomes from the parent cell.

segregation (seg"rĕ-ga'shun) The separation and movement of homologous chromosomes to the poles of the cell.

sex chromosomes (seks kro'mo-sōmz) Chromosomes that carry the genes that determine the sex of the individual.

sexual reproduction (sek'shu-al re"pro-duk'shun) The propagation of organisms involving the union of gametes from two parents.

sperm cells (spurm sels) The haploid sex cells produced by sexually mature males.

synapsis (sin-ap'sis) The condition in which the two members of a pair of homologous chromosomes come to lie close to one another.

testes (tes'tēz) The male sex organs that produce haploid cells—the sperm.

trisomy (tris'-oh-me) An abnormal number of chromosomes resulting from the nondisjunction of homologous chromosomes during meiosis; for example, as in Down syndrome.

zygote (zi'gōt) A diploid cell that results from the union of an egg and a sperm.

THE DYNAMIC HUMAN Correlations to Chapter Ten:

Reproductive System → Explorations → (*a*) Female → Oogenesis; (*b*) Male → Spermatogenesis

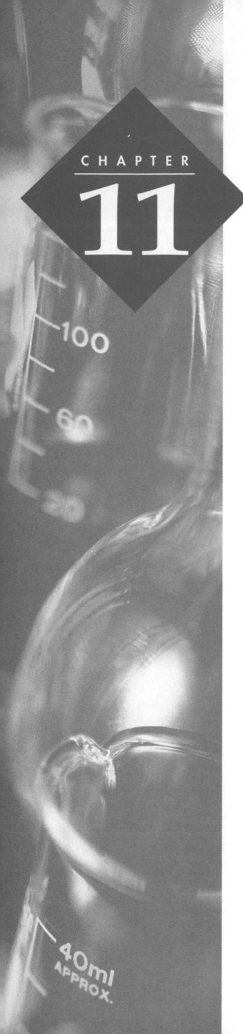

Mendelian Genetics

CHAPTER OUTLINE

PURPOSE

This chapter considers the fundamentals of inheritance. In previous chapters we introduced the concept of DNA as a molecule for storing the genetic information used to manufacture proteins and to guide the processes of mitosis and meiosis. Here we will describe how characteristics are passed from one generation to the next, using many human characteristics to illustrate these patterns of inheritance.

CLINICAL VIEWPOINT

The field of bioengineering is advancing as quickly as the electronics industry. The first bioengineering efforts focused on the development of genetically altered crops that displayed improvements over past varieties, such as increased resistance to infectious disease. The second wave of research involved manipulating DNA, which resulted in improved food handling and processing, such as the slowing of ripening in tomatoes. Currently, crops are being genetically manipulated to manufacture large quantities of specialty chemicals and biopolymers. While some of these products have been produced from genetically engineered microorganisms, crops of turnips, potatoes, and tobacco can generate tens or hundreds of kilograms of specialty product per year. Researchers have shown, for example, that turnips can produce interferon (an antiviral agent), tobacco can create antibodies to fight human disease, oilseed rape plants can serve as a source of human brain hormones, and potatoes can synthesize human serum albumin that is indistinguishable from the genuine human blood protein.

LEARNING OBJECTIVES

- Be able to work single-factor and double-factor genetic problems dealing with traits that show dominance, recessiveness, and lack of dominance
- Be able to work genetic problems dealing with multiple alleles, polygenic inheritance, and X-linked characteristics
- Explain how environmental conditions influence an organism's phenotype

Why do you have a particular blood type or hair color? Why do some people have the same skin color as their parents, while others have a skin color different from that of their parents? These questions can be better answered if you understand how genes work. A **gene** is a portion of DNA that determines a characteristic. Through meiosis and reproduction, these genes can be transmitted from one generation to another. The study of genes, how genes produce characteristics, and how the characteristics are inherited is the field of biology called **genetics.** The first person to systematically study inheritance and formulate laws about how characteristics are passed from one generation to the next was an Augustinian monk named Gregor Mendel (1822–1884). However, his work was not generally accepted until 1900, when three men, working independently, rediscovered some of the ideas that Mendel had formulated over thirty years earlier. Because of his early work, the study of the pattern of inheritance that follows the laws formulated by Gregor Mendel is often called **Mendelian genetics.**

To understand this chapter, you need to know some basic terminology. One term that you have already encountered is *gene.* Mendel thought of a gene as a particle that could be passed from the parents to the **offspring** (children, descendants, progeny). Today we know that genes are actually composed of specific sequences of DNA nucleotides. The particle concept is not entirely inaccurate though, because genes are located on specific portions of chromosomes; however, they are not like beads on a string.

Another important idea to remember is that all sexually reproducing organisms have a diploid stage. Since gametes are haploid and most organisms are diploid, the conversion of diploid to haploid cells during meiosis is an important process. The diploid cells have two sets of chromosomes—one set inherited from each parent. Therefore, they have two chromosomes of each kind and two genes for each characteristic. When sex cells are produced by meiosis, reduction division occurs, and the diploid number is reduced to haploid. Therefore, the sex cells produced by meiosis have only one chromosome of each of the homologous pairs that was in the diploid cell that began meiosis. Diploid organisms usually result from the fertilization of a haploid egg by a haploid sperm. Therefore, they inherit one gene of each type from each parent. For example, each of us has two genes for earlobe shape: one came with our father's sperm, the other with our mother's egg (figure 11.1).

Each diploid organism has two genes for each characteristic. There may be several alternative forms or **alleles** of each gene within the population. In people, there are two alleles for earlobe shape. One allele produces an earlobe that is fleshy and hangs free, while the other allele produces a lobe that is attached to the side of the face and does not hang free. The type of earlobe that is present is determined by the type of allele (gene) received from each parent and the way in which these alleles interact with one another. Alleles are always located on the pair of homologous chromosomes—one allele on each chromosome. These alleles are also always at the same specific **locus** (location) (figure 11.2).

The **genome** is a set of all the genes necessary to specify an organism's complete list of characteristics. A diploid (2*n*) cell has two genomes and a haploid cell (*n*) has one genome. The **genotype** of an organism is a listing of the genes present in that organism. It consists of the cell's DNA code; therefore, you cannot see the genotype of an organism. It is impossible to know the complete genotype of most organisms, but it is often possible to figure out the genes present that determine a particular characteristic. For example, there are three possible genotypic combinations of the two alleles for earlobe shape. A person's genotype could be (1) two alleles for attached earlobes, (2) one allele for attached and one allele for free earlobes, or (3) two alleles for free earlobes.

How would individuals with each of these three genotypes appear? The way each combination of alleles expresses itself is known as the **phenotype** of the

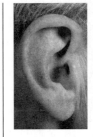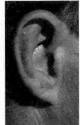

(a)   (b)

FIGURE 11.1 *Genes control structural features.*
Whether your earlobe is free (a), or attached (b) depends on the genes you have inherited. As genes express themselves, their actions affect the development of various tissues and organs. Some people's earlobes do not separate from the side of their head in the same fashion as do those of others. How genes control this complex growth pattern and why certain genes function differently than others is yet to be clarified.

GENES AND CHARACTERISTICS

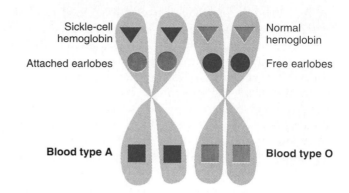

FIGURE 11.2 ⬛ A pair of homologous chromosomes. Homologous chromosomes contain genes for the same characteristics at the same place. Note that the attached-earlobe allele is located at the ear-shape locus on one chromosome, and the free-earlobe allele is located at the ear-shape locus on the other member of the homologous pair of chromosomes. The other two genes are for hemoglobin structure (alleles normal and sickled) and blood type (alleles type A and type O). The examples presented here are for illustrative purposes only. We do not really know if these particular genes are on these chromosomes. It is hoped that the Human Genome Project described in chapter 10 will resolve this problem.

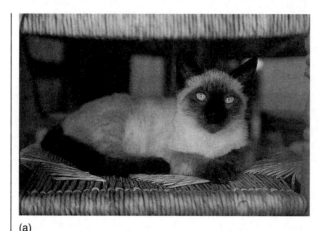

(a)

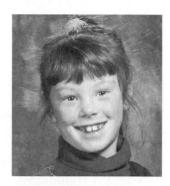

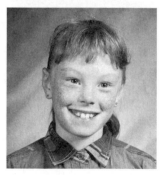

(b)

FIGURE 11.3 The environment and gene expression. The expression of many genes is influenced by the environment. (a) The gene for dark hair in the cat is sensitive to temperature and expresses itself only in the parts of the body that stay cool. (b) The gene for freckles expresses itself more fully when a person is exposed to sunlight.

organism. A person with two alleles for attached earlobes will have earlobes that do not hang free. A person with one allele for attached earlobes and one allele for free earlobes will have a phenotype that exhibits free earlobes. An individual with two alleles for free earlobes will also have free earlobes. Notice that there are three genotypes, but only two phenotypes. The individuals with the free-earlobe phenotype can have different genotypes.

Often where two alleles are present within a given cell, one may not express itself or its effect may be masked or hidden by a more dominant allele. Sometimes, the physical environment determines whether or not certain genes function. For example, some cats have coat-color genes that do not reveal themselves unless the temperature of the skin is below a certain point. Often, the only parts of a cat that become cool enough to allow the genes to express themselves are the tips of the ears and the feet (figure 11.3a). Consequently these areas will differ in color from the rest of the cat's body. An example in humans is the presence of genes for freckles that do not show themselves fully unless the person's skin is exposed to sunlight (figure 11.3b).

The expression of some genes is directly influenced by the presence of other alleles in the organism. For any particular pair of alleles in an individual organism, the two alleles from the two parents are either identical or not identical. The organism is **homozygous** for a trait when it has two identical alleles for that particular characteristic. A person with two alleles for freckles is said to be homozygous for that trait. A person with two alleles for no freckles is also homozygous. If an organism is homozygous, the characteristic expresses itself in a specific manner. A person homozygous for free earlobes has free earlobes, and a person homozygous for attached earlobes has attached earlobes.

An individual is designated as **heterozygous** when it has two different allelic forms of a particular gene. The heterozygous individual received one form of the gene from one parent and a different allele from the other parent. For instance, a person with one allele for freckles and one allele for no freckles is heterozygous. If an organism is heterozygous, these two different alleles interact to determine a characteristic.

Often, one allele expresses itself more than the other. A **dominant allele** expresses itself and masks the effect of other alleles for the trait. For example, if a person has one allele for free earlobes and one allele for attached earlobes, that person has a phenotype of free earlobes. The allele for free earlobes is dominant. A **recessive allele** is one that, when present with another allele, does not express itself; it is masked by the effect of the other allele. Having attached earlobes is a recessive characteristic. A person with one allele for free earlobes and one allele for attached earlobes has a phenotype of free earlobes. Recessive traits only express themselves when the organism is homozygous for the recessive alleles. If you have attached earlobes, you have two alleles for that trait. Recessive genes are not necessarily bad. The term *recessive* has nothing to do with the significance of the gene—it simply describes how it can be expressed. Recessive alleles are not less likely to be inherited but must be present in a homozygous condition to express themselves.

Mendelian genetics involves the study of the transfer of genes from one generation to another and the ways in which the genes received from the parents influence the traits of the offspring. Before you go on, be certain that you understand how meiosis works and how the gametes formed from this process are combined by fertilization. It is in meiosis that the two alleles in a pair of genes segregate. Although we will talk about the segregation of genes in this chapter, remember that it is the chromosomes and not the individual genes that actually segregate.

Notice that the chromosomes in figure 11.2 have two different alleles for hemoglobin: one for sickle-cell hemoglobin and one for normal hemoglobin. By meiosis, the parent may contribute a gamete containing an allele for sickle-cell hemoglobin or an allele for normal hemoglobin. By fertilization, the offspring will receive two alleles for hemoglobin production, but only one from each parent. For most of the remainder of this chapter, we will deal with how to determine which genes are passed on by the parents and how to determine the genetic makeup of the offspring resulting from fertilization.

MENDEL'S LAWS OF HEREDITY

Heredity problems are concerned with determining which alleles are passed from the parents to the offspring and how likely it is that various types of offspring will be produced. The first person to develop a method of predicting the outcome of inheritance patterns was Mendel, who performed experiments concerning the inheritance of certain characteristics in sweet pea plants. From his work, Mendel concluded which traits were dominant and which were recessive. Some of his results follow.

Characteristic	Dominant Allele	Recessive Allele
plant height	tall	dwarf
pod shape	full	constricted
pod color	green	yellow
seed surface	round	wrinkled
seed color	yellow	green
flower color	purple	white

What made Mendel's work unique was that he studied only one trait at a time. Previous investigators had tried to follow numerous traits at the same time. When this was attempted, the total set of characteristics was so cumbersome to work with that no clear idea could be formed of how the offspring inherited traits. Mendel used traits with clear-cut alternatives, such as purple or white flower color, yellow- or green-colored seed pods, and tall or dwarf pea plants. He was very lucky to have chosen pea plants in his study because they naturally self-pollinate. When self-pollination occurs in pea plants over many generations, it is possible to develop a population of plants that is homozygous for a number of characteristics. Such a population is known as a *pure line.*

Mendel took a pure line of pea plants having purple flower color, removed the male parts (anthers), and discarded them so that they could not self-pollinate. He then took anthers from a pure-breeding white-flowered plant and pollinated the antherless purple flowers. When the pollinated flowers produced seeds, Mendel collected, labeled, and planted them. When these seeds germinated and grew, they eventually produced flowers. You might be surprised to learn that all of the plants resulting from this cross had purple flowers. One of the prevailing hypotheses of Mendel's day would have predicted that the purple and white colors would have blended together, resulting in flowers that were lighter than the parental purple flowers. Another hypothesis would have predicted that the offspring would have had a mixture of white and purple flowers. The unexpected result—all of the offspring produced flowers like those of one parent and no flowers like those of the other—caused Mendel to examine other traits as well and form the basis for much of the rest of his work. He repeated his experiments using pure strains for other traits. Pure-breeding tall plants were crossed with pure-breeding dwarf plants. Pure-breeding plants with yellow pods were crossed with pure-breeding plants with green pods. The results were all the same: the offspring showed the characteristic of one parent and not the other.

Next, Mendel crossed the offspring of the white-purple cross (all of which had purple flowers) with each other to see what the third generation would be like. Had the characteristics of the original white-flowered parent been lost completely? This second-generation cross was made by pollinating these purple flowers that had one white parent among themselves. The seeds produced from this cross were collected and grown. When these plants flowered, three-fourths of them produced purple flowers and one-fourth produced white flowers.

After analyzing his data, Mendel formulated several genetic laws to describe how characteristics are passed from one generation to the next and how they are expressed in an individual.

Mendel's law of dominance   When an organism has two different alleles for a given trait, the allele that is expressed, overshadowing the expression of the other allele, is said to be *dominant.* The gene whose expression is overshadowed is said to be *recessive.*

Mendel's law of segregation   When gametes are formed by a diploid organism, the alleles that control a trait separate from one another into different gametes, retaining their individuality.

Mendel's law of independent assortment   Members of one gene pair separate from each other independently of the members of other gene pairs.

At the time of Mendel's research, biologists knew nothing of chromosomes or DNA or of the processes of mitosis and meiosis. Mendel assumed that each gene was separate from other genes. It was fortunate for him that most of the characteristics he picked to study were located on a separate chromosome. If two or more of these genes had been located on the same chromosome (*linked genes*),

BOX 11.1

Cystic Fibrosis—What's the Probability?

One in every twenty persons has a defective gene that causes cystic fibrosis. Cystic fibrosis, the most common lethal genetic disorder, affects nearly 30,000 people in North America. In order for a person to have this disorder they must inherit a gene for cystic fibrosis from each parent. Persons with two genes for cystic fibrosis suffer from respiratory infections and have a life expectancy of twenty years.

Until recently the test used to detect this gene in people with a history of cystic fibrosis was only 50% accurate and could not detect the gene in persons with no family history of the disease. A new test is 75% accurate in detecting people with the gene regardless of their family history. This new test enables prospective parents to better determine the probability that they will have an offspring with cystic fibrosis.

he probably would not have been able to formulate his laws. The discovery of chromosomes and DNA have led to modifications of Mendel's laws. However, it was Mendel's work that formed the foundation for the science of genetics.

PROBABILITY VERSUS POSSIBILITY

In order to solve heredity problems, you must have an understanding of probability. **Probability** is the chance that an event will happen, and is often expressed as a percent or a fraction. *Probability* is not the same as *possibility*. It is possible to toss a coin and have it come up heads. But the probability of getting a head is more precise than just saying it is possible to get a head. The probability of getting a head is one out of two (1/2 or 0.5 or 50%) because there are two sides to the coin, only one of which is a head (box 11.1). Probability can be expressed as a fraction:

$$\text{Probability} = \frac{\text{the number of events that can produce a given outcome}}{\text{the total number of possible outcomes}}$$

What is the probability of cutting a deck of cards and getting the ace of hearts? The number of times that the ace of hearts can occur is one. The total number of possible outcomes (number of cards in the deck) is fifty-two. Therefore, the probability of cutting an ace of hearts is 1/52.

What is the probability of cutting an ace? The total number of aces in the deck is four, and the total number of cards is fifty-two. Therefore, the probability of cutting an ace is 4/52 or 1/13.

It is also possible to determine the probability of two independent events occurring together. *The probability of two or more events occurring simultaneously is the product of their individual probabilities.* If you throw a pair of dice, it is possible that both will be fours. What is the probability that they both will be fours? The probability of one die being a four is 1/6. The probability of the other die being a four is also 1/6. Therefore, the probability of throwing two fours is

$$1/6 \times 1/6 = 1/36$$

STEPS IN SOLVING HEREDITY PROBLEMS— SINGLE-FACTOR CROSSES

The first type of problem we will work is the easiest type, a single-factor cross. A **single-factor cross** is a genetic cross or mating in which a single characteristic is followed from one generation to the next. Sometimes a single-factor cross is also referred to as a *monohybrid* (*mono* = one, *hybrid* = combination) cross.

In humans, the allele for free earlobes is dominant and the allele for attached earlobes is recessive. If both parents are heterozygous (have one allele for free earlobes and one allele for attached earlobes), what is the probability that they can have a child with free earlobes? with attached earlobes?

In solving a heredity problem there are five basic steps:

Step 1: Assign a symbol for each allele.
Usually a capital letter is used for a dominant allele and a small letter for a recessive allele. Use the symbol *E* for free earlobes and *e* for attached earlobes.

	Genotype	**Phenotype**
E = free earlobes	*EE*	free earlobes
e = attached earlobes	*Ee*	free earlobes
	ee	attached earlobes

Step 2: Determine the genotype of each parent and indicate a mating.
Since both parents are heterozygous, the male genotype is *Ee*. The female genotype is also *Ee*. The × between them is used to indicate a mating.

$$Ee \times Ee$$

Step 3: Determine all the possible kinds of gametes each parent can produce.
Remember that gametes are haploid; therefore, they can only have one allele instead of the two present in the diploid cell. Since the male has both the free-earlobe allele and the attached-earlobe allele, half of his gametes will contain the free-earlobe allele and the other half will contain the attached-earlobe allele. Since the female has the same genotype, her gametes will be the same as his.

For genetic problems, a *Punnett square* is used. A **Punnett square** is a box figure that allows you to determine the probability of genotypes and phenotypes of the offspring of a particular cross. Remember, because of the process of meiosis, each gamete receives only one allele for each characteristic listed. Therefore, the male will give either an *E* or *e*; the female will also give either an *E* or *e*. The possible gametes produced by the male parent are listed on the left side of the square, while the female gametes are listed on the top. In our example, the Punnett square would show a single dominant allele and a single recessive allele from the male on the left side. The alleles from the female would appear on the top.

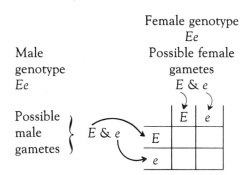

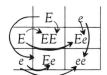

Step 4: Determine all the gene combinations that can result when these gametes unite.
To determine the possible combinations of alleles that could occur as a result of this mating, simply fill in each of the empty squares with the alleles that can be donated from each parent. Determine all the gene combinations that can result when these gametes unite.

Step 5: Determine the phenotype of each possible gene combination.
In this problem, three of the offspring, *EE, Ee,* and *Ee,* have free earlobes. One offspring, *ee,* has attached earlobes. Therefore, the answer to the problem is that the probability of having offspring with free earlobes is 3/4; for attached earlobes, it is 1/4.

Take the time to learn these five steps. All single-factor problems can be solved using this method; the only variation in the problems will be the types of alleles and the number of possible types of gametes the parents can produce. Now let's work a problem with one parent heterozygous and the other homozygous for a trait.

Some people are unable to convert the amino acid phenylalanine into the amino acid tyrosine. Such individuals suffer from phenylketonuria (PKU) and may become mentally retarded. The normal condition is to convert phenylalanine to tyrosine. It is dominant over the condition for PKU. If one parent is heterozygous and the other parent is homozygous for PKU, what is the probability that they will have a normal child? one with PKU?

Step 1:
Use the symbol N for normal and n for PKU.

	Genotype	**Phenotype**
N = normal	NN	normal metabolism of phenylalanine
n = PKU	Nn	normal metabolism of phenylalanine
	nn	PKU disorder

Step 2:

$$Nn \times nn$$

Step 3:

	n
N	
n	

Step 4:

	n
N	Nn
n	nn

Step 5:
In this problem, one-half of the offspring will be normal, and one-half will have PKU.

THE DOUBLE-FACTOR CROSS

A **double-factor cross** is a genetic study in which two pairs of alleles are followed from the parental generation to the offspring. Sometimes this type of cross is referred to as a *dihybrid* (*di* = two, *hybrid* = combination) cross. This problem is worked in basically the same way as a single-factor cross. The main difference is that in a double-factor cross you are working with two different characteristics from each parent.

It is necessary to use Mendel's law of independent assortment when working double-factor problems. Recall that according to this law, members of one allelic pair separate from each other independently of the members of other pairs of alleles. This happens during meiosis when the chromosomes segregate. (Mendel's law of independent assortment applies only if the two pairs of alleles are located on separate chromosomes. We will use this assumption in double-factor crosses.)

In humans, the allele for free earlobes is dominant over the allele for attached earlobes. The allele for dark hair dominates the allele for light hair. If both parents are heterozygous for earlobe shape and hair color, what types of offspring can they produce, and what is the probability for each type?

Step 1:

Use the symbol *E* for free earlobes and *e* for attached earlobes. Use the symbol *D* for dark hair and *d* for light hair.

	Genotype	Phenotype
E = free earlobes	*EE*	free earlobes
e = attached earlobes	*Ee*	free earlobes
D = dark hair	*ee*	attached earlobes
d = light hair	*DD*	dark hair
	Dd	dark hair
	dd	light hair

Step 2:

Determine the genotype for each parent and show a mating. The male genotype is *EeDd*, the female genotype is *EeDd*, and the × between them indicates a mating.

$$EeDd \times EeDd$$

Step 3:

Determine all the possible gametes each parent can produce and write the symbols for the alleles in a Punnett square. Since there are two pairs of alleles in a double-factor cross, each gamete must contain one allele from each pair—one from the earlobe pair (either *E* or *e*) and one from the hair color pair (either *D* or *d*). In this example, each parent can produce four different kinds of gametes. The four squares on the left indicate the gametes produced by the male; the four on the top indicate the gametes produced by the female.

To determine the possible gene combinations in the gametes, select one allele from one of the pairs of alleles and match it with one allele from the other pair of alleles. Then match the second allele from the first pair of alleles with each of the alleles from the second pair. This may be done as follows:

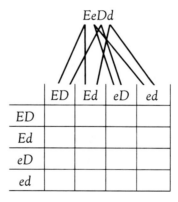

Step 4:

Determine all the gene combinations that can result when these gametes unite. Fill in the Punnett square.

	ED	Ed	eD	ed
ED	EEDD	EEDd	EeDD	EeDd
Ed	EEDd	EEdd	EeDd	Eedd
eD	EeDD	EeDd	eeDD	eeDd
ed	EeDd	Eedd	eeDd	eedd

Step 5:

Determine the phenotype of each possible gene combination. In this double-factor problem there are sixteen possible ways in which gametes could combine to produce offspring. There are four possible phenotypes in this cross. They are represented in the chart below.

Genotype		Phenotype		Symbol
EEDD or EEDd or EeDD or EeDd	=	free earlobes and dark hair	=	*
EEdd or Eedd	=	free earlobes and light hair	=	∧
eeDD or eeDd	=	attached earlobes and dark hair	=	″
eedd	=	attached earlobes and light hair	=	+

	ED	Ed	eD	ed
ED	EEDD *	EEDd *	EeDD *	EeDd *
Ed	EEDd *	EEdd ∧	EeDd *	Eedd ∧
eD	EeDD *	EeDd *	eeDD ″	eeDd ″
ed	EeDd *	Eedd ∧	eeDd ″	eedd +

The probability of having a given phenotype is

9/16 free earlobes, dark hair
3/16 free earlobes, light hair
3/16 attached earlobes, dark hair
1/16 attached earlobes, light hair

For our next problem, let's say a man with attached earlobes is heterozygous for hair color and his wife is homozygous for free earlobes and light hair. What can they expect their offspring to be like?

This problem has the same characteristics as the previous problem. Following the same steps, the symbols would be the same, but the parental genotypes would be as follows:

$$eeDd \times EEdd$$

The next step is to determine the possible gametes that each parent could produce and place them in a Punnett square. The male parent can produce two different kinds of gametes, *eD* and *ed*. The female parent can only produce one kind of gamete, *Ed*.

	Ed
eD	
ed	

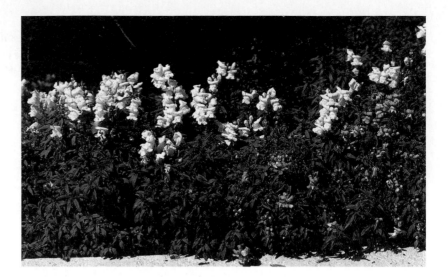

If you combine the gametes, only two kinds of offspring can be produced:

	Ed
eD	EeDd
ed	Eedd

They should expect either a child with free earlobes and dark hair or a child with free earlobes and light hair.

REAL-WORLD SITUATIONS

So far we have considered a few simple cases in which a characteristic is determined by simple dominance and recessiveness between two alleles. Other situations, however, do not fit these patterns. Some genetic characteristics are determined by more than two alleles; moreover, some traits are influenced by gene interactions and some traits are inherited differently, depending on the sex of the offspring.

Lack of (Incomplete) Dominance

In the cases that we have considered so far, one allele of the pair was clearly dominant over the other. Although this is common, it is not always the case. In some combinations of alleles, there is a **lack of dominance** or **incomplete dominance.** This is a situation in which two unlike alleles both express themselves, neither being dominant. A classic example involves the color of the petals of snapdragons. There are two alleles for the color of these flowers. Because neither allele is recessive, we cannot use the traditional capital and small letters as symbols for these alleles. Instead, the allele for white petals is given the symbol F^W, and the one for red petals is given the symbol F^R (figure 11.4). There are three possible combinations of these two alleles:

Genotype	**Phenotype**
F^{W}F^W	white flowers
F^{R}F^R	red flowers
F^{R}F^W	pink flowers

Notice that there are only two different alleles, red and white, but there are three phenotypes, red, white, and pink. Both the red-flower allele and the white-flower allele partially express themselves when both are present, and this results in pink.

Heredity problems dealing with lack of dominance are worked according to the five steps used in other problems. In the following lack-of-dominance problem, only one trait is involved; therefore, it is worked as a single-factor problem.

If a pink snapdragon is crossed with a white snapdragon, what phenotypes can result, and what is the probability of each phenotype?

Step 1:

	Genotype	**Phenotype**
F^W = white flowers	$F^W F^W$	white flower
F^R = red flowers	$F^W F^R$	pink flower
	$F^R F^R$	red flower

Step 2:

$$F^R F^W \times F^W F^W$$

Step 3:

	F^W
F^R	
F^W	

Step 4:

	F^W
F^R	$F^W F^R$ pink
F^W	$F^W F^W$ white

Step 5:

This cross results in two different phenotypes—pink and white. No red flowers can result because this would require that both parents be able to contribute at least one red allele. The white flowers are homozygous for white, and the pink flowers are heterozygous.

Multiple Alleles

So far we have discussed only those traits that are determined by two alleles. However, there can be more than two different alleles for a trait. The fact that some characteristics are determined by several different alleles for a particular characteristic is called **multiple alleles.** However, an individual can have only a maximum of two of the alleles for the characteristic. A good example of a characteristic that is determined by multiple alleles is the ABO blood type. There are three alleles for blood type:

I^A = blood type A
I^B = blood type B
i = blood type O

(The symbols, I and i, stand for the technical term for the antibody proteins in the blood serum, the *immunoglobulins.*)

Locus 1	d^1d^1	d^1D^1	d^1D^1	D^1D^1	D^1d^1	D^1d^1	D^1D^1
Locus 2	d^2d^2	d^2d^2	d^2D^2	D^2d^2	D^2d^2	D^2D^2	D^2D^2
Locus 3	d^3d^3	d^3d^3	d^3d^3	d^3d^3	D^3D^3	D^3D^3	D^3D^3
Total number of dark-skin genes	0	1	2	3	4	5	6

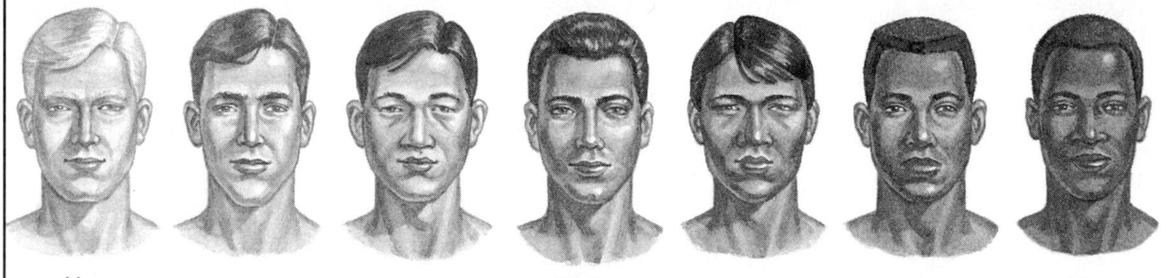

Very light — Medium — Very dark

FIGURE 11.5 Polygenic inheritance.
Skin color in humans is an example of polygenic inheritance. The darkness of the skin is determined by the number of dark-skin genes a person inherits from his or her parents.

A and B show *codominance* when they are together in the same individual, but both are dominant to the O allele. These three alleles can be combined as pairs in six different ways, resulting in four different phenotypes:

Genotype	Phenotype
I^AI^A	blood type A
I^Ai	blood type A
I^BI^B	blood type B
I^Bi	blood type B
I^AI^B	blood type AB
ii	blood type O

Multiple-allele problems are worked as single-factor problems. Some examples are in the practice problems at the end of this chapter.

Polygenic Inheritance

Thus far we have considered phenotypic characteristics that are determined by alleles at a specific, single place on homologous chromosomes. However, some characteristics are determined by the interaction of genes at several different loci (on different chromosomes or at different places on a single chromosome). This is called **polygenic inheritance** (*poly* = many). A number of different pairs of alleles may combine their efforts to determine a characteristic. Skin color in humans is a good example of this inheritance pattern. According to some experts, genes for skin color are located at a minimum of three different loci. At each of these loci, the allele for dark skin is dominant over the allele for light skin. Therefore, a wide variety of skin colors is possible, depending on how many dark-skin alleles are present (figure 11.5). Polygenic inheritance is very common in determining characteristics that are quantitative in nature. In the skin-color example, and in many others as well, the characteristics cannot be categorized in terms of *either/or*, but the variation in phenotypes can be classified as *how much* or *what amount* (*see* box 11.2). For instance, people show great variations in height. There are not just tall and short

Box 11.2   The Inheritance of Eye Color

It is commonly thought that eye color is inherited in a simple dominant/recessive manner. Brown eyes are considered to be dominant over blue eyes. The real pattern of inheritance, however, is considerably more complicated than this. Eye color is determined by the amount of a brown pigment, known as *melanin*, that is present in the iris of the eye. If there is a large quantity of melanin present on the anterior surface of the iris, the eyes are dark. Black eyes have a greater quantity of melanin than brown eyes.

If there is not a large amount of melanin present on the anterior surface of the iris, the eyes will appear to be blue, not because of a blue pigment but because blue light is returned from the iris. The iris appears blue for the same reason that deep bodies of water tend to appear blue. There is no blue pigment in the water, but blue wavelengths of light are returned to the eye from the water. People appear to have blue eyes because the blue wavelengths of light are reflected from the iris.

Just as black and brown eyes are determined by the amount of pigment present, colors such as green, gray, and hazel are produced by the various amounts of melanin in the iris. If a very small amount of brown melanin is present in the iris, the eye tends to appear green, whereas relatively large amounts of melanin produce hazel eyes.

Several different genes are probably involved in determining the quantity and placement of the melanin and, therefore, in determining eye color. These genes interact in such a way that a wide range of eye color is possible. Eye color is probably determined by polygenic inheritance, just as skin color and height are. Some newborn babies have blue eyes that later become brown. This is because they have not yet begun to produce melanin in their irises at the time of birth.

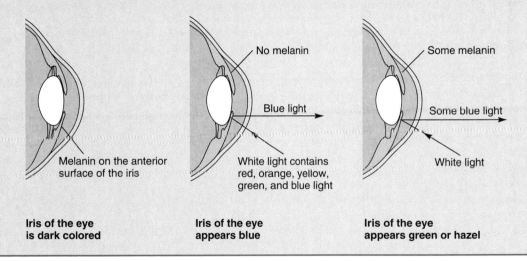

Iris of the eye is dark colored

Melanin on the anterior surface of the iris

Iris of the eye appears blue

No melanin

Blue light

White light contains red, orange, yellow, green, and blue light

Iris of the eye appears green or hazel

Some melanin

Some blue light

White light

people—there is a wide range. Some people are as short as one meter, and others are taller than two meters. This quantitative trait is probably determined by a number of different genes. Intelligence also varies significantly, from those who are severely retarded to those who are geniuses. Many of these traits may also be influenced by outside environmental factors, such as diet, disease, accidents, and social factors. These are just some examples of polygenic inheritance patterns.

Pleiotropy

A gene often has a variety of effects on the phenotype of an organism. This is called *pleiotropy*. **Pleiotropy** (*pleio-* = changeable) is a term used to describe the multiple effects that a gene may have on the phenotype of an organism. For example, the gene for sickle-cell hemoglobin has two major effects. One is good and one is bad. Having the allele for sickle-cell hemoglobin can result in abnormally shaped red blood cells. This occurs because the hemoglobin molecules are synthesized with the wrong amino acid sequence. These abnormal hemoglobin molecules tend

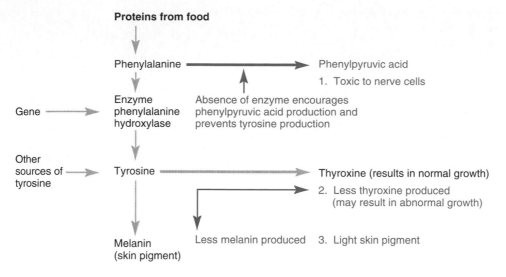

Proteins from food

Phenylalanine ——————→ Phenylpyruvic acid
                                 1. Toxic to nerve cells

Gene ——————→ Enzyme phenylalanine hydroxylase

Absence of enzyme encourages phenylpyruvic acid production and prevents tyrosine production

Other sources of tyrosine ——→ Tyrosine ══════→ Thyroxine (results in normal growth)
                              2. Less thyroxine produced (may result in abnormal growth)

Melanin (skin pigment)   Less melanin produced   3. Light skin pigment

Figure 11.6 Pleiotropy.

Pleiotropy is a condition in which a single gene has more than one effect on the phenotype. This diagram shows how the normal pathways work (these are shown in black). If the enzyme phenylalanine hydroxylase is not produced because of an abnormal gene, there are three major results: (1) mental retardation because phenylpyruvic acid kills nerve cells, (2) abnormal body growth because less of the growth hormone thyroxine is produced, and (3) pale skin pigmentation because less melanin is produced (abnormalities are shown in color). It should also be noted that if a woman who has PKU becomes pregnant, her baby is likely to be born retarded. While the embryo may not have the genetic disorder, the phenylpyruvic acid produced by the pregnant mother will damage the developing brain cells. This is called *maternal PKU*.

to attach to one another in long, rodlike chains when oxygen is in short supply. These rodlike chains distort the shape of the red blood cells into a sickle shape. When these abnormal red blood cells change shape, they clog small blood vessels. The sickled red cells are also destroyed more rapidly than normal cells. This results in a shortage of red blood cells, causing anemia, and an oxygen deficiency in the tissues that have become clogged. People with sickle-cell anemia may experience pain, swelling, and damage to organs such as the heart, lungs, brain, and kidneys.

Although sickle-cell anemia is usually lethal in the homozygous condition, it can be beneficial in the heterozygous state. A person with a single sickle-cell allele is more resistant to malaria than a person without this allele. A heterozygous person may not demonstrate any ill effects, but under laboratory conditions with low oxygen, there is a change in the red blood cells. Three genotypes can exist (Hb^A = normal hemoglobin, Hb^S = sickle-cell hemoglobin):

Genotype	Phenotype
$Hb^A\ Hb^A$	normal hemoglobin and nonresistance to malaria
$Hb^A\ Hb^S$	normal hemoglobin and resistance to malaria
$Hb^S\ Hb^S$	resistance to malaria but death from sickle-cell anemia

Originally, sickle-cell anemia was found at a high frequency in parts of the world where malaria was common. Today, however, this genetic disease can be found anywhere in the world. In the United States, it is most common among black populations whose ancestors came from equatorial Africa.

Let's look at another example of pleiotropy. In this example, a single gene affects many different chemical reactions that depend on the way a cell metabolizes the amino acid phenylalanine commonly found in many foods (figure 11.6). People normally have an allele for the production of an enzyme that converts the amino acid phenylalanine to tyrosine. If this allele is functioning properly, phenylalanine will be converted to tyrosine, which will be available to be converted into thyroxine and melanin by other enzymes. If the enzyme that normally converts phenylalanine to tyrosine is absent or not functioning properly, toxic materials can accumulate and result in a loss of nerve cells, causing mental retardation. Because less tyrosine is produced, there is also less of the growth hormone, thyroxine, resulting in abnormal body growth. Because tyrosine is necessary to form the pigment melanin, people who have this condition will have lighter skin color because of an absence of this pigment. These effects can be limited by reducing the amount of phenylalanine in the diet, a difficult thing to do since this amino acid is very common. The one abnormal allele produces three different phenotypic effects: mental retardation, abnormal growth, and light skin.

Linkage

Pairs of alleles located on nonhomologous chromosomes separate independently of one another during meiosis when the chromosomes separate into sex cells. Since each chromosome has many genes on it, these genes tend to be inherited as a group. Genes located on the same chromosome that tend to be inherited together are called a **linkage group.** The closer two genes are to each other on a chromosome, the more probable it is that they will be inherited together. The process of crossing-over, which occurs during prophase I of meiosis, may split up these linkage groups. Crossing-over happens between homologous chromosomes donated by the mother and the father, and results in a mixing of genes.

Sex-Linked Genes

Many organisms have two types of chromosomes. Autosomes are not involved in sex determination and have the same genes on both members of the homologous pair of chromosomes. Sex chromosomes are a pair of chromosomes in mammals and some other animals that control the sex of an organism. In humans, and some other animals, there are two types of sex chromosomes—the X chromosome and the Y chromosome. The Y chromosome is much shorter than the X chromosome and has no genes for traits found on the X chromosome. One portion of the Y chromosome contains the male-determining gene. Females are normally produced when two X chromosomes are present. Males are usually produced when one X chromosome and one Y chromosome are present.

Genes found on the X chromosome are said to be **X-linked.** Because the Y chromosome is shorter than the X chromosome, it does not have many of the alleles that are found on the comparable portion of the X chromosome. Therefore, in a man, the presence of a single allele on his only X chromosome will be expressed, regardless of whether it is dominant or recessive. The only confirmed Y-linked trait in humans is the SRY gene. This gene controls the differentiation of the embryonic gonad to a male testis. By contrast, more than one hundred genes are on the X chromosome. Some of these X-linked genes can result in abnormal traits such as color blindness, hemophilia, brown teeth, and a form of muscular dystrophy. To better understand an X-linked gene, let's now use the five steps of solving genetics problems to work an X-linked problem.

In humans the gene for normal color vision is dominant and the gene for color blindness is recessive. Both genes are X-linked. A male who has normal vision mates with a female who is heterozygous for normal color vision. What type of children can they have in terms of these traits, and what is the probability for each type?

Step 1:
Because this condition is linked to the X chromosome, it has become traditional to symbolize the allele as a superscript on the letter X. Since the Y chromosome does not contain a homologous allele, only the letter Y is used.

	Genotype	Phenotype
X^N = normal color vision	$X^N Y$	male, normal color vision
X^n = color-blind	$X^n Y$	male, color-blind
Y = male (no gene present)	$X^N X^N$	female, normal color vision
	$X^N X^n$	female, normal color vision
	$X^n X^n$	female, color-blind

Step 2:
Male's genotype = $X^N Y$ (normal color vision)
Female's genotype = $X^N X^n$ (normal color vision)

$$X^N Y \times X^N X^n$$

Step 3:

	X^N	X^n
X^N		
Y		

Step 4:
The genotypes of the probable offspring are listed in the body of the Punnett square:

	X^N	X^n
X^N	$X^N X^N$	$X^N X^n$
Y	$X^N Y$	$X^n Y$

Step 5:
The phenotypes of the offspring are determined:

normal female	carrier female
normal male	color-blind male

A **carrier** is any individual who is heterozygous for a trait. In this situation, the recessive allele is hidden. In X-linked situations, only the female can be heterozygous because the males lack one of the X chromosomes. Heterozygous females will exhibit the dominant trait (normal vision in this problem), but have the recessive allele hidden. If a male has a recessive allele on the X chromosome, it will be expressed because there is no other allele on the Y chromosome to dominate it. If a heterozygous carrier (must be female) has sons, there is a probability that she should expect half of them to be color-blind and half to have normal color vision. For these reasons, there are many more color-blind males than there are color-blind females.

The specific phenotype an organism exhibits is determined by the interplay of the genotype of the individual and the conditions the organism encounters as it develops. Therefore, it is possible for two organisms with identical genotypes (identical twins) to differ in their phenotypes. All genes must express themselves through the manufacture of proteins. These proteins may be structural or enzymatic, and the enzymes may be more or less effective, depending on the specific biochemical conditions when the enzyme is in operation. The expression of the genes will vary depending on the environmental conditions while the gene is operating.

Maybe you assumed that the dominant allele would always be expressed in a heterozygous individual. It is not so simple! Here, as in other areas of biology, there are exceptions. For example, the allele for six fingers is dominant over the allele for five fingers in humans. Some people who have received the allele for six fingers have a fairly complete sixth finger; in others, it may appear as a little stub. In another case, a dominant allele causes the formation of a little finger that cannot be bent as a normal little finger. However, not all people who are believed to have inherited that allele will have a stiff little finger. In some cases, this dominant characteristic is not expressed or perhaps only shows on one hand. Thus, there may be variation in the degree to which a dominant allele expresses itself, and in some cases it may not be expressed. Other genes may be interacting with these dominant alleles, causing the variation in expression. It is important to recognize that the environment affects the expression of our genes in many ways.

Both internal and external environmental factors can influence the expression of genes. For example, at conception, a male receives genes that will eventually determine the pitch of his voice. However, these genes are expressed differently after puberty. At puberty, male sex hormones are released. This internal environmental change results in the deeper male voice. A male who does not produce these hormones retains a higher-pitched voice in later life. A comparable situation in females occurs when an abnormally functioning adrenal gland causes the release of large amounts of male hormones. This results in a female with a deeper voice. Also recall the genetic disease PKU. The effects of the abnormal metabolism can be limited by reducing the amount of phenylalanine in a person's diet.

Another influence on gene expression is called *gene imprinting.* This occurs when a gene donated by one of the parents has its expression altered by a gene donated by the other parent. Certain genes donated by the father affect those donated by the mother, and certain genes donated by the mother affect those donated by the father. It is also true that certain genes only function properly when donated by the father, and other genes only function properly when donated by the mother. Although the mechanics of the process are not yet well understood, it is known that paternal and maternal genes contribute in different ways to the developing embryo. Two forms of mental retardation illustrate gene imprinting in humans—Angelman and Prader-Willi syndromes. Prader-Willi is transmitted from the mother and Angelman from the father. Patients with Angelman syndrome display excessive laughter, jerky movements, and other symptoms of physical and mental retardation. Those with Prader-Willi syndrome show mental retardation, extreme obesity, short stature, and unusually small hands and feet. Both are disorders of chromosome 15.

Many external environmental factors can influence the phenotype of an individual. One such factor is diet. Diabetes mellitus, a metabolic disorder in which glucose is not properly metabolized and is passed out of the body in the urine, has a genetic basis. Some people who have a family history of diabetes are thought to have inherited the trait for this disease. Evidence indicates that they can delay the onset of the disease by reducing the amount of sugar in their diet. This change in the external environment influences gene expression in much the same way that temperature influences the expression of color production in cats or sunlight affects the expression of freckles in humans (*see* figure 11.3).

SUMMARY

Genes are units of heredity composed of specific lengths of DNA that determine the characteristics an organism displays. Specific genes are at specific loci on specific chromosomes. The phenotype displayed by an organism is the result of the effect of the environment on the ability of the alleles to express themselves. Diploid organisms have two genes for each characteristic. The alternative forms of genes for a characteristic are called alleles. There may be many different alleles for a particular characteristic. Those organisms with two identical alleles are homozygous for a characteristic; those with different alleles are heterozygous for a characteristic. Some alleles are dominant over other alleles that are said to be recessive.

Sometimes two alleles both will express themselves, and often a gene will have more than one recognizable effect on the phenotype of the organism. Some characteristics may be determined by several different pairs of alleles. In humans and some other animals, males have an X chromosome with a normal number of genes and a Y chromosome with fewer genes. Although they are not identical, they behave as a pair of homologous chromosomes. Since the Y chromosome is shorter than the X chromosome and has fewer genes, many of the recessive characteristics present on the X chromosome appear more frequently in males than in females, who have two X chromosomes.

QUESTIONS

1. How many kinds of gametes are possible with each of the following genotypes?
    a. *Aa*
    b. *AaBB*
    c. *AaBb*
    d. *AaBbCc*

2. What is the probability of getting the gamete *ab* from each of the following genotypes?
    a. *aabb*
    b. *Aabb*
    c. *AaBb*
    d. *AABb*

3. What is the probability of each of the following sets of parents producing the given genotypes in their offspring?

Parents	Offspring genotype
a. *AA × aa*	*Aa*
b. *Aa × Aa*	*Aa*
c. *Aa × Aa*	*aa*
d. *AaBb × AaBB*	*AABB*
e. *AaBb × AaBB*	*AaBb*
f. *AaBb × AaBb*	*AABB*

4. If an offspring has the genotype *Aa*, what possible combinations of parental genotypes can exist?

5. In humans, the allele for albinism is recessive to the allele for normal skin pigmentation.
    a. What is the probability that a child of a heterozygous mother and father will be an albino?
    b. If a child is normal, what is the probability that it is a carrier of the recessive albino allele?

6. In certain pea plants, the allele *T* for tallness is dominant over *t* for shortness.
    a. If a homozygous tall and homozygous short plant are crossed, what will be the phenotype and genotype of the offspring?
    b. If both individuals are heterozygous, what will be the phenotypic and genotypic ratios of the offspring?

7. Smoos are strange animals with one of three shapes: round, cuboidal, or pyramidal. If two cuboidal smoos mate, they always have cuboidal offspring. If two pyramidal smoos mate, they always produce pyramidal offspring. If two round smoos mate, they produce all three kinds of offspring. Assuming only one locus is involved, answer the following questions.
    a. How is smoo shape determined?
    b. What would be the phenotypic ratio if a round and cuboidal smoo were to mate?

8. What is the probability of a child having type AB blood if one of the parents is heterozygous for A blood and the other is heterozygous for B? What other genotypes are possible in these children?

9. A color-blind woman marries a man with normal vision. They have ten children—six boys and four girls.

   a. How many are expected to be normal?

   b. How many are expected to be color-blind?

10. A light-haired man has blood type O. His wife has dark hair and blood type AB, but her father had light hair.

   a. What is the probability that this couple will have a child with dark hair and blood type A?

   b. What is the probability that they will have a light-haired child with blood type B?

   c. How many different phenotypes could their children show?

11. Certain kinds of cattle have two alleles for coat color: *R* = red, and *r* = white. When an individual cow is heterozygous, it is spotted with red and white (roan). When two red alleles are present, it is red. When two white alleles are present, it is white. The allele *L*, for lack of horns, is dominant over *l*, for the presence of horns.

   a. If a bull and a cow both have the genotype *RrLl*, how many possible phenotypes of offspring can they have?

   b. How probable is each phenotype?

12. Hemophilia is a disease that prevents the blood from clotting normally. It is caused by a recessive allele located on the X chromosome. A boy has the disease; neither his parents nor his grandparents have the disease. What are the genotypes of his parents and grandparents?

ANSWERS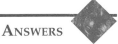

1. a. 2—*A,a*
  b. 2—*AB, aB*
  c. 4—*AB, Ab, aB, ab*
  d. 8—*ABC, ABc, Abc, AbC, aBC, aBc, abC, abc*

2. a. 100%—only, *ab* is possible
  b. 50%—*Ab* and *ab* are equally possible
  c. 25%—*AB, Ab, aB,* and *ab* are equally possible
  d. 0%—*ab* not possible

3. a. 100%
  b. 1/2 or 50%
  c. 1/4 or 25%
  d. 1/8 or 12.5%
  e. 1/4 or 25%
  f. 1/16 or 6.25%

4. *AA × aa*
  AA × Aa
  Aa × Aa
  Aa × aa

5. a. 1/4 or 25%
  b. 2/3 or 67%

6. a. Tall, *Tt*
  b. Phenotypic ratio—3 tall to 1 short
    Genotypic ratio—1 homozygous tall, 2 heterozygous tall, 1 homozygous short

7. a. This is a case of lack of dominance
  b. 50% or 1/2 round, 50% or 1/2 cuboidal

8. 1/4 or 25%
  $I^A i, I^B i, ii$

9. a. (4) All the girls have the normal phenotype but are carriers
  b. (6) All the boys are color-blind

10. a. 1/4 or 25%
  b. 1/4 or 25%
  c. 4

11. a. Six possible phenotypes:
  b. Red with horns—*RRll* = 1/16 or 6.25%
    Roan with horns—*Rrll* = 2/16 or 12.5%
    White with horns—*rrll* = 1/16 or 6.25%
    Red, hornless—*RRLL* or *RRLl* = 3/16 or 18.75%
    Roan, hornless—*RrLL* or *RrLl* = 6/16 or 37.5%
    White, hornless—*rrLL* or *rrLl* = 3/16 or 18.75%

12. Father $X^N Y$
    Mother $X^N X^n$
    Mother's father $X^N Y$
    Mother's mother $X^N X^n$
    Father's father $X^N Y$
    Father's mother $X^N X^?$

CHAPTER GLOSSARY

alleles (al'lēlz) Alternative forms of a gene for a particular characteristic (e.g., attached-earlobe allele and free-earlobe allele are alternative alleles for ear shape).

autosomes (aw'to-sōmz) Chromosomes that are not involved in determining the sex of an organism.

carrier (kar're-er) Any individual having a hidden, recessive allele.

dominant allele (dom'in-ant al'lēl) An allele that expresses itself and masks the effect of other alleles for the trait.

double-factor cross (dub'l fak'tur kros) A genetic study in which two pairs of alleles are followed from the parental generation to the offspring (dihybrid cross).

gene (jēn) A unit of heredity located on a chromosome and composed of a sequence of DNA nucleotides.

genetics (jĕ-net'iks) The study of genes, how genes produce characteristics, and how the characteristics are inherited.

genome (je'nōm) A set of all the genes necessary to specify an organism's complete list of characteristics.

genotype (je'no-tīp) The catalog of genes of an organism, whether or not these genes are expressed.

heterozygous (hĕ"ter-o-zi'gus) Describes a diploid organism that has two different alleles for a particular characteristic.

homozygous (ho"mo-zi'gus) Describes a diploid organism that has two identical alleles for a particular characteristic.

lack of dominance (lak uv dom'in-ans) The condition of two unlike alleles both expressing themselves, neither being dominant.

law of dominance (law uv dom'in-ans) When an organism has two different alleles for a trait, the allele that is expressed and overshadows the expression of the other allele is said to be dominant. The allele whose expression is overshadowed is said to be recessive.

law of independent assortment (law uv in"de-pen'dent ă-sort'ment) Members of one allelic pair will separate from each other independently of the members of other allele pairs.

law of segregation (law uv seg"rĕ-ga'shun) When gametes are formed by a diploid organism, the alleles that control a trait separate from one another into different gametes, retaining their individuality.

linkage group (lingk'ij grūp) Genes located on the same chromosome that tend to be inherited together.

locus (loci) (lo'kus) (lo'si) The spot on a chromosome where an allele is located.

Mendelian genetics (Men-dĕ'le-an jĕ-net'iks) The pattern of inheriting characteristics that follows the laws formulated by Gregor Mendel.

multiple alleles (mul'tĭ-pul al'lēlz) A term used to refer to conditions in which there are several different alleles for a particular characteristic, not just two.

offspring (of'spring) Descendants of a set of parents.

phenotype (fēn'o-tīp) The physical, chemical, and behavioral expression of the genes possessed by an organism.

pleiotropy (pli-ot'ro-pe) The multiple effects that a gene may have on the phenotype of an organism.

polygenic inheritance (pol"e-jen'ik in-her'ĭ-tans) The concept that a number of different pairs of alleles may combine their efforts to determine a characteristic.

probability (prob"a-bil'ĭ-te) The chance that an event will happen, expressed as a percent or fraction.

Punnett square (pun'net sqwār) A method used to determine the probabilities of allele combinations in a zygote.

recessive allele (re-sĕ'siv al'lēl) An allele that, when present with its homolog, does not express itself and is masked by the effect of the other allele.

sex chromosomes (seks kro'mo-sōmz) A pair of chromosomes that determine the sex of an organism.

single-factor cross (sing'ul fak'tur kros) A genetic study in which a single characteristic is followed from the parental generation to the offspring (monohybrid cross).

X-linked gene (eks-lingt jēn) A gene located on one of the sex-determining X chromosomes.

THE DYNAMIC HUMAN Correlations to Chapter Eleven:

Immune and Lymphatic Systems → Clinical Concepts → Blood Type

Glossary

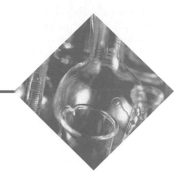

absorption (ab-sorp'shun) Energy that enters an intercepting object and stops.

acetyl (ă-sēt'l) The 2-carbon remainder of the carbon skeleton of pyruvic acid that is able to enter the mitochondrion.

acid (ă'sid) Any compound that releases a hydrogen ion (or other ion that acts like a hydrogen ion) in a solution.

activation energy (ak''tĭ-va'shun en'ur-je) Energy required to start a reaction.

active site (ak'tiv sīt) The place on the enzyme that causes the substrate to change.

active transport (ak'tiv trans-port) Use of a carrier molecule to move molecules across a cell membrane in a direction opposite that of the concentration gradient. The carrier requires an input of energy other than the kinetic energy of the molecules.

adenine (ad'ĕ-nēn) A double-ring nitrogenous-base molecule in DNA and RNA. It is the complementary base of thymine or uracil.

adenosine triphosphate (ATP) (uh-den'o-sēn tri-fos'fāt) A molecule formed from the building blocks of adenine, ribose, and phosphates. It functions as the primary energy carrier in the cell.

aerobic cellular respiration (a-ro'bik sel'yu-lar res''pĭ-ra'shun) The biochemical pathway that requires oxygen and converts food, such as carbohydrates, to carbon dioxide and water. During this conversion, it releases the chemical-bond energy as ATP molecules; a series of reactions in the mitochondria involved in the release of usable energy from food molecules by combining them with oxygen molecules.

alcoholic fermentation (al''ko-hol'ik fer''men-ta'shun) The anaerobic respiration pathway in yeast cells. During this process, pyruvic acid from glycolysis is converted to ethanol and carbon dioxide.

alleles (al-lēlz') Alternative forms of a gene for a particular characteristic (e.g., attached-earlobe alleles and free-earlobe alleles are alternative alleles for ear shape).

amino acid (ah-mēn'o ă'sid) A short carbon skeleton that contains an amino group, a carboxylic acid group, and one of various side groups.

anaerobic cellular respiration (an'uh-ro''bik sel'yu-lar res''pĭ-ra'shun) A biochemical pathway that does not require oxygen for the production of ATP and does not use O_2 as its ultimate hydrogen ion acceptor.

anaphase (an'ă-fāz) The third stage of mitosis, characterized by dividing the centromeres and movement of the chromosomes to the poles.

Angstrom (ang'strem) (Å) Unit of measurement of wavelengths of energy in the electromagnetic spectrum; one 100 millionth (10^{-8}) of a centimeter.

antibiotics (an-te-bi-ot'iks) Drugs that selectively kill or inhibit the growth of a particular cell type.

anticodon (an''te-ko'don) A sequence of three nitrogenous bases on a tRNA molecule capable of forming hydrogen bonds with three complementary bases on an mRNA codon during translation.

assimilation (a-sim'i-la'shun) The physiological process that takes place in a living cell when converting nutrients in food into specific molecules required by the organism.

atom (ă'tom) The smallest part of an element that still acts like that element.

atomic mass unit (AMU) (ă-tom'ik mas yu-nit) A unit of measure used to describe the mass of atoms and is equal to 1.67 × 10^{-24} grams, approximately the mass of one proton.

atomic nucleus (ă-tom'ik nu'kle-us) The central region of the atom.

atomic number (ă-tom'ik num'ber) The number of protons in an atom.

attachment site (uh-tatch'munt sīt) A specific point on the surface of the enzyme where it can physically attach itself to the substrate; also called **binding site.**

autosomes (aw'to-sōmz) Chromosomes not involved in determining the sex of individuals.

base (bās) Any compound that releases a hydroxyl group in a solution (or other ion that acts like a hydroxyl group).

binding site (bīn'ding sīt) See **attachment site.**

biochemical pathway (bi''o-kem'ĭ-kal path'wā) A major series of enzyme-controlled reactions linked together.

biochemistry (bi''o-kem'iss-tre) The chemistry of living things, often called biological chemistry.

biotechnology (bi''o-tek-nol'uh-je) The science of gene manipulation.

buffer (bŭ'fer) A mixture of a weak acid and the salt of a weak acid that operates to maintain a constant pH.

calorie (kal'o-re) The amount of heat necessary to raise the temperature of one gram of water one degree Celsius.

cancer (kan'sur) A tumor that is malignant.

carbohydrate (kar-bo-hi'drāt) One class of organic molecules composed of carbon, hydrogen, and oxygen in a ratio of 1:2:1 in most monosaccharides. The basic building block of a carbohydrate is a simple sugar (= monosaccharide).

carbon skeleton (kar'bon skel'uh-ton) Central portion of an organic molecule composed of rings or chains of carbon atoms.

carrier (kar're-er) Any individual having a hidden, recessive allele.

catalyst (cat'uh-list) A chemical that speeds up a reaction but is not used up in the reaction.

cell (sel) The basic structural unit that makes up all living things.

cellular membranes (sel'yu-lar mem'brāns) Thin sheets of material composed of phospholipids and proteins. Some of the proteins have attached carbohydrates or fats.

cellular respiration (sel′yu-lar res″pĭ-ra′shun) A major biochemical pathway along which cells release the chemical-bond energy from food and convert it into a usable form (ATP).

Celsius (sel′se-us) Scale of measuring temperature (abbreviated ° C).

centrioles (sen′tre-ōls) Organelles containing 2 sets of 9 short microtubules located just outside the nucleus and arranged in a cylinder.

centromere (sen′tro-mēr) The unreplicated region where two chromatids are joined.

chemical bonds (kem′ĭ-kal bonds) Forces that combine atoms or ions and hold them together.

chemical formula (kem′ĭ-kal form′yu-lah) Symbols used to represent each of the component atoms when we designate a compound.

chemical reaction (kem′ĭ-kal re-ak′shun) The formation or rearrangement of chemical bonds, usually indicated in an equation by an arrow from the reactants to the products.

chemical symbol (kem′ĭ-kal sim′bol) "Shorthand" used to represent 1 atom of an element, such as Al for aluminum or C for carbon.

chromatid (kro′mah-tid) One of two component parts of a chromosome formed by replication and attached at the centromere.

chromatin (kro′mah-tin) Areas or structures within the nucleus of a cell composed of long molecules of deoxyribonucleic acid (DNA) in association with proteins. See **nucleoproteins.**

chromosomal mutation (kro-mo-sōm′al miu-ta′shun) A change in the gene arrangement in a cell as a result of breaks in the DNA molecule.

chromosomes (kro′mo-sōmz) Tightly coiled complex structures within the nucleus composed of various kinds of histone proteins and DNA that contains the cell's genetic information.

cilia (sil′e-ah) Numerous short, hairlike structures projecting from the cell surface that enable locomotion.

codon (ko′don) A sequence of 3 nucleotides of an mRNA molecule that directs the placement of a particular amino acid during translation.

coenzyme (ko-en′zīm) A molecule that works with an enzyme to enable the enzyme to function as a catalyst.

colloid (kol′oid) A mixture that contains dispersed particles larger than molecules but small enough that they do not settle out.

competitive inhibition (kum-pet′ĭ-tiv in″hĭ-bĭ′shun) The formation of a temporary enzyme-inhibitor complex that interferes with the normal formation of enzyme-substrate complexes, resulting in a decreased turnover.

complementary base (kom″plĕ-men′tahre bās) A base that can form hydrogen bonds with another base of a specific nucleotide.

complete protein (kom-plēt pro′te-in) Protein molecules that provide all the essential amino acids.

complex carbohydrates (kom′pleks kar′bo-hi′drāts) Macromolecules composed of simple sugars combined by dehydration synthesis to form a polymer.

compound (kom′pound) A kind of matter that consists of a specific number of atoms (or ions) joined to each other in a particular way and held together by chemical bonds.

concentration gradient (kon″sen-tra′shun gra″de-ent) The gradual change in the number of molecules per unit of volume over distance.

conductor (kon-duk′tor) Connector of 2 areas that allows the flow of electrons.

control group (con-trōl′ grup) The situation used as the basis for comparison in a controlled experiment.

control processes (con-trōl′pro′ses-es) Mechanisms that ensure that an organism will carry out all metabolic activities in the proper sequence (coordination) and at the proper rate (regulation).

controlled experiment (con-trōl′d eksper′i-ment) An experiment that allows for a comparison of two events that are identical in all but one respect.

covalent bond (ko-va′lent bond) The attractive force formed between two atoms that share a pair of electrons.

cristae (krĭs′te) Folded surfaces of the inner membranes of mitochondria.

crossing-over (kros-sing o-ver) The exchange of a part of a chromatid from one chromosome with an equivalent part of a chromatid from a homologous chromosome.

cycles per second (si′kls) Numbers of waves of energy in regard to the electromagnetic spectrum.

cytokinesis (si-to-kĭ-ne′sis) Division of the cytoplasm of 1 cell into 2 new cells.

cytoplasm (si″to-plazm) The more fluid portion of the protoplasm that surrounds the nucleus.

cytosine (si′to-sēn) A single-ring nitrogenous-base molecule in DNA and RNA. It is complementary to guanine.

daughter cells (daw′tur sels) Two cells formed by cell division.

daughter chromosomes (daw′tur kro′mo-sōmz) Chromosomes produced by DNA replication that contain identical genetic information; formed after chromosome division in anaphase.

daughter nuclei (daw′tur nu′kle-i) Two nuclei formed by mitosis.

dehydration synthesis reaction (de-hi-dra′shun sin′thuh-sis re-ak′shun) A reaction that results in the formation of a macromolecule when water is removed from between the two smaller component parts.

denature (de-nā′chur) Irreversible change of the chemical and physical properties of a protein or other organic molecule.

density (den′sĭ-te) The weight of a certain volume of a material.

deoxyribonucleic acid (DNA) (de-ok″se-ri-bo-nu-kle′ik ă′sid) A polymer of nucleotides that serves as genetic information. In prokaryotic cells, it is a duplex DNA (double-stranded) loop and contains attached HU proteins. In eukaryotic cells, it is found in strands with attached histone proteins. When tightly coiled, it is known as a chromosome.

deoxyribose (de-ok″se-ri′bōs) A 5-carbon sugar molecule; a component of DNA.

diet (di-et) The amount of food and drink consumed by a person from day to day.

differentiation (dif″fur-ent-she-a′shun) The process of forming specialized cells within a multicellular organism.

diffusion (di″fiu′zhun) Net movement of a kind of molecule from an area of higher concentration to an area of lower concentration.

diffusion gradient (di″fiu′zhun gra″de-ent) The difference in the concentration of diffusing molecules over distance.

diploid (dip′loid) Having two sets of chromosomes: one set from the maternal parent and one set from the paternal parent.

dissociation (dis-so′she-a′shun) The separation of ions from an ionically bonded compound when it is mixed with water to form a solution.

DNA code (D-N-A cōd) A sequence of three nucleotides of a DNA molecule.

DNA polymerase (po-lim′er-ās) An enzyme that bonds DNA nucleotides together when they base pair with an existing DNA strand.

DNA replication (rep″lĭ-ka′shun) The process by which the genetic material (DNA) of the cell reproduces itself prior to its distribution to the next generation of cells.

dominant allele (dom'in-ant al'lēl) An allele that expresses itself and masks the effect of other alleles for the trait.

double bond (dubl bond) A pair of covalent bonds between two atoms formed when they share two pairs of electrons.

double-factor cross (dub'l-fak'tur kros) A genetic study in which two pairs of alleles are followed from the parental generation to the offspring (dihybrid cross).

Down syndrome (down sin'drōm) A genetic disorder resulting from the presence of an extra chromosome number 21. Symptoms include slightly slanted eyes, flattened facial features, a large tongue, and a tendency toward short stature and fingers. Some individuals also display mental retardation.

duplex DNA (du'pleks) DNA in a double-helix shape.

dynamic equilibrium (di-nam'ik e"kwĭ-lib're-um) A state of balance reached when molecules are completely dispersed and their movement is equal in all directions.

egg cells (eg selz) The haploid sex cells produced by sexually mature females.

electrolyte (e-lek'tro-līt) Solutions containing dissolved inorganic ions, such as sodium, potassium, and chloride, and capable of conducting electricity.

electromagnetic spectrum (e-lek"tro-mag'net-ik spek'trum) Wavelike forms of energy such as radio waves, X rays, and light.

electron transport system (ETS) (e-lek'tron trans'port sis'tem) The series of oxidation-reduction reactions in aerobic cellular respiration in which the energy is removed from hydrogens and transferred to ATP.

electrons (e-lek'trons) The negatively charged particles moving at a distance from the nucleus of an atom that balance the positive charges of the protons.

elements (el'ĕ-ments) Matter consisting of only one kind of atom.

empirical evidence (em-pir'-ĭ-cal ev-ĭ-dens) The information gained by observing an event.

empirical formula (em-pir'ĭ-kal for'miu-lah) A symbol that will tell what elements are in a compound and also how many atoms of each element are required.

endoplasmic reticulum (ER) (en"do-plaz'mik re-tĭk'yu-lum) Folded membranes and tubes throughout the eukaryotic cell that provide a large surface upon which chemical activities take place.

energy (en'er-je) The property of an object that enables it to do work.

enzymatic competition (en-zi-mă-tik com-pĕ-tĭ'shun) Competition among several different available enzymes to combine with a given substrate material.

enzymes (en'zīms) Protein molecules produced by organisms that are able to control the rate at which chemical reactions occur.

enzyme-substrate complex (en'zīm-sub'strāt kom'pleks) A temporary molecule formed when an enzyme attaches itself to a substrate molecule.

essential amino acids (e-sen'shal ah-mēn'o ă'sids) Those amino acids that are unable to be synthesized by the human body and must be part of the diet, such as lysine, tryptophan, and valine.

essential fatty acid (e-sen'shal fat-te ă'sid) The fatty acid linoleic acid; it is unable to be synthesized by the human body and must be part of the diet.

eukaryotic cells (yu'ka-re-ah"tik sels) One of the two major types of cells; characterized by cells that have a true nucleus, as in plants, fungi, protists, and animals.

experiment (ek-sper'ĭ-ment) A re-creation of an event in a way that enables a scientist to gain valid and reliable empirical evidence.

experimental group (ek-sper'ĭ-men'tal grūp) The situation in a controlled experiment that is identical to the control group in all respects but one.

faciliated diffusion (fah-sil'ĭ-ta"ted dĭ"fiu'zhun) Diffusion assisted by carrier molecules.

FAD (flavin adenine dinucleotide) (fla-ven ădd-ă-nen die-new-cle-o-tid) A hydrogen carrier used in respiration.

fat (fat) A class of water-insoluble macromolecules composed of a glycerol and 3 fatty acids.

fatty acid (fat-te ă'sid) One of the building blocks of a fat, composed of a long-chain carbon skeleton with a carboxylic acid functional group.

fermentation (fir-men-ta-shun) Pathways that oxidize glucose to generate ATP energy using something other than O_2 as the ultimate hydrogen ion acceptor.

fertilization (fer"tĭ-lĭ-za'shun) The joining of haploid nuclei, usually from an egg and a sperm cell, resulting in a diploid cell called the zygote.

First Law of Thermodynamics (furst law uv ther"mo-di-nam'iks) Also known as the **Law of Conservation of Energy** states that the total amount of energy in the universe remains constant; it can neither be created nor destroyed but only transferred and transformed.

flagella (flah-jel'luh) Long, hairlike structures projecting from the cell surface that enable locomotion.

fluid-mosaic model (flu'id mo-za'ik mod'l) The concept that the cell membrane is composed primarily of protein and phospholipid molecules that are able to shift and flow past one another.

force (fors) Anything that has the potential to make an object move or alter its movement.

formula (form'yu-lah) The group of chemical symbols that indicate what elements are in a compound and the number of each kind of atom present. Two types are used: empirical and structural.

frequency (fre'kwen-se) The number of waves of energy produced per second.

functional groups (fung"shun-al grūps) Specific combinations of atoms attached to the carbon skeleton that determine specific chemical properties.

gamete (gam'ēt) A haploid sex cell.

gametogenesis (gă-me"to-jen'ĕ-sis) The generating of gametes; the meiotic cell-division process that produces sex cells; oogenesis and spermatogenesis.

gas (gas) The state of matter in which the molecules are more energetic than the molecules of a liquid, resulting in only slight attraction for each other.

gene (jēn) Any molecule, usually a segment of DNA, located on a chromosome that is able to (1) replicate by directing the manufacture of copies of itself; (2) mutate, or chemically change, and transmit these changes to future generations; (3) store information that determines the characteristics of cells and organisms; and (4) use this information to direct the synthesis of structural and regulatory proteins.

generative processes (jen'uh-ra"tiv pros'es-es) Actions that increase the size of an individual organism (growth), or increase the number of individuals in a population (reproduction).

gene-regulator proteins (jēn-reg'yu-la-tor pro'te-ins) Chemical messengers within a cell that inform the genes as to whether protein-producing genes should be turned on or off or whether they should have their protein-producing activities increased or decreased; for example, gene-repressor proteins and gene-activator proteins.

genetics (jĕ-net′iks) The study of genes, how genes produce characteristics, and how the characteristics are inherited.

genome (je′nōm) A set of all the genes necessary to specify an organism's complete list of characteristics.

genotype (je′no-tīp) The catalog of genes of an organism, whether or not these genes are expressed.

glycerol (glis′er-ol) One of the building blocks of a fat, composed of a carbon skeleton that has three alcohol groups (OH) attached to it.

glycolysis (gli-kol′ĭ-sis) The anaerobic first stage of cellular respiration, consisting of the enzymatic breakdown of a sugar into 2 molecules of pyruvic acid.

Golgi apparatus (gōl′je ap″pah-rat′us) A stack of flattened, smooth, membranous sacs; the site of synthesis and packaging of certain molecules in eukaryotic cells.

gonad (go-nad) A generalized term for the organs in which meiosis occurs; ovaries and testes.

granules (gran′yūls) Materials whose structure is not as well defined as that of other organelles. See **inclusions.**

grounding (grownd′ing) Connecting an area with the ground (earth), which then acts as the ultimate receptor of displaced electrons.

guanine (gwah′nēn) A double-ring nitrogenous-base molecule in DNA and RNA. It is the complementary base of cytosine.

haploid (hap′loid) Having a single set of chromosomes resulting from the reduction division of meiosis.

heat (hēt) A form of energy produced by the random motion of atoms and molecules.

heterozygous (hĕ″ter-o-zi′gus) Describes a diploid organism that has 2 different alleles for a particular characteristic.

high-energy phosphate bond (hi-en′ur-je fos-fāt bond) The bond between two phosphates in an ADP or ATP molecule that readily releases its energy for cellular processes.

homologous chromosomes (ho-mol′o-gus kro′mo-sōmz) A pair of chromosomes in a diploid cell that contain similar genes at corresponding loci throughout their length.

homozygous (ho″mo-zi′gus) Describes a diploid organism that has two identical alleles for a particular characteristic.

hydrogen bond (hi′dro-jen bond) Weak attractive forces between molecules; important in determining how groups of molecules are arranged.

hydrolysis (hi-drol′ĭ-sis) A process that occurs when a large molecule is broken down into smaller parts by the addition of water.

hydrophilic (hi″dro-fil′ik) Readily absorbing or dissolving in water.

hydrophobic (hi″dro-fo′bik) Tending not to combine with, or incapable of dissolving in, water.

hydroxyl ion (hi-drok′sil i′on) A negatively charged particle (OH⁻) composed of oxygen and hydrogen atoms released from a base when dissolved in water.

hypertonic (hi-pur-tŏn′ik) A comparative term describing one of two solutions. The hypertonic solution is the one with the higher amount of dissolved material.

hypothesis (hi-poth′e-sis) A possible answer to or explanation of a question that accounts for all the observed facts and is testable.

hypotonic (hi″po-tŏn′ik) A comparative term describing one of two solutions. The hypotonic solution is the one with the lower amount of dissolved material.

inclusions (in-klu′zhuns) A general term referring to materials inside a cell that are usually not readily identifiable; stored materials.

incomplete protein (in-kom-plēt pro′te-in) Protein molecules that do not provide all the essential amino acids.

independent assortment (in″de-pen′dent ă-sort′ment) The segregation, or assortment, of one pair of homologous chromosomes, independently of the segregation, or assortment, of any other pair of chromosomes.

inhibitor (in-hib′ĭ-tōr) A molecule that temporarily attaches itself to an enzyme, thereby interfering with the enzyme's ability to form an enzyme-substrate complex.

initiation code (ĭ-nĭ′she-a″shun cōd) The code on DNA with the base sequence TAC that begins the process of transcription.

inorganic molecules (in-or-gan′ik mol-uh-kiuls) Molecules that do not contain carbon atoms in rings or chains.

insulators (in′su-la″tors) Material that prohibits the flow of electrons.

interphase (in′tur-fāz) The stage between cell divisions in which the cell is engaged in metabolic activities.

ionic bond (i-on′ik bond) The attractive force between ions of opposite charge.

ions (i′ons) Electrically unbalanced or charged atoms.

isomers (i′so-meers) Molecules that have the same empirical formula but different structural formulae.

isotonic (i′so-tŏn′ik) A term used to describe two solutions that have the same concentration of dissolved material.

isotopes (i′so-tōps) Atoms of the same element that differ only in the number of neutrons.

kilocalorie (kcalorie) (kil′o-kal″o-re) The amount of heat energy required to raise the temperature of one kilogram of water one degree Celsius.

kinetic energy (kĭ-net′ik en′er-je) Energy of motion.

Krebs cycle (krebz si′kl) The series of reactions in aerobic cellular respiration, resulting in the production of two carbon dioxides, the release of four pairs of hydrogens, and the formation of an ATP molecule.

lack of dominance (lak uv dom′in-ans) The condition of two unlike alleles both expressing themselves, neither being dominant.

law of dominance (law uv dom′in-ans) When an organism has two different alleles for a trait, the allele that is expressed and overshadows the expression of the other allele is said to be dominant. The allele whose expression is overshadowed is said to be recessive.

law of independent assortment (law uv in″de-pen′dent ă-sort′ment) Members of one allelic pair will separate from each other independently of the members of other allele pairs.

law of segregation (law uv seg″rĕ-ga′shun) When gametes are formed by a diploid organism, the alleles that control a trait separate from one another into different gametes, retaining their individuality.

linkage group (lingk′ij grūp) Genes located on the same chromosome that tend to be inherited together.

lipids (lǐ′pids)   Large organic molecules that do not easily dissolve in water; classes include fats, phospholipids, and steroids.

liquid (lik′wid)   The state of matter in which the molecules are strongly attracted to each other, but because they are farther apart than in a solid, they move past each other more freely.

locus (loci) (lo′kus) (lo′si)   The spot on a chromosome where an allele is located.

lysosome (li′so-sōm)   A specialized organelle that holds a mixture of hydrolytic enzymes.

mass (mas)   Resistance to forces.

mass number (mas num′ber)   The weight of an atomic nucleus expressed in atomic mass units (the sum of the protons and neutrons).

matter (mat′er)   Anything that has weight (mass) and also takes up space (volume).

meiosis (mi-o′sis)   The specialized pair of cell divisions that reduce the chromosome number from diploid (2n) to haploid (n).

Mendelian genetics (Men-dě′le-an jě-net′iks)   The pattern of inheriting characteristics that follows the laws formulated by Gregor Mendel.

messenger RNA (mRNA) (mes′en-jer)   A molecule composed of ribonucleotides that functions as a copy of the gene and is used in the cytoplasm of the cell during protein synthesis.

metabolic processes (mě-tă-bol′ik pros′es-es)   The total of all chemical reactions within an organism; for example, nutrient uptake and processing, and waste elimination.

metaphase (me′tah-fāz)   The second stage in mitosis, characterized by alignment of the chromosomes at the equatorial plane.

microfilaments (mi′′kro-fil′ah-ments)   Long, fiberlike structures made of actin protein and found in cells, often in close association with the microtubules; provide structural support and enable movement.

microscope (mi′kro-skōp)   An instrument used to make an object appear larger than it appears to the naked eye.

microtubules (mi′kro-tū′′byuls)   Small, hollow tubes of protein that function throughout the cytoplasm to provide structural support and enable movement.

minerals (min′er-als)   Inorganic elements that are not able to be manufactured by the body but are required in low concentrations; essential to metabolism.

mitochondrion (mi-to-kahn′dre-on)   A membranous organelle resembling a small bag with a larger bag inside that is folded back on itself; serves as the site of aerobic cellular respiration.

mitosis (mi-to′sis)   A process that results in equal and identical distribution of replicated chromosomes into two newly formed nuclei.

mixture (miks′chur)   Matter that contains two or more substances NOT in set proportions.

molecule (mol′ě-kūl)   The smallest particle of a chemical compound; also the smallest naturally occurring part of an element or compound.

multiple alleles (mul′tĭ-pul al′lēlz)   A term used to refer to conditions in which there are several different alleles for a particular characteristic, not just two.

mutagenic agent (miu-tah-jen′ik a-jent)   Anything that causes permanent change in DNA.

mutation (miu-ta′shun)   Any change in the genetic information of a cell.

NAD⁺ (nicotinamide adenine dinucleotide) (nik′′o-tin′ah-mid ăd′ă-nen die-new-klě-o-tid)   An electron acceptor and hydrogen carrier used in respiration.

nanometers (na′′no-me′ters)   A billionth of a meter.

negative-feedback inhibition (neg′ă-tiv-fēd′băk in′′hĭ-bish′un)   A metabolic control process that operates at the surfaces of enzymes. This process occurs when one of the end products of the pathway alters the three-dimensional shape of an essential enzyme in the pathway and interferes with its operation long enough to slow its action.

net movement (net muv′ment)   Movement in one direction minus the movement in the other.

neutralization (nu′tral-ĭ-za′′shun)   A chemical reaction involved in mixing an acid with a base; results in formation of a salt and water.

neutrons (nu′trons)   Particles in the nucleus of an atom that have no electrical charge; they were named *neutrons* to reflect this lack of electrical charge.

nitrogenous base (ni-trah′jen-us bās)   A category of organic molecules found as components of the nucleic acids. There are five common types: thymine, guanine, cytosine, adenine, and uracil.

nonconductors (non′′kon-duk′tors)   Material that prohibits the flow of electrons.

nondisjunction (non′′dis-junk′shun)   An abnormal meiotic division that results in sex cells with too many or too few chromosomes.

nuclear membrane (nu′kle-ar mem′brān)   The structure surrounding the nucleus that separates the nucleoplasm from the cytoplasm.

nucleic acids (nu′kle-ik ă′sids)   Complex molecules that store and transfer information within a cell. They are constructed of fundamental monomers known as nucleotides.

nucleolus (plural nucleoli) (nu′′kle-o′lus)   Nuclear structures composed of completed or partially completed ribosomes and the specific parts of chromosomes that contain the information for their construction.

nucleoplasm (nu′kle-o-plazm)   The liquid matrix of the nucleus composed of a mixture of water and the molecules used in the construction of the rest of the nuclear structures.

nucleoproteins (nu-kle-o-pro′te-inz)   The duplex DNA strands with attached proteins; also called chromatin fibers.

nucleosomes (nu′kle-o-sōmz)   Histone clusters with their encircling DNA.

nucleotide (nu′kle-o-tīd)   The building block of the nucleic acids. Each is composed of a 5-carbon sugar, a phosphate, and a nitrogenous base.

nucleus (nu′kle-us)   The central body that contains the information system for the cell.

nutrients (nu′tre-ents)   Molecules required by organisms for growth, reproduction, and/or repair.

nutrition (nu′trish-un)   Processes involved in taking in, assimilating, and utilizing nutrients.

observation (ob′′sir-va′-shun)   The process of using the senses or extensions of the senses to record events.

offspring (of′spring)   Descendants of a set of parents.

orbital (or′bĭ-tal)   The area of an atom able to hold a maximum of two electrons.

organ (or′gun)   A structure composed of two or more kinds of tissues.

organelles (or-gan-elz′)   Cellular structures that perform specific functions in the cell. The function of an organelle is directly related to its structure.

organ system (or′gun sis′tem)   A group of organs that perform a particular function.

organic molecules (or-gan'ik mol'uh-kiuls) Complex molecules whose basic building blocks are carbon atoms in chains or rings.

organism (or'gah-nizm) An independent living unit.

osmosis (os-mo'sis) The net movement of water molecules through a selectively permeable membrane.

osteoporosis (os'te-o-por-o'sis) A disease condition resulting from the demineralization of the bone resulting in pain, deformities, and fractures. Related to a loss of calcium.

ovaries (o'var-ēz) The female sex organs that produce haploid sex cells—the eggs or ova.

oxidation-reduction reactions (ok''sǐ-da'shun-re-duk'shun re-ak'shuns) Electron transfer reactions in which the molecules losing electrons become oxidized and those gaining electrons become reduced.

peptide bond (pep'tīd bond) A covalent bond between amino acids in a protein.

periodic table of the elements (pēr-e-od'ik ta-bul uv the el'ě-ments) A list of all of the elements in order of increasing atomic number (number of protons).

pH A scale used to indicate the strength of an acid or base.

phagocytosis (fǎ''jo-si-to'sis) The process by which the cell wraps around a particle and engulfs it.

phenotype (fēn'o-tīp) The physical, chemical, and behavioral expression of the genes possessed by an organism.

phosphate (fos-fāt) Part of a nucleotide; composed of phosphorus and oxygen atoms.

phospholipid (fos''fo-lī'pid) A class of water-insoluble molecules that resemble fats but contain a phosphate group (PO_4) in their structure.

photosynthesis (fo-to-sin'thuh-sis) A major biochemical pathway in green plants, resulting in the manufacture of food molecules.

pinocytosis (pǐ''no-si-to'sis) The process by which a cell engulfs some molecules dissolved in water.

plasma membrane (plaz'muh mem'brān) The outer-boundary membrane of the cell; also known as the cell membrane.

pleiotropy (pli-ot'ro-pe) The multiple effects that a gene may have on the phenotype of an organism.

point mutation (point miu-ta'shun) A change in the DNA of a cell as a result of a loss or change in a nitrogenous-base sequence.

polygenic inheritance (pol''e-jen'ik inher'ǐ-tans) The concept that a number of different pairs of alleles may combine their efforts to determine a characteristic.

polypeptide chain (pǒ''le-pep'tīd chān) A macromolecule composed of a specific sequence of amino acids.

polysome (pah'le-sōm) A sequence of several translating ribosomes attached to the same mRNA.

potential energy (po-ten'shal en'er-je) The energy an object has because of its position.

pressure (presh'ur) The force of the collisions of molecules on the surface of an area.

probability (prob''a-bil'ǐ-te) The chance that an event will happen, expressed as a percent or fraction.

products (prǒ'dukts) New molecules resulting from a chemical reaction.

prokaryotic cells (pro'ka-re-ot''ik sels) One of the two major types of cells. They do not have a typical nucleus bound by a nuclear membrane and lack many of the other membranous cellular organelles; for example, bacteria.

promoter (pro-mo'ter) A region of DNA at the beginning of each gene, just ahead of an initiator code.

prophase (pro'fāz) The first phase of mitosis during which individual chromosomes become visible.

protein (pro'te-in) Macromolecules made up of one or more polypeptides attached to each other by bonds.

protein-sparing (pro'te-in-spar-ing) The conservation of proteins by first oxidizing carbohydrates and fats as a source of ATP energy.

protein synthesis (pro'te-in sin'thě-sis) The process whereby the tRNA utilizes the mRNA as a guide to arrange the amino acids in their proper sequence according to the genetic information in the chemical code of DNA.

protons (pro'tons) Particles in the nucleus of an atom that have a positive electrical charge.

protoplasm (pro'to-plazm) The living portion of a cell as distinguished from the nonliving cell wall.

pseudoscience (su-do-si'ens) The use of the appearance of science to mislead. The assertions made are not valid or reliable.

Punnett square (pun'net sqwār) A method used to determine the probabilities of allele combinations in a zygote.

pyruvic acid (pi-ru'vik as'id) A 3-carbon carbohydrate that is the end product of the process of glycolysis.

radioactive (ra-de-o-ak'tiv) A term used to describe the property of releasing energy or particles from an unstable atom.

reactants (re-ak'tants) Materials that will be changed in a chemical reaction.

recessive allele (re-sě'siv al'lēl) An allele that, when present with its homolog, does not express itself and is masked by the effect of the other allele.

recombinant DNA (re-kom'bǐ-nant) DNA that has been constructed by inserting new pieces of DNA into the DNA of another organism, such as a bacterium.

reduction division (re-duk'shun dǐ-vǐ'zhun) A type of cell division in which daughter cells get only half the chromosomes from the parent cell.

reflection (re-flek'shun) Energy that bounces off of the object it intersects.

refraction (re-frak'shun) Energy that passes through an object and leaves in a direction different from the direction that it entered.

regulator proteins (reg'yu-la-tor pro'te-ins) Proteins that influence the activities that occur in an organism—for example, enzymes and some hormones.

reliable (re-li'a-bul) Giving the same result on successive trials.

responsive processes (re-spon'siv pros'es-es) Those abilities to react to external and internal changes in the environment; for example, irritability, individual adaptation, and evolution.

ribonucleic acid (ri-bo-nu-kle'ik ǎ'sid) A polymer of nucleotides formed on the template surface of DNA by transcription. Three forms that have been identified are mRNA, rRNA, and tRNA.

ribose (ri'bōs) A 5-carbon sugar molecule that is a component of RNA.

ribosomal RNA (rRNA) (ri-bo-sōm'al) A globular form of RNA; a part of ribosomes.

ribosomes (ri'bo-sōmz) Small structures composed of two protein and ribonucleic acid subunits involved in the assembly of proteins from amino acids.

RNA polymerase (po-lim'er-ās) An enzyme that attaches to the DNA at the promoter region of a gene when the genetic information is transcribed into RNA.

salts (salts) Ionic compounds formed from a reaction between an acid and a base.

saturated (sat'yu-ra-ted) Carbon skeleton of a fatty acid that contains no double bonds between carbons.

science (si'ens) A process or way of arriving at a solution to a problem or understanding an event in nature involving hypotheses formation and testing.

scientific law (si-en-tif'ik law) A uniform or constant feature of nature supported by several theories.

scientific method (si-en-tif'ik method) A way of gaining information (facts) about the world around you involving observation, hypothesis formation, experimentation, theory formation, and law formation.

Second Law of Thermodynamics (sek'ond law uv ther"mo-di-nam'iks) Basic principle that states that one form of energy can be converted to a second form of energy, but in doing so, a third form, heat, is also produced.

segregation (seg"rĕ-ga'shun) The separation and movement of homologous chromosomes to the poles of the cell.

selectively permeable (sĕ-lek'tiv-le per'me-ah-b'l) The property of a membrane that allows certain molecules to pass through it but interferes with the passage of others.

sex chromosomes (seks kro'mo-sōmz) Chromosomes that carry genes that determine the sex of the individual.

sexual reproduction (sek'shu-al re"pro-duk'shun) The propagation of organisms involving the union of gametes from two parents.

sickle-cell anemia (sĭ-kul-sel ah-ne'me-ah) A disease caused by a point mutation. This malfunction produces sickle-shaped red blood cells.

single-factor cross (sing'ul-fak'tur kros) A genetic study in which a single characteristic is followed from the parental generation to the offspring (monohybrid cross).

solid (sol'id) The state of matter in which the molecules are packed tightly together; they vibrate in place.

solution (so-lu'shun) Homogenous mixtures in which the particles are the size of atoms or small molecules.

specific gravity (spĕ-sif'ik grav'ĭ-te) Density of a substance compared to the density of water.

sperm cells (spurm selz) The haploid sex cells produced by sexually mature males.

spindle (spin'dul) An array of microtubules extending from pole to pole; used in the movement of chromosomes.

states of matter (stātes uv mat'er) Physical conditions of matter (solid, liquid, and gas) determined by the relative amounts of energy of the molecules.

steroid (stēr'oid) One of the three kinds of lipid molecules characterized by their arrangement of interlocking rings of carbon.

structural formula (struk'chu-ral for'miu-lah) A drawing that shows the number and spacial arrangement of the atoms within a molecule.

structural proteins (struk'chu-ral pro'te-ins) Proteins that are important for holding cells and organisms together, such as the proteins that make up the cell membrane, muscles, tendons, and blood.

substrate (sub'strāt) A reactant molecule with which the enzyme combines.

suspension (sus-pen'shun) Similar to a solution, but the dispersed particles are larger than molecular size.

synapsis (sin-ap'sis) The condition in which the two members of a pair of homologous chromosomes come to lie close to one another.

telophase (tel'uh-fāz) The last phase in mitosis characterized by the formation of daughter nuclei.

temperature (tem'per-ah-tūr) A measure of molecular kinetic energy.

template (tem'plet) A model from which a new structure can be made. This term has special reference to DNA as a model for both DNA replication and transcription.

termination code (ter-mŭ-na'shun cōd) The DNA nucleotide sequence just in back of a gene with the code ATT, ATC, or ACT that signals "stop here."

testes (tes'tēz) The male sex organs that produce haploid cells—the sperm.

theory (the'-o-re) A plausible, scientifically acceptable generalization supported by several hypotheses and experimental trials.

thymine (thi'mēn) A single-ring nitrogenous-base molecule in DNA but not in RNA. It is complementary to adenine.

tissue (tish'u) A group of similar cells that performs a specific function; ex., bone.

transcription (tran-skrip'shun) The process of manufacturing RNA from the template surface of DNA. Three forms of RNA that may be produced are mRNA, rRNA, and tRNA.

transfer RNA (tRNA) (trans-fur) A molecule composed of ribonucleic acid. It is responsible for transporting a specific amino acid into a ribosome for assembly into a protein.

translation (trans-la'shun) The assembly of individual amino acids into a polypeptide.

transparency (trans-par'en-sē) Property of material that allows the transmission of energy through it.

triglyceride (tri-glis'er-ide) A form of lipid composed of a glycerol molecule that has three attached fatty acids.

trisomy (tris'-oh-me) An abnormal number of chromosomes resulting from the nondisjunction of homologous chromosomes during meiosis; for example, as in Down syndrome.

turnover number (turn'o-ver num'ber) The number of molecules of substrate that a single molecule of enzyme can react with in a given time.

unsaturated (un-sat'yu-ra-ted) A carbon skeleton of a fatty acid containing carbons that are double-bonded to each other at one or more points.

uracil (yu'rah-sil) A single-ring nitrogenous-base molecule in RNA but not in DNA. It is complementary to adenine.

vacuole (vak'yu-ōl) A large sac within the cytoplasm of a cell, composed of a single membrane.

valid (va'-lid) Meaningful data that fits into the framework of scientific knowledge.

variable (var'e-ă-bul) The single factor that is allowed to be different.

vesicles (vĕ'sĭ-kuls) Small, intracellular, membrane-bound sacs in which various substances are stored.

vitamins (vi-tah-mins) Organic molecules that are not able to be manufactured by the body, but are required in very low concentrations.

wavelength (wāv'length) Distance from one crest to the next crest of a wave of energy in the electromagnetic spectrum.

weight (wāt) The force of gravity on an object.

X-linked gene (eks-lingt jēn) A gene located on one of the sex-determining X chromosomes.

zygote (zi'gōt) A diploid cell that results from the union of an egg and a sperm.

Credits

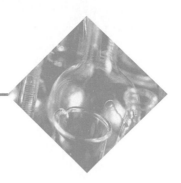

Index

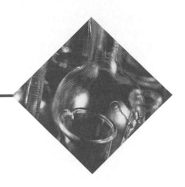

An *italicized* page number indicates where the term is defined in the chapter glossary. A **boldface** page number indicates where the term appears boldfaced in the text. References to figures, tables, and boxes are designated after the page number.

ABO blood types, multiple alleles for, 203–4
Absorption, **43**, 43(fig.), *49*
Acetyl, 118–19, **123**, *137*
Acids, 25, **31**–32, *35*
  and pH scale, **31**, 32(fig.)
Acquired immunodeficiency syndrome (AIDS), 147(box)
Activation energy, **98**, 99(fig.), *108*
Active transport, 74, **79**, 80(fig.), *95*
Adaptation, 15, 17(table)
Adenine, 66, **139**, 140(fig.), 141–42, *158*
Adenosine, 141
Adenosine diphosphate (ADP), 112, 112(fig.), 113, 113(fig.)
Adenosine monophosphate (AMP), 113, 113(fig.), 141
Adenosine triphosphate (ATP), 112(fig.), 112–14, 117(fig.), *137*
  in chemiosmosis, 119, 121(fig.)
  in electron-transport system, 119–20, 120(fig.), 124, 125
  in fermentation, 126, 127(fig.)
  in glycolysis, 117–18, 121–23, 125
  in Krebs cycle, 119, 123(fig.), 124, 125
  structure of, 113, 113(fig.)
Aerobic cellular respiration, **84**, 85(fig.), *95*, **114**–125, *137*
  electron-transport system in, 119–20, 124, 125
  of glucose, 115–18, 121–23
  Krebs cycle in, 118–19, 123–24, 125
Age, and nondisjunction of chromosomes, 187–88, 188(fig.)

AIDS, and reverse transcriptase, 147(box)
Alanine, 63(box), 150(table)
Alcohol
  fermentation of, 126, *137*
  metabolism of, 97, 101
Alleles, **193**, 194–95, *212*
  dominant, **195**, 196, 202, *212*
    lack of, 202(fig.), 202–3, *212*
    variable expression of, 209
  in double-factor cross, 199–202
  multiple, **203**–4, *212*
  recessive, **195**, 196, *212*
    carrier of, **208**, *212*
  in single-factor cross, 197–99
Amino acids, **61**, *68*, 150(table)
  essential, 133, 133(table), *137*
  and nucleic acid dictionary, 150–51, 151(table)
  peptide bond of, **61**, 61(fig.)
  and protein synthesis, 62–65, 151–54
  sequence of, 62–65, 152(fig.), 153, 154
  in sickle-cell anemia, 63, 155(fig.), 155–56
  structure of, 61, 61(fig.), 62–63(box)
Amylase, 101
Anaerobic respiration, **118**, **121**, **126**–28, *137*
Anaphase
  in meiosis, 177–78, 178(fig.), 179, 180(fig.)
  in mitosis, **164**–65, 165(fig.), *171*
Anemia
  iron deficiency, 135
  sickle-cell, 63, 155(fig.), **155**–56, *159*
    genetic factors in, 155, 194(fig.), 195, 205–6
    and malaria resistance, 206
Angelman syndrome, 209
Angstrom units, **40**, *49*
Animals
  haploid and diploid cells in, 175, 175(table), 176(fig.)
  mitosis in, 166–67(fig.)
  sex determination in, 189(box)
Anorexia nervosa, 109–10

Antibiotic drugs, 92, 92(table), *95*, 107
Antibodies, 50, 62
Anticodon, **148**, *158*
Antigens, 69
Arginine, 63(box), 133(table), 150(table)
Arginine aminase, 101
Asparagine, 63(box), 150(table)
Aspartic acid, 63(box), 150(table)
Assimilation, **131**, *137*
Atherosclerosis, 59, 60(box)
Atom, **21**, *35*
  Bohr model, 25(fig.), 26
  chemical bonds of, 30–34
  electron distribution in, 25–28
  in functional group, **54**, 55(fig.), *68*
  inert or noble, 29
  ions of, 28–30
  isotopes of, 22, 23, 23(fig.)
  mass number of, **22**, 23, *36*
  modern model of, 26–28
  nucleus of, **21**–22, 22(fig.), *35*
  structure of, 21–23, 22(fig.)
Atomic mass unit (AMU), **22**, 23(table), *35*
Atomic number, **22**, 23, *35*
ATP. *See* Adenosine triphosphate
Autosomes, **188**, *191, 212*

Bacteria
  and antibiotic drugs, 92, 92(table), *95*, 107
  as prokaryotic cells, 71, 91–92
Barr body, 189
Basal body, 88
Base, 25, **31**–32, *35*
  complementary, 141–**42**, *158*
  and pH scale, **31**, 32(fig.)
Biochemistry, **51**, *68*, 109–37
  adenosine triphosphate as energy source in, 112–14
  cellular respiration in, 111, 112, 114–31
  chemical reactions in, 98–99. *See also* Chemical reactions